# Human Diseases

## A Systemic Approach

**Sixth Edition**

**Mary Lou Mulvihill, PhD**
Professor Emeritus
William Rainey Harper College
Palatine, Illinois

**Mark Zelman, PhD**
Associate Professor
Aurora University
Aurora, Illinois

**Paul Holdaway, MA**
Professor
William Rainey Harper College
Palatine, Illinois

**Elaine Tompary, PharmD**
Outcomes Research
McNeil Consumer and Specialty Pharma
Fort Washington, Pennsylvania

**Jill Raymond, PhD**
Associate Professor
Rock Valley College
Rockford, Illinois

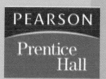

PEARSON

Prentice
Hall

Upper Saddle River, New Jersey 07458

**Library of Congress Cataloging-in-Publication Data**

Human diseases : a systemic approach / Mary Lou Mulvihill
   . . . [et al.].—6th ed.
      p. ; cm.
   Includes bibliographical references and index.
   ISBN 0-13-152749-5
   1.  Pathology.
   [DNLM: 1.   Clinical Medicine. 2.   Disease.   WB 100
   H9182 2006]   I. Mulvihill, Mary L. RB111.M83 2006
   616—dc22
                                2005008254

To Mary Lou Mulvihill,
friend, colleague, and
educator, whose vision
began this work

and

To our students who inspired
us to continue it

Notice:
The authors and the publisher of this volume have taken care that the information and technical recommendations contained herein are based on research and expert consultation, and are accurate and compatible with the
standards generally accepted at the time of publication. Nevertheless, as new information becomes available,
changes in clinical and technical practices become necessary. The reader is advised to carefully consult manufacturers' instructions and information material for all supplies and equipment before use, and to consult with a
health care professional as necessary. This advice is especially important when using new supplies or equipment
for clinical purposes. The authors and publisher disclaim all responsibility for any liability, loss, injury, or damage
incurred as a consequence, directly or indirectly, of the use and application of any of the contents of this volume.

**Publisher:** Julie Levin Alexander
**Assistant to Publisher:** Regina Bruno
**Executive Editor:** Mark Cohen
**Associate Editor:** Melissa Kerian
**Editorial Assistant:** Jaquay Felix
**Media Editor:** John J. Jordan
**Development Editor:** Andrea Edwards, Triple
   SSS Press
**Director of Production and Manufacturing:**
   Bruce Johnson
**Managing Production Editor:** Patrick Walsh
**Production Liaison:** Christina Zingone
**Production Editor:** Jessica Balch, Pine Tree
   Composition

**Manufacturing Manager:** Ilene Sanford
**Manufacturing Buyer:** Pat Brown
**Design Director:** Cheryl Asherman
**Design Coordinator:** Christopher Weigand
**Interior Designer:** Amanda Kavanagh
**Cover Designer:** Michael Ginsberg
**Director of Marketing:** Karen Allman
**Channel Marketing Manager:** Rachele Strober
**Manager of Media Production:** Amy Peltier
**New Media Project Managers:** Stephen Hartner and
   Tina Rudowski
**Composition:** Pine Tree Composition, Inc.
**Printer/Binder:** Courier Kendallville
**Cover Printer:** Phoenix Color Corp.

Pearson Prentice Hall™ is a trademark of Pearson Education, Inc.
Pearson® is a registered trademark of Pearson plc.
Prentice Hall® is a registered trademark of Pearson Education, Inc.
Pearson Education Ltd., *London*
Pearson Education Australia Pty. Limited, *Sydney*
Pearson Education Singapore, Pte. Ltd.
Pearson Education North Asia Ltd., *Hong Kong*
Pearson Education Canada, Ltd., *Toronto*
Pearson Educación de Mexico, S.A. de C.V.
Pearson Education—Japan, *Tokyo*
Pearson Education Malaysia, Pte. Ltd.
Pearson Education, Upper Saddle River, New Jersey

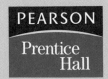

10 9 8 7 6 5 4 3 2 1
ISBN 0-13-152749-5

# Table of Contents

# Welcome to the Sixth Edition

Thoroughly updated and featuring a new eye-catching visual design, the sixth edition of *Human Diseases: A Systemic Approach* is enhanced by several new features. Additionally, a complete set of multimedia ancillaries combine with this authoritative textbook to provide a true multidimensional teaching and learning experience. Inclusive of these improvements, the book remains grounded in the logical organization and engaging, readable style that have made it a success throughout the years.

# Hallmark Features

The text organization remains similar to that of the fifth edition. Part I, *Mechanisms of Disease,* introduces students to the major concepts essential to the study and understanding of disease, including terminology, immunity and inflammation, nutrition, inheritance, neoplasia, and infectious diseases. Part II, *Diseases of the Systems,* discusses the major diseases of the body systems. Also returning is the popular *Side by Side* feature, substantially improved with new photographs comparing normal and disease states; *Prevention Plus!,* which presents common-sense disease prevention strategies; *Diseases at a Glance* charts, a key study aid that lists major facts about each disease and improved by the addition of etiology; and expanded *Interactive Activites,* including case studies and multiple-choice, true/false, and fill-in-the-blank exercises.

# Enhancements to the Sixth Edition

- **New Mental Illness Chapter.** The most substantial and important addition to the sixth edition is the new chapter, *Mental Illness,* which discusses the nature of mental illness and explains the etiology, signs and symptoms, diagnosis, and treatment of major disorders. Readers will learn that mental illness is highly prevalent and, if left untreated, causes a significant amount of morbidity and adversely affects quality of life. Like the other diseases in this text, mental illness has a biological basis and therefore may be diagnosed and treated.

- **Age-Related Diseases.** Readers should recognize that the risk, and therefore incidence, of diseases changes over the lifespan. Hence, we have added *Age-Related Diseases* at the end of each system chapter as a reminder of the normal changes and common diseases associated with aging.

- **Disease Chronicles.** These chapter-opening passages provide an interesting context and relevance to the study of disease.

- **Integrated Pharmacology.** Common pharmacologic treatments of disease have been incorporated throughout the text. Readers will recognize the names and uses of common over-the-counter and prescription medicines.

- **Resources Listings.** Articles, books, and organizations are identified to help readers further their study of disease.

- **Updated Chapters.** Chapter 2, Chapter 4 and Chapter 6 have been significantly updated and revised to improve currency and accuracy. All chapters were scrutinized and revised. Some passages benefited from substantial rewriting.

- **Logical Consolidation of Content.** We also responded to student and instructor comments by consolidating, but not reducing, certain material: all digestive system diseases have been combined into Chapter 10; Chapter 7 combines diseases of the heart and blood vessels.

- **Addition of Diseases of the Eyes and Ears.** This material has been included in an expanded Chapter 14, *Diseases of the Nervous System and Special Senses.*

- **A Better Fit for One-Semester Courses.** By incorporating aging and wellness topics throughout, the sixth edition now has 17 chapters, making this text adaptable to most semester-long courses.

## ▶ Teaching and Learning Package

### Student CD-ROM

An interactive student CD-ROM is packaged in the back of the book and contains a host of interactive study aids. The videos and animations help the students to visualize the content they are learning. Interactive exercises, games, and activities provide students with extra practice to master the chapter content.

### Companion Website and Syllabus Manager®

The **free** companion website (www.prenhall .com/mulvihill) is a text-specific, interactive, online workbook that provides student activities and practice quizzes—complete with instant scoring and immediate feedback. This website may be used to enrich the students' learning, and comes complete with Internet links, an audio glossary, and case studies. The website scores the student's results and allows those results to be sent to instructors via e-mail. Adoption of this textbook provides the instructor with online access to the Syllabus Manager®, which includes features to facilitate student use of the website and allow faculty to post their syllabi.

### Instructor's Resource Manual

This manual contains a wealth of material to help faculty plan and manage the human disease course. It includes lecture suggestions and content abstracts, learning objectives, a 693-question test bank and more for each chapter.

### Instructor's Resource CD-ROM

The CD-ROM packaged along with this Instructor's Resource Manual provides many resources in an electronic format. It includes the complete 693-question test bank that allows instructors to design customized quizzes and exams. It also includes a PowerPoint lecture package that contains key discussion points along with color images, animations, and videos. This package allows instructors to customize the materials to meet their specific course needs.

### Image Library

A collection of 198 images is available for instructors to download for presentation purposes. This library encompasses each of the high-quality images contained in the text and may be used in any way that instructors wish. This collection is free to all adopters and can be found on the Instructor's Resource CD-ROM as well as the Companion Website. To register for online access, instructors may visit www.prenhall .com/mulvilhill and click on the image library link.

### Online Course Management Systems

**OneKey® Online Course Options in Blackboard and WebCT** are available for schools using course management systems. The online course solutions feature interactive assessment modules, electronic test bank, PowerPoint lectures, animations and video clips, and more. OneKey® is the one location for all your text resources. For more information about adopting an online course management system to accompany **Human Diseases, 6/e,** please contact your local Prentice Hall representative or go to the website: www.prenhall.com/onekey.

The reviewers of *Human Diseases: A Systemic Approach, Sixth Edition* have provided many excellent suggestions and ideas for improving the text. The quality of the reviews has been outstanding, and the reviews have been a major aid in the preparation of the manuscript. Their assistance provided by these experts is deeply appreciated.

**Deborah Bedford**
Program Coordinator and Instructor
Health and Human Services
North Seattle Community College
Everett, Washington

**Sue Boulden, BSN, CMA**
Director
Medical Assisting Program
Mount Hood Community College
Gresham, Oregon

**Barbara Gresham, PT, MS**
PTA Program Instructor
McLennan Community College
Waco, Texas

**Angela Kennedy**
Head and Professor
Department of Health Information Management
Louisiana Tech University
Ruston, Louisiana

**Winifred Benchoff Khalil, RN, MA**
Professor
Department of Allied Health
San Diego Mesa College
San Diego, California

**Litta Dennis, BSN, MS, CAN**
Illinois Central College
East Peoria, Illinois

**Jennifer Lamé, MPH, BS, RHIT**
Instructor
Health Information Technology
Idaho State University
Pocatello, Idaho

**Dorothy Larson, MS, BS**
Instructor
Department of Biological Sciences
Ridgewater College
Willmor, Minnesota

**Norma Longoria**
Instructor
Medical Information Program
South Texas Community College
McAllen, Texas

**Sue Moe, RN**
Faculty
Health Division
Northwest Technical College
East Grand Forks, Minnesota

**Lisa Nagle, CMA, BSED**
Department Head
Medical Assisting Department
Augusta Technical College
Augusta, Georgia

**Robert M. Pilewski, MD**
Professor
Department of Clinical Pathology
University of Pittsburgh—Titusville
Pittsburgh, Pennsylvania

**Patricia L. Schrull, MBA, MSN, MEd, RN**
Assistant Professor
Department of Allied Heath and Nursing
Lorain County Community College
Elyria, Ohio

**Jacqueline M. Stephens**
Associate Professor
Department of Biological Sciences
Louisiana State University
Baton Rouge, Louisiana

**Tova Wiegand-Green**
Program Chair and Assistant Professor
Medical Assisting Program
Ivy Tech State College
Fort Wayne, Indiana

## ▶ Supplement Reviewers

### Student CD-ROM

**Marsha Hemby, BA, RN, CMA**
Department Chair
Medical Assisting
Pitt Community College
Greenville, North Carolina

**Irma Rodriguez, RHIA, CCS**
Program Chair
Health and Medical Administration Services
South Texas College
McAllen, Texas

### Test Bank

**Rose Goeden, RHIA**
Instructor
Department of Health
Information Management
Dakota State University
Madison, South Dakota

**Cosette Hardwick, PT**
Assistant Professor
Department of Biology
Missouri Western State College
St. Joseph, Missouri

**Cathy Russo, BSN, RN, MA**
Department of Health Sciences
City College of San Francisco
San Francisco, California

### Companion Website

**Anne Carpenter, RN, MSN**
Adjunct Faculty
Marshall University
Huntington, West Virginia

**Cosette Hardwick, PT**
Assistant Professor
Department of Biology
Missouri Western State College
St. Joseph, Missouri

**Ellen M. Smith, NRCMA-A**
Instructor
Medical Assisting Program
Berks Technical Institute
Wyomissing, Pennsylvania

**Mark Zelman, PhD,** is Associate Professor of Biology and Chair of Natural Sciences and Mathematics at Aurora University in Aurora, Illinois. After earning his BS in biology from Rockford College, Dr. Zelman received his PhD in microbiology and immunology from Loyola University Chicago, where he studied mechanisms of streptococcal infection-related autoimmune diseases, and completed postdoctoral studies in cell physiology at the University of Chicago. Dr. Zelman teaches a variety of biology courses, and pursues a wide range of interests in biology and science education. He enjoys writing, running, bicycling, and watching his sons, Joe and Tom, grow up. He could not have completed this marathon without loving support and cheers from his dear wife, Lisa.

**Paul Holdaway, MA,** a native Hoosier, is a graduate of Indiana State University and was an instructor there for two years. He is currently the senior member of the Biology Department at Harper College in Palatine, Illinois, where Dr. Mary Lou Mulvihill was an admired fellow biologist and friend. Dr. Zelman and Dr. Tompary are also former departmental colleagues and longstanding friends. Upon Dr. Mulvihill's retirement, Professor Holdaway assumed the teaching schedule of Dr. Mulvihill, and he has been involved in the anatomy, physiology and human disease curriculum since that time. Paul takes pleasure in a wide range of biological and clinical interests, as well as sports and family activities.

**Elaine Tompary, PharmD,** received her Doctor of Pharmacy Degree from the University of Illinois at Chicago. Dr. Tompary taught courses in pharmacology, pathophysiology, pharmacy law, and pharmaceutical calculations at William Rainey Harper College and the College of Lake County in Illinois. She has served as mentor and preceptor for pharmacy students at the University of Illinois and Drake University. She currently works for McNeil Consumer and Specialty Pharmaceuticals as a manager of medical science and outcomes research. She is a dedicated wife to Drew and mother and teacher to her children, Christopher and Andriana.

**Jill Raymond, PhD,** received her PhD in Microbiology from the University of California at Davis. She received and completed a postdoctoral fellowship in infectious diseases at the University of California at San Diego, where she studied the parasite *Giardia lamblia*. Dr. Raymond has published several scientific papers, as well as a non-majors and a majors laboratory manual. She has been teaching for ten years, the last nine have been at Rock Valley College, Rockford, Illinois. Dr. Raymond teaches a variety of biology courses including Biology for majors, Biology for non-majors, Human Disease, Microbiology, and Anatomy and Physiology. Dr. Raymond would like to thank her wonderful husband and family for their continuing support through the craziness of writing a textbook.

# Part I

# Mechanisms of Disease

How do we define and describe disease? What causes disease? In Part I, we discuss the manifestations, terminology, diagnosis, and mechanisms of disease.

## Chapters

# Introduction to Disease

CHAPTER

1

## Learning Objectives

After studying this chapter, you should be able to

- Define disease
- Name and define the manifestations of disease
- Understand terms used to describe disease
- Explain diagnosis of disease
- Name and define the chief causes of disease

## Fact or Fiction?

Plague does not occur in the United States.

*Fiction: Plague first reached the western United States around 1900. Plague now occurs at low levels in the American southwest, particularly in Arizona, Colorado, and New Mexico. Rats, mice, foxes, squirrels, marmots, prairie dogs, and even house cats have been identified as carriers.*

# Disease Chronicle

## The Black Death

... if one were to seek to establish one generalization ... to catch the mood of the Europeans in the second half of the fourteenth century, it would be that they were enduring a crisis of faith. Assumptions which had been taken for granted for centuries were now in question, the very framework of men's reasoning seemed to be breaking up. And though the Black Death was far from being the only cause, the anguish and disruption which it had inflicted made the greatest single contribution to the disintegration of an age.

—P. Ziegler, *The Black Death*

The Black Death, also known as the plague, has killed and terrified many people through the ages. For much of human history, understanding of disease, indeed knowledge of normal human physiology, was extremely limited. Effective control and treatment of most diseases awaited a systematic, scientific approach and a body of medical knowledge and technology.

## MedMedia
www.prenhall.com/mulvihill

Use the web address to the left to access the free, interactive Companion Website created for this textbook. It features chapter-specific exercises, Internet links, news links, and an audio glossary. Additionally, explore the CD-ROM that accompanies this book to discover Disease Focus videos and a rich array of activities that accompany this chapter.

## ▶ Introduction

Changes constantly occur within the body, and yet a steady state called homeostasis is generally maintained. Although pH, temperature, blood composition, and fluid levels fluctuate, organ systems normally correct these changes before they threaten the body's health. A significant disturbance in the homeostasis of the body triggers a variety of responses that often produce disease. If we consider homeostasis to be a state of equilibrium, disease can be defined as a state of functional disequilibrium, a change in function or structure that is considered to be abnormal. Clearly, knowledge of normal structure (anatomy) and normal function (physiology) are essential to pathology, the study of disease.

## ▶ Manifestations of Disease

A disease manifests itself through certain signs and symptoms. Signs are objective evidence of disease observed on physical examination, such as abnormal pulse or respiratory rate, fever, sweating, and pallor; symptoms are subjective indications of disease reported by the patient, such as pain, dizziness, and itching. Certain sets of signs and symptoms occur concurrently in some diseases, and their combination is called a syndrome.

## ▶ Diagnosis

Diagnosis, the determination of the nature of a disease, is based on many factors, including the signs, symptoms, and, often, laboratory results. Laboratory tests include such familiar procedures as urinalysis, blood chemistry, electrocardiography, and radiography. Diagnostic-imaging techniques such as computed tomography (CT scan), magnetic resonance imaging (MRI), ultrasound, and nuclear medicine allow physicians to visualize structural and functional changes. A biopsy, surgical removal and analy-

sis of tissue samples, yields information about changes at the cellular level. A physician also derives information for making a diagnosis from a physical examination, from interviewing the patient or a family member, and from a medical history of the patient and family.

## ▶ Describing Disease

The physician, having made a diagnosis, may state the prognosis of the disease, or the predicted course and outcome of the disease. The prognosis may state the chances for complete recovery, predict the permanent loss of function, or give probability of survival. The course of a disease varies; it may have a sudden onset and short term, in which case it is an acute disease. Influenza, measles, and the common cold are examples. A disease may begin insidiously and be long-lived, or chronic. Such diseases include diabetes, cancers, and osteoarthritis. Diseases that will end in death are called terminal.

The signs and symptoms of a chronic disease at times subside, during a period known as remission. They may recur in all their severity in a period of exacerbation. Certain diseases, leukemia and ulcerative colitis, for example, are characterized by periods of remission and exacerbation. A relapse occurs when a disease returns weeks or months after its apparent cessation.

A complication is a disease or other abnormal state that develops in a person already suffering from a disease. The complication may negatively affect the prognosis or course of the original disease. For example, a person confined to bed with a serious fracture may develop pneumonia as a complication of the inactivity. Infection of the testes may be a complication of mumps, particularly after puberty. Anemia generally accompanies leukemia, cancer, and chronic kidney disease. The aftermath of a particular disease is called the sequela, a sequel. The permanent damage to the heart after rheumatic fever is an example of a sequela, as is the paralysis of polio. The sterility resulting from severe inflammation of the fallopian tubes is also a sequela.

| Table 1–1 | Ten Leading Causes of Death, 2001, U.S. |
| --- | --- |
| **Disease** | **Number of Deaths** |
| Heart disease | 699,697 |
| Cancer | 553,251 |
| Stroke | 163,601 |
| Chronic lower respiratory disease | 123,974 |
| Accidents | 97,707 |
| Diabetes | 71,252 |
| Pneumonia/influenza | 62,123 |
| Alzheimer's disease | 53,679 |
| Nephritis, nephrotic syndrome, and nephrosis | 39,661 |
| Septicemia | 32,275 |

*Source:* CDC National Vital Statistic Report, vol. 51, no. 5

| Table 1–2 | Major Causes of Disease |
| --- | --- |
| **Cause** | **Diseases** |
| Inflammation/ autoimmunity/allergy | Asthma, systemic lupus erythematosus |
| Infection | Tuberculosis, influenza |
| Neoplasm | Lung cancer, malignant melanoma |
| Heredity | Sickle cell anemia, cystic fibrosis |
| Malnutrition | Pernicious anemia, iron-deficiency anemia |
| Stress | Hypertension, heart disease |

Public health agencies monitor the impact diseases have on populations by gathering mortality and morbidity data. Mortality is a measure of the number of deaths attributed to a disease in a given population over a given period of time. Morbidity is a measure of the disability and extent of illness caused by a disease. Each gives public health officials and physicians an idea of how serious a disease is and thus helps direct resources toward prevention and cure. Table 1–1 lists the 10 leading causes of death in the United States.

## ▶ Causes of Disease

An important aspect of any disease is its etiology, or cause. The source or cause of a disease, together with its development, is its pathogenesis. If the cause of a disease is not known, it is said to be idiopathic. Most causes of disease fall into one or more categories. At the root of most causes, however, is a lesion of some sort. A lesion could be a damaged gene or enzyme, or abnormal cells, tissues, or organs. The

## Prevention ✚ Plus!

### Handwashing: A Healthy Habit

Infection can often be prevented by the simple task of thorough handwashing with soap, rubbing vigorously for at least 10 seconds. Disease-causing microorganisms may be present on the skin surface, but proper handwashing prevents ingesting them or passing them on to others. Hands should always be washed before handling or eating food, before exiting the bathroom, after playing with pets, and after handling money. Health-care professionals must wash their hands after working with patients.

major causes and mechanisms of disease are discussed in the remaining chapters in Part I of the text. These causes include inflammatory or immune disorders, including allergy; infection; abnormal cell growth (neoplasms); heredity; nutrition; environmental; and stress. Table 1–2 lists these major causes and examples of associated diseases.

## CHAPTER SUMMARY

The body attempts to maintain homeostasis in the midst of ever-changing conditions. Disease is a state of functional disequilibrium that may be resolved by recovery or death. The definition, description, diagnosis, and causes of disease were discussed.

## RESOURCES

Centers for Disease Control and Prevention: www.cdc.gov

United States Department of Health and Human Services: www.dhhs.gov

# Interactive Activities

## Cases for Critical Thinking

1. Some athletes may develop abnormally high red blood cell counts. Why? In the athlete's case, is this a sign of disease?

2. A patient reports to her physician that she feels weak and dizzy. Is this enough information to make a diagnosis? What other sources of information can her physician consult?

3. Consult Table 1–1. How can this information be used to direct health-care research and resources? What is the significance of the information about accidents?

4. Table 1–2 lists heart disease as an example of a disease caused by stress. Discuss the link between heart disease and other causes listed in this table.

## Multiple Choice

1. A skin rash is an example of a _____.

   a. sign
   b. symptom
   c. laboratory result
   d. syndrome

2. A(n) _____ disease has a sudden onset and short course.

   a. acute
   b. terminal
   c. chronic
   d. idiopathic

3. The cause of a disease is known as its _____.

   a. pathogensis
   c. sequela
   b. complication
   d. etiology

4. A steady state maintained within the body is called _____.

   a. homeostasis
   b. disease
   c. disequilibrium
   d. pathology

5. Signs and symptoms recur and become worse during _____.

   a. remission
   b. exacerbation
   c. relapse
   d. complication

## True or False

_____ 1. Anatomy is the study of normal body function.

_____ 2. Mortality refers to the number of deaths caused by a disease.

_____ 3. Symptoms are objective evidence of a disease.

_____ 4. Signs may be perceived by the physician.

_____ 5. Exacerbation and remission may characterize a chronic disease.

## Fill-Ins

1. The predicted outcome of a disease is its _____.

2. Damaged tissue, DNA, or enzymes are examples of _____ that cause a disease.

3. If the cause of a disease is not known, it is said to be _____.

4. Return of symptoms after their apparent cessation is _____.

5. The signs and symptoms of a chronic disease at times subside during a period known as _____.

# MedMedia Wrap-Up

**www.prenhall.com/mulvihill**
Remember to visit this website for extra study practice, including exercises, Internet links, news updates, and an audio glossary.

**Activity CD-ROM**
Check out the CD-ROM in the back of this book. You will find games, exercises, puzzles, and videos to help enhance your understanding of this chapter.

In these renal glomeruli, there is proliferation of cells representing proliferative glomerulonephritis. (Courtesy of the National Toxicology Program.)

# Immunity, Inflammation, and Immune Disorders

**CHAPTER**

# 2

## Learning Objectives

After studying this chapter, you should be able to

- List and discuss nonspecific defenses
- List and discuss the signs and symptoms of inflammation
- List and discuss specific defenses
- Describe hypersensitivity
- Describe autoimmunity
- Describe AIDS as it relates to immunodeficiency
- Compare and contrast active and passive immunity

## Fact or Fiction?

HIV can be transmitted through saliva.

*Fiction:* HIV is found in saliva, but in such small concentrations that it is estimated a person would have to ingest a bucket of saliva to become infected.

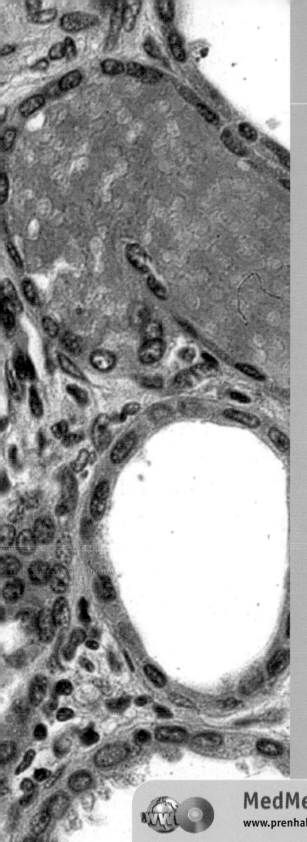

# Disease Chronicle

## Inflammation

Throughout history, humans undoubtedly have observed the inflammatory response even if they understood little of its causes or treatment. One of the early systemic descriptions of inflammation came from the Roman physician Celsus, who listed its cardinal signs: heat, redness, swelling, and pain. Ancient Greeks used the bark of willow trees to decrease inflammation. Today, the active ingredient in aspirin, acetylsalicylic acid, is derived from a related anti-inflammatory chemical in willow tree bark.

## ▶ Defense Mechanisms

The immune system has the daunting task of protecting the body against foreign attack. Immunity is the ability of the body to defend itself against infectious agents, foreign cells, and even abnormal body cells, such as cancer cells. Immunity includes nonspecific and specific defenses. Nonspecific defense mechanisms are effective against any foreign agent that enters the body and are referred to as innate immunity. Specific defense mechanisms are effective against particular identified foreign agents and are referred to as acquired immunity.

### Nonspecific Defense and Innate Immunity

**Physical and Chemical Barriers**  Intact skin is the body's first line of defense. A physical barrier, skin also produces chemical barriers to infection. Secretions such as tears, saliva, sweat, and oil contain chemicals that destroy foreign invaders. Mucous membranes that line body passages open to the exterior produce mucus, which traps foreign material and forms a barrier to invasion. Microscopic cilia hairs that line the respiratory tract sweep out debris and impurities trapped in mucus.

**Phagocytosis**  White blood cells (leukocytes) can destroy infectious agents through phagocytosis. In phagocytosis, which means cell eating, leukocytes engulf and digest bacteria or other material. This process is fairly nonspecific, unable to discriminate among or remember past encounters with various types of infectious agents. While some leukocytes travel in the blood to target foreign material, others remain in tissues.

**Natural Killer Cells**  Natural killer cells are a type of leukocyte that recognizes body cells with abnormal membranes. Cell membranes can become altered from cells being infected with foreign invaders like viruses. Natural killer cells can destroy abnormal cells on contact by secreting a protein that destroys the cell membrane.

**Fever**  Fever can be a sign that the body is defending itself. When phagocytes find and destroy foreign invaders, they release substances that raise body temperature. Fever aids the immune system by stimulating phagocytes, increasing metabolism, and inhibiting the multiplication of some microorganisms. Hence, fever is a symptom arising from the normal interplay between the immune system and microorganisms, and can be beneficial. Fever should not always be eliminated; however, fever should be monitored closely.

**Interferon**  Interferon is a group of substances that stimulate the immune system. Because interferon boosts the immune system, it has been used to treat infections and cancer. Interferon was first found in cells infected with the flu virus and was named for its ability to interfere with viral multiplication. Virus-infected cells and other agents produce interferon.

### Inflammation

The cause of the inflammation may be a trauma or injury, such as a sprained ankle or a severe blow. A physical irritant in the tissue—a piece of glass, a wasp sting, or an ingrown toenail—will trigger the response. Pathogenic organisms—bacteria, viruses, fungi, or parasites—will do the same. Figure 2–1 shows various agents that are capable of stimulating an inflammatory response.

The cardinal signs and symptoms of inflammation are redness, swelling, heat, and pain. Inflammation is a protective tissue response to injury or invasion.

Vascular changes occur when tissue is traumatized or irritated. Local blood vessels, arterioles, and capillaries dilate, increasing blood flow to the injured area. This increased amount of blood, hyperemia, causes the heat and redness associated with inflammation. As the blood flow to the site of the injury or infection increases, more and more leukocytes reach the area. Leukocytes called neutrophils or polymorphs line up within the capillary walls. The polymorphs are specialized cells that defend the body against invading microorganisms and speed

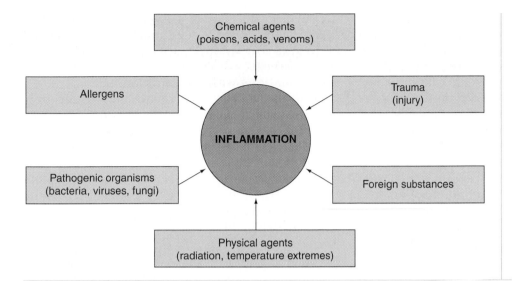

**Figure 2–1**
Agents capable of stimulating an inflammatory response.

healing by engulfing cell debris in injured tissues.

The damaged tissue releases a substance called **histamine** that causes the capillary walls to become more permeable. This increased permeability enables plasma and neutrophils to move out of the blood vessels into the tissue. Figure 2–2 shows the vascular changes that occur with inflammation and the movement of polymorphs to the infected site. The attraction of the white blood cells to the site of inflammation is called **chemotaxis**.

The plasma and white blood cells that escape from the capillaries comprise the **inflammatory exudate**. This exudate in the tissues causes the swelling associated with inflammation. The excess of fluid in the tissues puts pressure on sensitive nerve endings, causing pain.

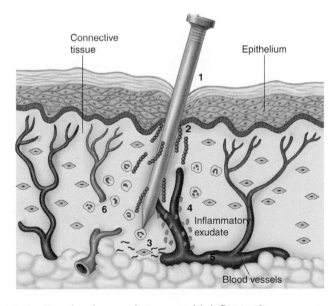

1. Dirty nail punctures skin.

2. Bacteria enter and multiply.

3. Injured cells release histamine.

4. Blood vessels dilate and become permeable, releasing inflammatory exudate.

5. Blood flow to the damaged site increases.

6. Neutrophils (polymorph) move toward bacteria (chemotaxis) and destroy them (phagocytosis).

**Figure 2–2** Vascular changes that occur with inflammation.

Bacterial infection may cause inflammation. The presence of toxin-producing bacteria such as staphylococci and streptococci triggers an inflammatory response. To increase the effectiveness of the inflammatory and immune response, the bone marrow and lymph nodes release very large quantities of leukocytes. The white cell count may rise to 30,000 or more from the normal range of 7000 to 9000 per cubic microliter of blood. The excessive production of white cells is called leukocytosis and is a sign of infection or inflammation, such as appendicitis.

The polymorphs die soon after ingesting bacteria and toxins, and release substances that liquefy the surrounding tissue, forming pus, a thick yellow fluid consisting of liquefied tissue, dead polymorphs, and inflammatory exudate. Other phagocytic white cells, the monocytes or macrophages, follow the polymorphs in the process of clearing debris. Inflammatory exudate contains a plasma protein, fibrin, essential for the blood-clotting mechanism. Fibrin forms a clot in the damaged tissue, walling off the infection and preventing its spread.

Bacteria that cause pus formation are called pyogenic bacteria. An inflammation associated with pus formation is a suppurative inflammation. Abscesses, boils, and styes are examples of inflammations with suppuration.

Wound healing and repair can occur only when bacteria have been destroyed. Cut edges of tissue grow together as connective tissue cells (fibroblasts) produce fibers that close the gap. Figure 2–3 shows the fibroblasts and their fibers healing a skin incision. The healed site consists of a meshwork of connective tissue fibers known as scar tissue. Sometimes the connective tissue fibers anchor together adjacent structures, causing adhesions, which can interfere with organ functions. The problems associated with adhesions are explained in later chapters.

A scar after surgery or a severe burn is often raised and hard. This development is known as keloid healing and is really a benign tumor (Figure 2–4). Surgery to remove such a scar is usually ineffective, as the subsequent incision will have a tendency to heal in the same way.

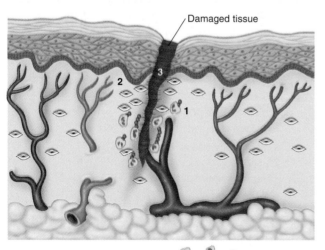

1. Neutrophils phagocytize bacteria.
2. Fibroblasts produce connective tissue fibers.
3. Fibers contract, drawing cut surfaces together.

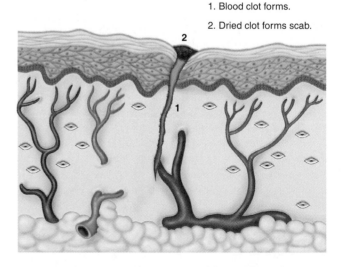

1. Blood clot forms.
2. Dried clot forms scab.

**Figure 2–3** Fibroblasts healing a wound.

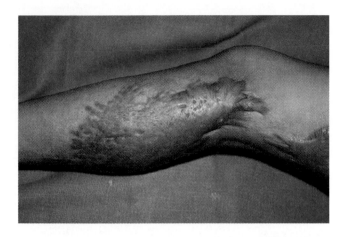

**Figure 2–4** Keloid. (© JCD/Custom Medical Stock Photo.)

## Specific Defenses and Acquired Immunity

While nonspecific defenses defend the body against infections in general, acquired immunity defends against specific types of microorganisms. Once established against a specific microorganism, acquired immunity also is able to respond specifically to future exposures to the same microorganism. Immunity can be acquired naturally by infection, as when chicken pox confers protection against acquiring it again. Immunity can be artificially acquired by immunization, as when the polio vaccine induces immunity against polio.

The foreign element that triggers the immune response is known as an antigen, which often is a protein from microorganisms or other foreign cells. Antigens differ from each other in structure and are unique. The specificity of acquired immunity is its ability to recognize these different antigens.

Specific defenses against antigens include humoral and cell-mediated immunity. Humoral immunity includes antibodies and cell-mediated immunity includes activated lymphocytes. Antibodies and activated lymphocytes comprise acquired immunity.

An important part of immunity is the body's lymphatic system. It consists of a complex network of thin-walled capillaries, lymph nodes, and lymphatic vessels that conduct and filter lymph. Lymph arises in tissue as a filtrate from blood capillaries. This pale watery fluid is returned via lymph capillaries and vessels to the blood. The lymph nodes filter the lymph, removing any microorganisms before they can enter the blood. Lymph nodes contain lymphocytes, monocytes, and plasma cells that destroy invading organisms. Organs such as the spleen, tonsils, and adenoids are comprised of lymphoid tissue and also function in the body's internal defense (Figure 2–5).

How do the tissues of the lymphatic system work with the components of acquired immunity to defend the body against infection? Remember that antibodies provide humoral immunity and activated lymphocytes provide cell-mediated immunity (Figure 2–6). Cells responsible for both humoral and cell-mediated immunity are found in lymph nodes and lymphoid tissue such as the spleen, bone marrow, tonsils, and adenoids. The lymphoid tissue is placed strategically in the body, such as in the throat and nasal cavity, to intercept invading organisms.

Both humoral and cell-mediated immunity can work together to fight a foreign invader. Both are activated by an antigen, such as Salmonella bacteria from an undercooked chicken breast. The antigen interacts with lymphocytes in tissues, in lymph, or in blood.

Two types of lymphocytes provide immunity: the T and B lymphocytes. The lymphocytes responsible for cell-mediated immunity are processed by the thymus gland; hence they are called T lymphocytes. The other type of lymphocytes, B lymphocytes, are responsible for humoral immunity. Antibodies and T lymphocytes are each highly specific for one type of antigen.

B cells can play different roles in humoral immunity. Some B cells interact with antigens and become activated. Some other activated B lymphocytes are transformed into plasma cells, which divide rapidly and produce large numbers of antibodies. These agents are secreted into the lymph and travel to the blood to be circulated through the body. The antibodies are plasma proteins, which are gamma globulins called immunoglobulins (Ig). Antibodies bind to antigens and tag the antigen for destruction by the immune system. There are several types of immunoglobulins, and each type has specialized

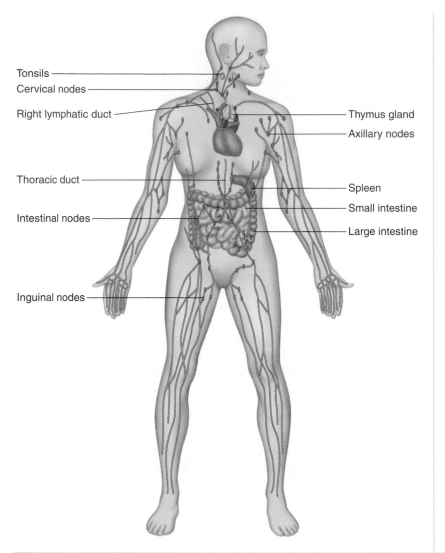

**Figure 2–5**
The lymphatic system.

Tonsils
Cervical nodes
Right lymphatic duct
Thoracic duct
Intestinal nodes
Inguinal nodes

Thymus gland
Axillary nodes
Spleen
Small intestine
Large intestine

functions. See Table 2–1 for a summary of their functions.

Other B lymphocytes do not become plasma cells but remain dormant until reactivated by the same antigen. These lymphocytes are called memory cells and are responsible for a more potent and rapid antibody response during subsequent exposures to the same antigen. This secondary response to the antigen produces antibodies faster and in larger quantities, and lasts longer than the initial response. This strong secondary response explains why a vaccine protects a person from a subsequent exposure to an infectious agent. The secondary immune response also is the basis for the effectiveness of booster shots, which are given at intervals after initial vaccinations in order to increase levels of memory cells (Figure 2–7).

There are several different kinds of T cells, each with different functions: cytotoxic T cells, helper T cells, and suppressor T cells.

The cytotoxic T cells are often called killer cells because they are capable of killing invading organisms. They have on their surfaces receptor proteins that bind tightly to cells or organisms that contain a specific antigen. Once bound, the cytotoxic T cells release poisonous substances into the attacked cell. Many organ-

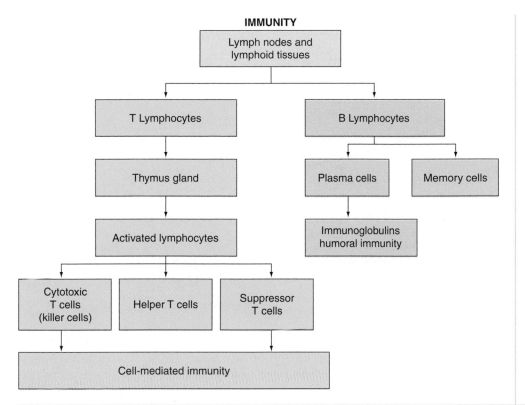

Figure 2–6
Cell-mediated immunity
versus humoral immunity.

isms can be killed by one killer cell. The cytotoxic cells are important in killing cells that have been invaded by viruses. These T cells also can destroy cancer cells

The helper T cells are named for their ability to help the immune system in many ways. They increase the activity of killer cells and stimulate B cells. Activated helper T cells secrete lymphokines that increase the response of other types of lymphoid cells to the antigen. In addition, lymphokines activate macrophages to destroy large numbers of invaders by phagocytosis.

## Table 2–1  Types of Immunoglobulins

| Type | Function | Location |
| --- | --- | --- |
| IgG | Produced in primary and secondary immune responses, neutralizes toxins and viruses | Blood plasma; crosses the placenta from mother to fetus |
| IgM | Protects newborns | Bound to B cells in circulation; usually the first to increase in the immune response |
| IgA | Localized protection at mucosal surfaces | Mucosal secretions, colostrum (early breast milk) |
| IgE | Allergy | Trace amounts in serum; secreted by sensitized plasma cells in tissues and locally attached to mast cells |
| IgD | Activates B cells | Attached to B cells |

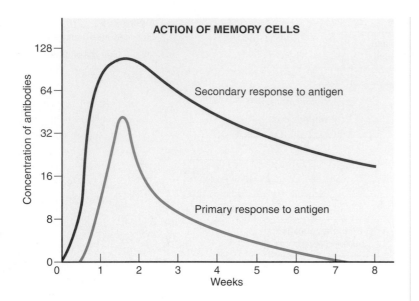

ACTION OF MEMORY CELLS

Concentration of antibodies

Secondary response to antigen

Primary response to antigen

Weeks

**Figure 2–7**
Secondary response begins more rapidly after exposure to antigen, produces more antibodies, and lasts for a longer time than initial exposure.

## ▶ Hypersensitivity—Allergies

Closely related to the concept of immunity is **allergy**, or **hypersensitivity**. Some diseases result from an individual's immune response, which causes tissue damage and disordered function rather than immunity. The immune phenomena are destructive rather than defensive in the individual who is hypersensitive or allergic (atopic) to an antigen. Hypersensitivity diseases or allergic diseases may manifest themselves locally or systemically.

Abnormal sensitivity to allergens such as pollens, dust, dog hair, and certain foods or chemicals is the result of overproduction of IgE and its interaction with the allergens. IgE attaches one end to cells called **basophils** and **mast cells**; its other end points away from the cells, where the IgE can bind to the allergens. Mast cells are found in connective tissue and contain the chemicals **heparin**, **serotonin**, **bradykinin**, and histamine.

When allergens enter the body and bind to the IgE antibodies located on the mast cells, the cells break down and release their chemicals. Histamine causes the dilation of the blood vessels, making them leak plasma into the tissues. This tissue fluid causes edema, or swelling, which when localized in the nasal

passages results in the familiar congestion and irritation of hay fever. If the tissue damage and edema are near the skin, the welts and itching of hives may appear. Antihistamines inhibit the effects of histamine and are quite effective in the treatment of hives but less so for hay fever. A typical allergic reaction is illustrated in Figure 2–8.

Skin tests can determine the specific cause of an allergy. This procedure involves injecting a minute amount of antigen intradermally and observing any redness, which indicates a positive skin reaction.

Allergy shots can desensitize the hypersensitive person. Small amounts of the offending allergen are administered, and concentrations are gradually increased. Desensitization inoculations work by causing an increase of IgG in the bloodstream. The IgG coats the allergen in the blood, blocking it from binding to IgE in the tissues, subsequently reducing the amount of tissue damage.

Local (atopic) allergies occur in confined areas such as skin and mucous membranes, and are exemplified by the development of a stuffy nose after inhaling pollen. In contrast, systemic allergy (**anaphylactic shock**) occurs throughout the body and may be life-threatening.

The underlying cellular mechanisms of the systemic anaphylactic reaction are the same as

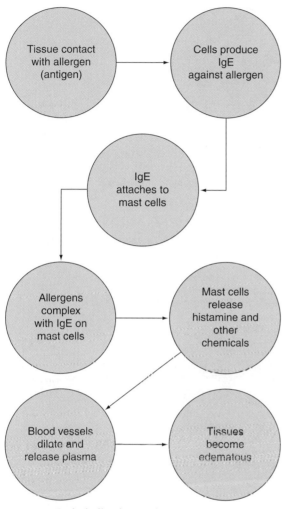

**Figure 2–8** Typical allergic reaction.

tress resembling asthma. Fluid in the larynx may obstruct the airways and necessitate a tracheotomy, a surgical opening into the trachea to facilitate passage of air or evacuation of secretions.

Less severe signs may include skin flush, hives, swelling of lips or tongue, wheezing, and abdominal cramps. Life-threatening signs include weakness and collapse due to low blood pressure, inability to breathe, and seizures.

Epinephrine, glucocorticoids, or cortisone derivatives may be used to reduce the immune response and stabilize the vascular system.

Four types of hypersensitivities are recognized. Type I hypersensitivities are labeled allergic or anaphylactic hypersensitivity. These are triggered by allergen binding to IgE on mast cells, which produces either local severe inflammation (atopic allergy) or systemic severe inflammation (anaphylactic shock) (Figure 2–9). These are produced by bee venom, foods, or pollen.

Type II hypersensitivities are labeled cytotoxic or cytolytic, and involve IgM or IgG interacting with foreign cells to cause their destruction. An example of a type II response is an incompatible blood transfusion. A person with type A blood has A antigens on the red cells and antibodies against type B blood in the serum. If such a person receives a type B transfusion, the antigens and antibodies interact. The red blood cells agglutinate, or clump together, and hemolyze (rupture). Massive hemolysis occurs (Figure 2–10).

Cross-matching for a blood transfusion must match blood type and Rh factor. In addition to antigens that determine blood type, Rh positive (Rh⁺) individuals have another antigen, the Rh factor, on their red blood cells. Rh negative (Rh⁻) individuals lack the Rh antigen. Another example of the cytolytic allergic response involves the transfusion of Rh⁺ blood to an Rh⁻ recipient. No

in the local response. However, during the systemic response, mast cells and basophils throughout the body become involved, triggering a generalized change in capillary permeability that leads to hypotension, low blood pressure, and shock. Smooth muscle contraction in the respiratory tract causes respiratory dis-

## Prevention ✚ PLUS!

### Epinephrine Treatment for Anaphylaxis

The most vital therapy for systemic anaphylaxis is prompt intramuscular injection of epinephrine (adrenalin). Certain allergic individuals must carry epinephrine at all times in an EpiPen®, which can be self-injected in an emergency.

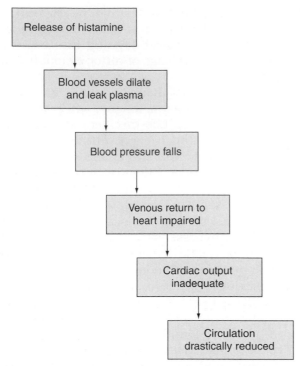

**Figure 2–9** Sequence of vascular events in anaphylactic shock.

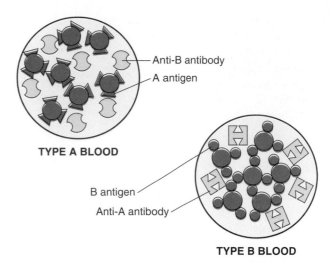

If type A blood receives a donation of type B, antibodies of the recipient react with antigens of the donor

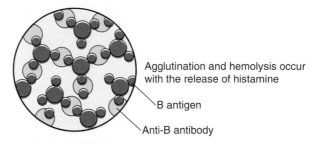

**Figure 2–10** Cytotoxic allergy (incompatible blood transfusion).

problems would arise for the Rh⁻ recipient if it were the first such transfusion received, but if the Rh⁻ recipient was previously exposed or sensitized to the Rh factor, the recipient may form antibodies against this foreign protein, causing clumping and rupture of red blood cells.

Rh incompatibility during pregnancy is also a type II hypersensitivity. An Rh⁻ mother can become sensitized to the Rh antigen if the fetus is Rh⁺. However, maternal antibodies do not form and damage the fetus during the first such pregnancy, because the maternal and fetal blood do not mix. But, during birth there may be mixing of blood, exposing the mother to the Rh⁺ antigen. The mother's immune system can recognize this antigen as foreign and produce antibodies against it, which would threaten subsequent pregnancies with an Rh⁺ fetus. To prevent this, RhoGAM®, an injectable medication, is given to Rh⁻ women after the delivery of Rh⁺ babies.

Type III hypersensitivities are labeled immune complex. In this type of hypersensitivity, antigens combine with antibodies, forming immune complexes. These immune complexes de-

posit in tissues and blood vessels, causing inflammation and tissue destruction. Immune complexes may form in the kidney (causing glomerulonephritis, triggered after a streptococcal infection) or the lung (causing farmer's lung, triggered by mold spore inhalation). Types I, II, and III are all immediate hypersensitivities; they develop within about 30 minutes of exposure to antigens or allergens.

Type IV hypersensitivities are called cell-mediated or delayed. Initial exposure to an antigen results in activation of a T-cell–mediated immune response, which is slow to develop (delayed). For example, no reaction occurs the first time one contacts the oil of poison ivy. However, T cells may become sensitized to it. On the next exposure, the typical rash and irritation appear, caused by T-cell secretion of cytokines that damage the tissues where the ivy oil has been absorbed. This delayed development is the type of reaction found in contact dermatitis and the positive tuberculin test (Figure 2–11).

Tissue and organ rejections are examples of type IV or delayed hypersensitivity reactions. Organs could be easily transplanted if it were not for the immune system. The immune system recognizes the transplanted organ as foreign, and lymphocytes attack it, eventually destroying the transplanted organ. Compounding the problem is that the transplanted organ carries with it donor lymphocytes that react against the recipient's tissues (a graft versus host reaction). For these reasons, donor and recipient antigens are matched as closely as possible to lessen possible rejection. Immunosuppressive medication must be taken prior to transplant surgery and possibly for the remainder of the recipient's life to suppress rejection. Table 2–2 summarizes the four types of hypersensitivities.

## ▶ Autoimmunity

The immune response normally recognizes the difference between the individual's own tissues and those of invaders; this is known as

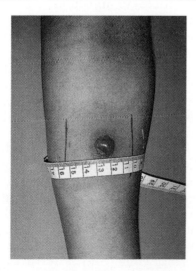

**Figure 2–11**  Positive tuberculin skin test. A Type IV hypersensitivity. (Courtesy of the CDC.)

tolerance. However, when tolerance fails, the immune system attacks the body's own tissue, causing autoimmune diseases. Autoimmune diseases occur when individuals develop antibodies to their own tissues or self-antigens. The antibodies produced are called autoantibodies because they attack the individual's tissues. Several of these autoimmune diseases, such as rheumatic fever, glomerulonephritis, myasthenia gravis, and rheumatoid arthritis, are described elsewhere in this book. Lupus erythematosus and scleroderma are considered here.

## Systemic Lupus Erythematosus

Systemic lupus erythematosus (SLE) is a noncontagious inflammatory disease that takes one of two forms: mild or severe. Young women are most frequently affected by systemic lupus, which may begin suddenly or insidiously. The skin develops a rash and becomes overly sensitive to sunlight. Joint and muscle pains may be accompanied by fever. The lymph nodes and spleen are frequently found to be enlarged. Periods of exacerbation and remission are characteristic of the disease. The discoid form is a minor disorder in which red, raised, itchy lesions develop. The lesions characteristically form the pattern of a butterfly over the nose and cheeks (Figure 2–12).

The severe form of lupus not only affects the skin but also causes the deterioration of collagenous connective tissue. Systemic lupus can affect the glomeruli of the kidney, causing abnormal excretion of albumin and blood as well as casts in the urine. The red cell, white cell, and platelet counts are low. The lining of the heart and the heart valves may deteriorate.

Hypersensitivity to an antigen is thought to be the cause of SLE. The antigen may be an allergen outside the body or the patient's own tissue to which the patient has become sensitized, and thus an example of autoimmunity. Consistent with the autoimmune hypothesis, antinuclear antibodies (ANA) have been observed in the blood of lupus patients. These antibodies attach to the body's own cell nuclei, destroying the RNA and DNA of the cell. Detection of ANA supports the diagnosis of lupus.

| Table 2–2 | Types of Hypersensitivities | |
|---|---|---|
| **Type** | **Mechanism** | **Effect** |
| I | Excess IgE bound to mast cells and activated by allergens | Inflammation |
| II | IgM or IgG cause destruction of foreign cells | Cell lysis |
| III | Immune complexes deposited in tissue and vessels | Inflammation and tissue destruction |
| IV | Sensitized T cells release cytokines | Inflammation and tissue damage |

Treatment of lupus is symptomatic and includes nonsteroidal anti-inflammatory, antipyretic, and analgesic medications. Life-threatening exacerbations are often treated with corticosteriods. The disease is chronic, with death frequently resulting from kidney or heart failure.

## Scleroderma

Scleroderma is a chronic, progressive autoimmune disorder of the skin. It is characterized by sclerosis or hardening, thickening, and shrinking of the skin and internal organs, including the heart, lungs, and kidneys. As tissues become hardened and thickened, function is often limited. Milder forms of scleroderma are limited to the skin, face, and extremities. The more severe form of scleroderma affects not only the skin but also internal organs.

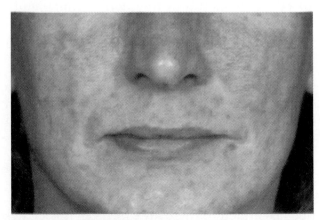

**Figure 2–12** Systemic lupus erythematosus rash. (© NMSB/Custom Medical Stock Photo.)

Treatment for scleroderma includes anti-inflammatory medications and immunosuppressive medication. Physical therapy helps to maintain muscle strength and joint mobility. Death usually results from cardiac, pulmonary, or renal failure.

## ▶ Immune Deficiency

### Acquired Immunodeficiency Syndrome (AIDS)

One of the most deadly diseases to affect today's population is acquired immunodeficiency syndrome (AIDS). AIDS destroys the individual's immune system, making the person remarkably susceptible to infection. AIDS was first noted among promiscuous homosexual and bisexual men and drug users who shared hypodermic needles.

AIDS is a global epidemic. As of the end of 2003, an estimated 37.8 million people worldwide were living with HIV/AIDS. Approximately two-thirds of these people live in sub-Saharan Africa. An estimated 4.8 million new HIV infections occurred worldwide during 2003; that is about 14,000 infections each day. Approximately 40,000 new HIV infections occur each year in the United States, about 70% among men and 30% among women. Of these newly infected people, half are younger than 25 years of age.

The causative agent of AIDS is the human immunodeficiency virus (HIV), a retrovirus; that is, it carries its genetic information as RNA rather than DNA. The virus infects primarily helper T$_4$

lymphocytes. The virus replicates within these lymphocytes, killing them and spreading to others. These lymphocytes normally activate B-cell lymphocytes; thus, the body's immune response is crippled, and the body is suceptible to infections and tumors that a healthy immune system could easily control.

The presence of HIV antibodies in the blood can be detected with the enzyme-linked immunosorbent assay (ELISA). If the ELISA test is positive, the test is usually repeated and the result confirmed using a Western blot test. A positive P24 antigen test indicates circulating HIV antigen. Anonymous free testing for HIV antibodies is available at local health departments.

HIV is transmitted via contaminated body fluids, including blood, semen, vaginal secretions, and breast milk. Therefore, HIV is transmitted by unprotected anal, oral, or vaginal intercourse, birth, breastfeeding, and the sharing of needles.

Before the law required that donated blood be screened, some recipients of blood transfusions developed AIDS. Reliable tests for the presence of the virus now minimize the risk of contracting it through contaminated blood transfusion. Blood donors do not contract the virus from giving blood because a new needle is used each time.

**HIV Infection** Even before full-blown AIDS develops, the virus destroys the immune system of the HIV-positive individual. Studies have shown that large amounts of the virus can be present during the asymptomatic stage of the disease. The virus resides in high concentration in lymph nodes, where it continues to increase.

There is a long and variable latent period of 2 to 8 years between HIV infection and the development of full-blown AIDS. An individual who tests positive for HIV may manifest some of the signs of AIDS, such as flulike symptoms, when first infected, but may recover and be symptom-free for some period of time. The long latent period increases the risk of spreading the infection because individuals are not aware they have the disease. Once infected, the patient is infected for life. Eventually, a threshold is crossed and the HIV-infected person develops AIDS. To move from an HIV-positive diagnosis to an AIDS diagnosis, one must have one of 23 indicator diseases and have a T4 (or CD4) cell count of less than 200.

**Precautions for Health-Care Professionals** Health-care professionals must exercise great precautions when handling blood or bodily secretions of AIDS patients. Several workers have contracted the virus by accidental needle sticks. The best protection against HIV exposure is consistent adherence to the Standard Precautions recommended by the Centers for Disease Control and Prevention (CDC) and the guidelines required by the Occupational Safety and Health Administration (OSHA).

OSHA requires employers to train employees who are at risk of exposure to blood-borne pathogens; training must be held during work hours and at no cost to employees. Appropriate instruction on handwashing; the use of gloves, gowns, and protective eye covering; and the proper disposal of sharps must be provided. Information must be given on the facility's exposure-control plan, blood-borne disease symptoms and modes of transmission, and use and limitations of risk-reduction methods. Employees must be informed of hepatitis B vaccination availability (Chapter 10), actions to take in case of emergencies, and procedures to follow if exposure incidents occur.

Warning labels bearing the biohazard symbol (Figure 2–13) in fluorescent orange or orange-red must be part of, or securely affixed to, containers used to store, transport, or dispose of potentially infectious material. Refrigerators and freezers used for such material must also be labeled. Red bags or red containers may be substituted for labels on containers of infectious wastes.

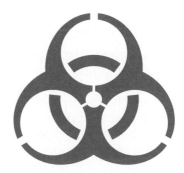

**BIOHAZARD**

**Figure 2–13** Required warning on potentially hazardous material.

**Treatment**  Development of a vaccine to prevent the spread of AIDS has not yet been possible. The genetic makeup of the AIDS virus varies greatly from strain to strain, and HIV tends to mutate quickly, which complicates the attempt to develop an AIDS vaccine.

Anti-HIV medications are used to control multiplication of the virus and to slow the progression of HIV-related disease. The sooner drug therapy begins after infection the better the chances are that the immune system will not be destroyed by HIV. While there is no cure for AIDS, a cocktail of drugs may hinder HIV multiplication to the extent that the viral load becomes undetectable in some individuals. Anti-HIV medications do not cure HIV infection, and individuals taking these medications can still transmit HIV to others.

Highly active antiretroviral therapy (HAART) is the recommended treatment for HIV infection. HAART combines three or more anti-HIV medications in a daily regimen. Anti-HIV medications fall into four classes. Nonnucleoside reverse transcriptase inhibitors bind to and disable reverse transcriptase, a protein that HIV needs to multiply. Nucleoside reverse transcriptase inhibitors are faulty versions of building blocks that HIV needs to multiply. When HIV uses a faulty building block replication of HIV is stalled. Protease inhibitors disable protease, a protein HIV needs to multiply. Fusion inhibitors prevent HIV entry into cells. It is important to realize that these drugs are very expensive, they cause side effects, and the regimen of pill-taking throughout the day is very demanding. If the drugs are not taken as prescribed or if the therapy is stopped, resistance or relapse may occur.

## Chronic Fatigue Syndrome

Chronic fatigue syndrome affects primarily young professionals in the prime of life. It has been dubbed "yuppie flu" because of the class of individuals affected. The flulike symptoms include severe and persistent fatigue, muscle and joint pain, and fever. The person experiences trouble with concentration and memory.

The cause and cure are unknown, although much research has been done on the disease. It was thought at first to be psychosomatic or the result of depression, but changes have been found in the patient's immune system. No virus has been proven to be the cause, but blood tests have shown an immune response consistent with a viral infection. Some, but not all, individuals have antibodies to Epstein-Barr virus. Other evidence points to herpes b virus.

## ▶ Vaccination

Two types of artificial immunity can be administered: active and passive immunity. In active immunity, the person receives a vaccine or a toxoid as the antigen, and he or she forms antibodies to counteract it. A vaccine consists of a low dose of dead or deactivated bacteria or viruses. Because the organisms have been specially treated to deactivate them, they cannot cause disease. As protein foreign to the body, these antigens do trigger antibody production against them. A toxoid works similarly. It consists of a chemically altered toxin, the poisonous material produced by a pathogenic organism. Having been treated chemically, the toxin will not cause disease. It will, however, stimulate the immune response. The newest types of vaccines insert genes for specific disease antigens into the genetic material of harmless organisms. The antigens produced by these organisms are extracted, purified, and used for immunization. The hepatitis B vaccine is produced in this manner.

Active immunity, in which cells are exposed to an antigen and begin to form the corresponding antibodies, is long-lived. Such protection prevents diseases such as polio and diphtheria. Time is required to build up immunity, and for some vaccines, a booster shot is necessary. Once cells have been sensitized to these viruses, bacteria, or toxins, they retain the ability to produce antibodies against them when encountered again.

What if a person is exposed to a serious disease such as hepatitis, tetanus, or rabies and has no immunity against it? It takes too much time to build antibodies in response to a vaccination. In this case, the person is given passive immunity, doses of preformed antibodies from immune serum of an animal, usually a horse. This type of immunity is short-lived but acts immediately. Table 2–3 contrasts active and passive immunity.

| Table 2–3 | Differences between Active and Passive Immunity |
| --- | --- |
| **Active Immunity** | **Passive Immunity** |
| Person forms antibodies | Preformed antibodies received |
| Vaccine (deactivated bacteria or virus) | Immune horse serum |
| or | or |
| Toxoid (chemically altered toxin) | Antibodies, cells in breast milk |
| Long-lived immunity (requires time to act) | Short-lived immunity (acts immediately) |

## ▶ Stress and the Immune System

Stressors such as trauma, infection, surgery, pain, and emotional distress all have significant effects on the immune system's ability to function. Stress causes an increased production of the hormone cortisol. Cortisol decreases production of antibodies and substances released by leukocytes that stimulate other cells of the immune system.

Cortisol production occurs when norepinephrine and epinephrine are released by the sympathetic nervous system, as happens during the fight-or-flight response. The combined effect of these three hormones increases the total number of neutrophils in the circulation.

Lymphocyte maturation in the lymph nodes stops because epinephrine decreases blood flow to the lymph nodes as it increases blood flow to the heart, lungs, brain, and muscles.

These changes in the immune response brought on by stress leave the body less capable of fighting off the effects of injury, disease, and other stress causes.

eign antigens and responds to counteract them with antibodies and activated lymphocytes. Antibodies produce humoral immunity, and activated lymphocytes produce cell-mediated immunity. Stimulated B cells turn into plasma cells that secrete the different types of immunoglobulins involved in humoral immunity. Several types of T cells, including killer cells, helper cells, and suppressor cells, are involved in cell-mediated immunity.

Allergies can be considered a side effect of immunity. Allergic diseases are the result of an immune response that causes tissue damage and disordered function rather than immunity. Hypersensitivity to harmless substances is the result of abnormally formed immunoglobulins in the allergic person. Allergies range in severity from local tissue damage, as in hay fever and hives, to a systemic anaphylactic reaction that can be life-threatening.

An abnormality in the immune system can cause disease when the body becomes hypersensitive to its own tissue and destroys it. This is known as autoimmunity. An example of deficiency in the immune system is acquired immunodeficiency syndrome, or AIDS. Artificial immunity can be provided by vaccination. In active immunity, the individual is given a vaccine or a toxoid and actively makes antibodies to counteract it. Preformed antibodies are given in passive immunity.

## CHAPTER SUMMARY

The immune system provides the body with strong defenses against invading organisms. These defenses can be specific or nonspecific.

Nonspecific defenses include physical and chemical barriers, phagocytosis, natural killer cells, fever, and inflammation. In specific defenses, the body recognizes for-

## RESOURCES

The National Institutes of Health: www.nih.org

The American Academy of Pediatrics: www.aap.org

Lupus Foundation of America: www.lupus.org

## Prevention ✚ PLUS!

### Disease Prevention through Vaccination

Without appropriate immunization, children are susceptible to many serious and life-threatening infections such as measles, whooping cough, hepatitis, and meningitis. Vaccines are effective, particularly when a high proportion of people in a population are immunized. Reactions to the vaccines are usually mild and rarely serious. The risks from these childhood diseases far outweigh the risk of a serious reaction from a vaccine. The chart below includes childhood immunization recommendations from the American Academy of Pediatrics.

| Vaccine ▼    Age ► | Birth | 1 mo | 2 mo | 4 mo | 6 mo | 12 mo | 15 mo | 18 mo | 24 mo | 4-6 y | 11-12 y | 13-18 y |
|---|---|---|---|---|---|---|---|---|---|---|---|---|
| | | Range of Recommended Ages | | | | Catch-up Immunization | | | | Preadolescent Assessment | | |
| Hepatitis B[1] | HepB #1 | only if motherHBsAg ( - ) | | | | | | | | | HepB series | |
| | | | HepB #2 | | | HepB #3 | | | | | | |
| Diphtheria, Tetanus, Pertussis[2] | | | DTaP | DTaP | DTaP | | DTaP | | | DTaP | Td | Td |
| Haemophilus influenzae Type b[3] | | | Hib | Hib | Hib | Hib | | | | | | |
| Inactivated Poliovirus | | | IPV | IPV | | IPV | | | | IPV | | |
| Measles, Mumps, Rubella[4] | | | | | | MMR #1 | | | | MMR #2 | MMR #2 | |
| Varicella[5] | | | | | | Varicella | | | | Varicella | | |
| Pneumococcal[6] | | | PCV | PCV | PCV | PCV | | | | PCV | PPV | |
| Influenza[7] | | | | | Influenza (Yearly) | | | | | Influenza (Yearly) | | |
| Hepatitis A[8] | | | | | | | | | | Hepatitis A Series | | |

*Vaccines below red line are for selected populations*

This schedule indicates the recommended ages for routine administration of currently licensed childhood vaccines, as of April 1, 2004, for children through age 18 years. Any dose not given at the recommended age should be given at any subsequent visit when indicated and feasible. ▨ Indicates age groups that warrant special effort to administer those vaccines not previously given. Additional vaccines may be licensed and recommended during the year. Licensed combination vaccines may be used whenever any components of the combination are indicated and the vaccine's other components are not contraindicated. Providers should consult the manufacturers' package inserts for detailed recommendations. Clinically significant adverse events that follow immunization should be reported to the Vaccine Adverse Event Reporting System (VAERS). Guidance about how to obtain and complete a VAERS form can be found on the Internet: www.vaers.org or by calling 800-822-7967.

# Interactive Activities

## Cases for Critical Thinking

1. Tetanus is caused by bacteria that enter the body through wounds in the skin. The bacteria produce a toxin that causes spastic muscle contraction. Death often results from failure of the respiratory muscles. A patient comes to the emergency room after stepping on a nail. If the patient has been vaccinated against tetanus, he is given a tetanus booster shot, which consists of the toxin altered so that it is harmless. If the patient has never been vaccinated against tetanus, he is given an antiserum shot against tetanus. Explain the rationale for this treatment.

2. Explain why identical twins are an ideal case for organ transplantation.

3. A crime scene investigator finds a body of a woman and discovers animal bites on the victim's body. The investigator examines the bites and sees they are not inflamed. Did the animal bites happen before or after the woman died?

## Multiple Choice

1. What are the signs and symptoms of inflammation?

   a. redness
   b. swelling
   c. heat
   d. pain
   e. all of the above

2. IgE is involved in _____.

   a. phagocytosis
   b. allergy
   c. mucosal immunity
   d. microbe destruction

3. _____ produce antibodies.

   a. T cells
   b. Plasma cells
   c. Neutrophils
   d. Eosinophils

4. Resistance of the skin to invading organisms is _____.

   a. innate immunity
   b. acquired immunity
   c. cellular immunity
   d. humoral immunity

5. Which is correct about active immunity?

   a. long lived
   b. short lived
   c. obtained with gamma globulin injections
   d. type of innate immunity

6. HIV is not transmitted via _____.

   a. blood
   b. semen
   c. vaginal secretions
   d. breast milk
   e. casual contact

7. Which is correct about fever?

   a. specific defense
   b. nonspecific disease
   c. harmful response to infection
   d. must be controlled

8. T cells that are capable of killing invading organisms are

   a. helper T cells
   b. suppressor T cells
   c. cytotoxic T cells
   d. memory T cells

9. Stress causes an increased production of what hormone?

   a. growth hormone
   b. histamine
   c. insulin
   d. cortisol

10. The attraction of white blood cells to the site of inflammation is called _____.

   a. agglutination
   b. edema
   c. hyperemia
   d. chemotaxis

## True or False

_____ 1. Activated lymphocytes provide humoral immunity.

_____ 2. Antibodies and T cells are specific for one antigen.

_____ 3. People immediately test positive for HIV antibodies.

_____ 4. Adrenalin is used to treat severe allergic reactions.

_____ 5. In autoimmune diseases, the body fails to recognize its own antigens.

_____ 6. Intact skin is the body's first line of defense.

_____ 7. Fever can be a sign that the body is defending itself.

_____ 8. Leukocytosis can be a sign of infection.

_____ 9. Allergy shots can desensitize a hypersensitive person.

_____ 10. Systemic anaphylaxis can be life-threatening.

## Fill-Ins

1. The virus responsible for AIDS destroys _____ cells.

2. The foreign element that triggers an immune response is known as an _____.

3. Some B cells remain dormant until reactivation by the same antigen. These are called _____.

4. _____ T cells can kill invading organisms.

5. A _____ consists of a low dose of dead or deactivated bacteria or viruses.

6. _____ is the ability of the body to defend itself against infectious agents, foreign cells, and abnormal body cells.

7. _____ defenses are effective against any foreign agent that enters the body.

8. Damaged tissue releases _____, which causes capillary walls to become permeable.

9. The _____ consists of a complex network of thin-walled capillaries carrying lymph fluid, nodes, and organs.

10. In _____, leukocytes take in and destroy foreign material.

## MedMedia
## Wrap-Up

**www.prenhall.com/mulvihill**

Remember to visit this website for extra study practice, including exercises, Internet links, news updates, and an audio glossary.

**Activity CD-ROM**

Check out the CD-ROM in the back of this book. You will find games, exercises, puzzles, and videos to help enhance your understanding of this chapter.

# Infectious Diseases

**CHAPTER**

# 3

## Learning Objectives

After studying this chapter, you should be able to

- Define infectious diseases
- Describe and compare the characteristics of bacteria, viruses, fungi, helminths, and arthropod vectors
- Explain the chief ways that infectious diseases are transmitted
- Explain the kinds of treatment for bacterial, viral, fungal, and parasitic infectious diseases
- Describe how vaccines work and the names and uses of common vaccines
- Understand the appropriate use of antibiotics and explain the problem of antibiotic resistance
- Describe examples and the causes of emerging infectious diseases

# Fact or Fiction?

Thanks to modern medicine, notorious infectious diseases like tuberculosis are things of the past.

*Fiction:* Antibiotic resistance, chronic disease, environmental changes, and other factors are responsible for the re-emergence of many infectious diseases, including tuberculosis.

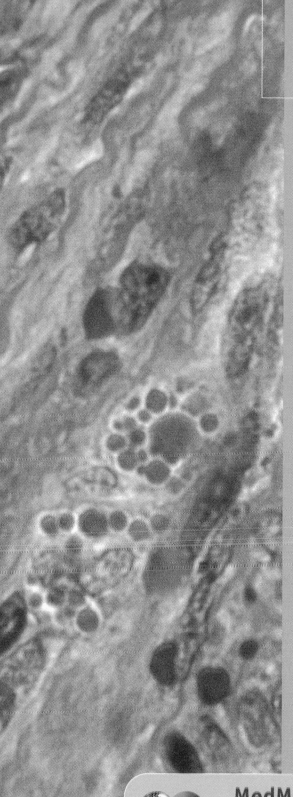

# Disease Chronicle

## West Nile Virus

**B**efore 1999, the American public had never heard of West Nile Virus; indeed, microbiologists had never detected the disease in the western hemisphere. In New York that spring and summer, tens of thousands of birds died suddenly and in the open: crows, blue jays, chickadees, and prized birds of the Bronx Zoo fell. Horses, which are susceptible to related encephalitis viruses, showed signs of infection. Humans too became sick, and some died. Gene testing soon demonstrated the cause to be West Nile Virus, named for the West Nile region of Uganda where it was first discovered. Transmitted by *Culex* mosquitoes and carried by infected birds, the virus efficiently swept across America. Fortunately, very few mosquitoes carry the virus. Of those people bitten, few become sick and fewer than 1%, mostly elderly and immune-compromised, become critically ill. Control measures, such as spraying and use of DEET repellents, appear to be effective in curtailing mosquito populations and preventing infection. Data suggest that, following the first waves of infection, some bird populations have acquired immunity to the virus.

## MedMedia
www.prenhall.com/mulvihill

Use the web address to the left to access the free, interactive Companion Website created for this textbook. It features chapter-specific exercises, Internet links, news links, and an audio glossary. Additionally, explore the CD-ROM that accompanies this book to discover Disease Focus videos and a rich array of activities that accompany this chapter.

## ▶ Introduction

What is the impact of infectious disease on human health? According to the World Health Organization, of 52 million deaths occurring worldwide each year, about 17 million are caused by infectious diseases. Of course, many more than 17 million people become ill each year with an infectious disease, and that suffering remains uncounted. As the world population grows, infectious disease will continue to grow in importance.

Some infectious diseases described in this book have been in existence for a long time, whereas others have emerged as new pathology. It is important to have a framework for understanding these infectious diseases. This chapter describes the nature of infectious diseases, surveys the types of microorganisms responsible for infections, explains their transmission, and outlines treatment and control strategies.

Infectious diseases are those diseases caused by pathogenic microorganisms. These diseases may be transmitted to humans by other humans or by some other element in the environment. Those diseases transmitted from human to human are said to be contagious or communicable. Measles and influenza are well-known contagious diseases. Infectious diseases are classified as noncommunicable if they cannot be transmitted directly from person to person. For example, rabies can be transmitted by the bite of a rabid raccoon, and cholera is transmitted by drinking fecal-contaminated water. In any case, some type of pathogenic microorganism causes these diseases.

## ▶ Pathogenic Microorganisms

Most microorganisms do not cause disease. Those that do cause disease are called pathogens. Humans can be infected by a variety of pathogens, ranging from tiny, single-celled bacteria to macroscopic, complex worms (Figure 3–1).

## Bacteria

Bacteria are microscopic, single-celled organisms. A simple structure (no nucleus or membranous organelles) and small size (1 to 10 μm) are key characteristics that differentiate bacteria from other single-celled organisms. Although often described as simple, they are far from primitive, for they have adapted to a wide variety of habitats and have evolved complex strategies for infecting and surviving in the human body.

Bacteria have cell walls, a rigid layer of organic material surrounding their delicate cell membranes. These walls give bacteria their characteristic shapes. Bacteria may have spherical, round cells called cocci, rod-shaped cells called bacilli, spiral-shaped cells called spirilla, corkscrew-shaped cells called spirochetes, or comma-shaped cells called vibrios. Figure 3–1 shows the cell structure of a rod-shaped bacterium. The walls protect these cells; should walls be disrupted, cells are susceptible to bursting. This is the action of the antibiotic penicillin. Penicillin interferes with correct cell wall construction of certain types of bacteria. The bacteria cell walls may be thick, thin, or absent. The thickness and chemical composition of the cell wall accounts for the way certain cells stain during the gram stain procedure. During the gram stain, thick-walled cells turn purple and thin-walled cells become red; thus, bacteria can be identified using this technique (Figure 3–2). Identification is critical to obtain an accurate diagnosis and effective treatment of an infection. Table 3–1 lists common gram-positive and gram-negative pathogens and the diseases associated with them. Other bacteria that do not fit into the above categories of shape and gram stain properties include the chlamydias and rickettsias, which are intracellular parasites. *Chlamydia trachomatis* causes a sexually transmitted infection. Rickettsias are transmitted by ticks and cause diseases such as typhus and Rocky Mountain spotted fever.

Bacteria grow rapidly and reproduce by splitting in half, a process known as binary fission. Under favorable conditions, this process may take only 30 minutes, which means that a small number of cells may increase to a very large number in a relatively short time. The reproduc-

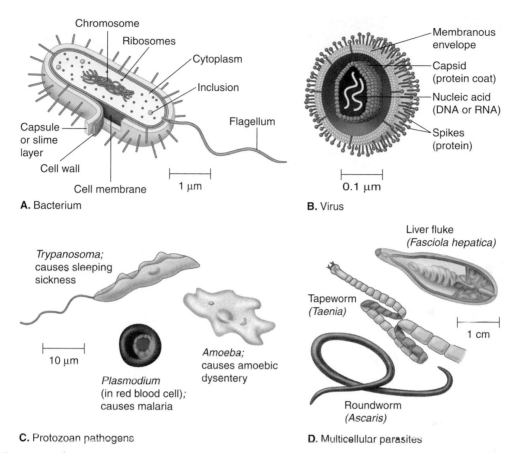

**Figure 3–1** Types of pathogenic organisms include bacteria (A), viruses (B), protozoa (C), and helminths, or worms (D).

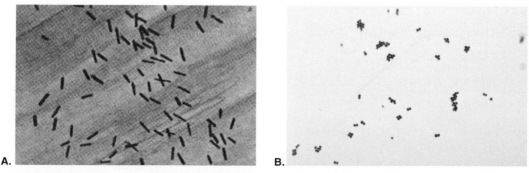

**Figure 3–2** Gram-stained bacteria on microscope slide. (A) Pink rod-shaped cells are *Escherichia coli.,* (Courtesy of the CDC, 1979.) (B) Purple cocci are *Staphylococcus aureus.* (© SIU BioMed/Custom Medical Stock Photo.)

## Table 3–1 Common Bacterial Pathogens and Associated Diseases

| Bacterial Pathogens | Disease(s) |
| --- | --- |
| **Gram-positive cocci** | |
| *Staphylococcus aureus* | Skin infections, food poisoning |
| *Streptococcus pyogenes* | Pharyngitis (strep throat) |
| *Streptococcus pneumoniae* | Lobar pneumonia |
| **Gram-positive bacilli** | |
| *Clostridium tetani* | Tetanus |
| *Clostridium botulinum* | Botulism |
| *Bacillus anthracis* | Anthrax |
| **Gram-negative cocci** | |
| *Neisseria gonorrhoeae* | Gonorrhea |
| **Gram-negative bacilli** | |
| *Salmonella typhimurium* | Salmonellosis |
| *Legionella pneumophila* | Legionellosis (Legionnaires' disease) |
| *Pseudomonas aeurginosa* | Urinary tract infections, burn infections |
| **Spirilla** | |
| *Campylobacter jejuni* | Acute enteritis, diarrhea |
| *Helicobacter pylori* | Gastritis, peptic ulcer |
| **Spirochetes** | |
| *Treponema pallidum* | Syphilis |
| *Borrelia burgdorferi* | Lyme disease |
| **Vibrios** | |
| *Vibrio cholerae* | Cholera |
| **Chlamydias and rickettsias** | |
| *Chlamydia trachomatis* | Trachoma, sexually transmitted chlamydia |
| *Rickettsia prowazekii* | Typhus |
| *Rickettsia rickettsii* | Rocky mountain spotted fever |

tion of a cell and its genetic material occurs with very few errors or mutations. Still, this rapid growth rate virtually guarantees that mutations will arise, and some of these will favor survival of the bacteria under certain conditions.

Some bacteria produce endospores, commonly called spores. The endospore contains the genetic material of the cell packaged in a tough outer coat that is resistant to desication, acid, extreme temperature, and even radiation. Endospores germinate and form growing cells when conditions are correct. Certain diseases, like tetanus and botulism, can be caused by endospores that contaminate food, water, or wounds.

Bacteria cause illness in humans in a variety of ways. A particularly potent toxin called endotoxin causes life-threatening shock. This toxin is released into tissues when gram-negative cells die. Some bacteria produce other types of toxins that interfere with normal physiology. For example, tetanus is caused by the toxin produced by the bacterium *Clostridium tetani*. The tetanus toxin interferes with the ability of muscle cells

to relax, resulting in frozen, rigid muscles characteristic of the disease. Other toxins are enzymes that enable the bacteria to spread through tissues and to obtain nutrients. Some signs and symptoms of bacterial infection are not generated by the bacteria themselves but rather by the immune response to the infection. Common characteristics of certain bacterial infections include swelling, redness, pain, fever, and pus.

## Viruses

Viruses are infectious particles made of a core of genetic material (either RNA or DNA) wrapped in a protein coat (capsid). Some viruses also have a lipid membrane surrounding their capsid (Figure 3–3). Viruses are not considered living organisms because they do not independently grow, metabolize, or reproduce. Viruses must carry out their life processes by entering cells and directing the cells' energy, materials, and organelles for these purposes.

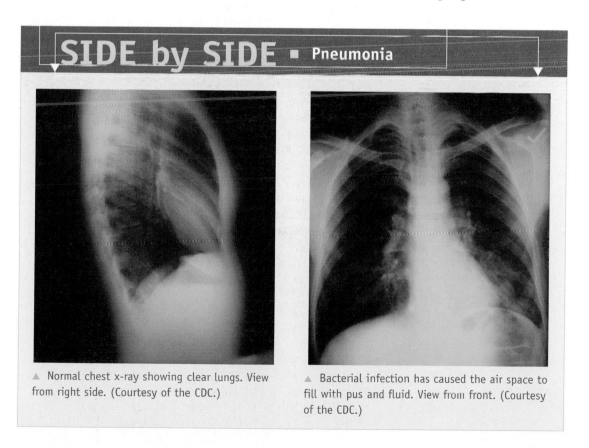

**SIDE by SIDE** ■ **Pneumonia**

▲ Normal chest x-ray showing clear lungs. View from right side. (Courtesy of the CDC.)

▲ Bacterial infection has caused the air space to fill with pus and fluid. View from front. (Courtesy of the CDC.)

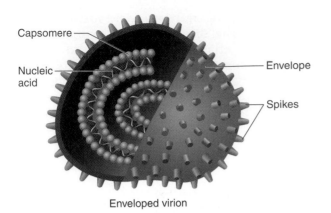

Capsomere

Nucleic acid

Envelope

Spikes

Enveloped virion

**Figure 3–3** Structure of an enveloped virus.

Certain viruses infect and grow in only certain types of human cells. Some viruses, like cold viruses, target only cells of the respiratory epithelium. Others, like herpes viruses, reproduce in nervous tissue. Signs and symptoms of infection result from the way these viruses reproduce in cells or from the way the immune system responds to viral infection. Some viruses cause the cells they infect to lyse, or rupture. This is the case when HIV infects and reproduces within T cells. The resultant T-cell deficiency leads to the immunodeficiency in AIDS. Other viruses sustain a latent infection, whereby the viruses insert themselves in cells and do not reproduce. At this time, no symptoms may be present. Later, a trigger such as stress, infection with another pathogen, or a weakened immune defense, activates the viruses. Symptoms of the disease then manifest themselves as the viruses reproduce. This pattern is seen in the waxing and waning of herpes infections. Other viruses cause abnormal cell growth because the viral genetic material interferes with the cell's growth-control genes. Abnormal growth of tissues is discussed further in Chapter 4. Such growth may be benign, as in a dermal wart. However, the result may be a malignant growth, that is, a cancer. For example, human papillomavirus infection is linked to cervical cancer. Table 3–2 lists examples of viruses and their associated diseases.

| Table 3–2 Viral Pathogens and their Diseases | |
| --- | --- |
| **Viruses** | **Diseases** |
| **DNA viruses** | |
| Herpes viruses | |
| Herpes simplex 1 | Cold sores and fever blisters |
| Herpes simplex 2 | Genital herpes |
| Varicella-Zoster | Chicken pox and shingles |
| Hepatitis B | Hepatitis ("serum hepatitis") |
| Epstein-Barr | Infectious mononucleosis |
| **RNA viruses** | |
| Influenza A, B, C | Influenza ("flu") |
| Hepatitis A, C, D, E | Infectious hepatitis |
| Rhinovirus | Common cold |
| Human immunodeficiency virus | HIV infection/AIDS |

## Protozoa

Protozoa are single-celled eukaryotic microorganisms. They are much larger than bacteria and have complex internal structures, including a nucleus and membranous organelles. Protozoa are found in nearly every habitat, and most do not cause disease. Protozoa are classified as amoeboids, flagellates, ciliates, and sporozoans.

Amoeboids move by means of cell membrane extensions called pseudopodia. These extensions may be familiar in another context—in human phagocytic leukocytes, which use pseudopodia to crawl about and ingest particles. An amoeba of great health concern is *Entamoeba histolytica*, the cause of amoebic dysentery (Chapter 10), an intestinal infection acquired from feces-contaminated food or water. The flagellates swim by using one or more whiplike appendages called flagella. Pathogens in this group include *Trypanosoma*, the cause of African sleeping sickness, and *Giardia*, the cause of giardiasis, an intestinal infection. Ciliates move by means of numerous short, hairlike projections called cilia. There are few pathogens among the ciliates. Sporozoans are not mobile. *Plasmodium* is the most notorious among them because it causes malaria. This diverse group of microorganisms causes disease in a variety of ways. Protozoa may invade and destroy certain tissues, or they may provoke damaging inflammatory responses.

## Fungi

Fungi are single-celled or multicelled organisms with cell walls that contain a special polysaccharide called chitin. Fungi use specialized filaments called mycelia to absorb nutrients from their surroundings. They also have reproductive structures bearing spores, which are known allergens.

Fungal infections are known as mycoses. Healthy human tissue is relatively resistant to fungal infections but may be susceptible under certain circumstances. Fungi can more easily infect damaged tissue than intact healthy tissue. Also, immunocompromised hosts may be unable to resist fungal infections. Fungi cause disease by producing toxins, interfering with normal organ structure or function, or inducing inflammation or allergy. Some common fungal diseases include candidiasis, an infection of skin or mucous membranes caused by the yeast *Candida*. Histoplasmosis is a respiratory infection caused by *Histoplasma*, which is inhaled in dust from soil contaminated with bird droppings. *Microsporum* and *Trichophyton* cause a variety of ringworm infections of the skin, hair, and nails (Chapter 17).

## Helminths

The wormlike animals, which include roundworms and flatworms, are called helminths. Like other animals, helminths are complex multicellular motile organisms. They often have well-developed reproductive systems capable of producing large numbers of offspring. Many helminths have also evolved complex life cycles and strategies for infecting new hosts. Infections with these organisms are often called infestations.

Roundworms are relatively round in cross section. They include filarial (threadlike) worms that infect the lymphatic system, like *Wuchereria*, the cause of elephantiasis. The human hookworm *Necator* (Figure 3–4) infects the small intestines, whereas the pinworm *Enterobius* infects the large intestine.

Flatworms, as the name suggests, have flattened bodies. *Schistosoma*, a type of helminth called a fluke, causes schistosomiasis, an infection of blood vessels. This infection is found in Southeast Asia, Africa, and parts of South America. Tapeworms like *Taenia* infect the intestines.

In some cases, transmission of helminths is relatively straightforward: *Ascaris* eggs can be swallowed in feces-contaminated food or water. In other cases, many pieces of a complex life cycle need to be in place to sustain infections. For example, although the juvenile *Schistosoma* can infect a person simply by swimming to a human foot and burrowing through the skin, the complete life cycle of *Schistosoma* depends on a particular snail as an intermediate host for development of other immature stages of the worm. The water in which the snails grow needs

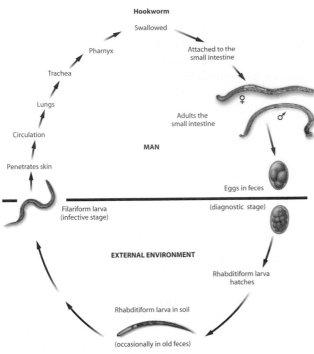

**Hookworm**

Swallowed

Pharnyx

Trachea

Attached to the small intestine

Lungs

Circulation

Adults the small intestine

**MAN**

Penetrates skin

Eggs in feces

Filariform larva (infective stage)

(diagnostic stage)

**EXTERNAL ENVIRONMENT**

Rhabditiform larva hatches

Rhabditiform larva in soil

(occasionally in old feces)

**Figure 3–4** The human hookworm lifecycle.

to be still and needs also to be contaminated with infested human urine or feces. Other helminths are transmitted by arthropod vectors, which are discussed later in this chapter.

Helminths cause disease by using the host's nutrients, as pinworms and tapeworms do when they infest the intestines. Others feed on blood, causing anemia. *Ascaris* can block or perforate the intestines when infestations become large, or the eggs or worms themselves can induce severe inflammatory responses.

## Arthropod Vectors

Animals with jointed legs and a hard exoskeleton are called arthropods. These include ticks, mites, lice, flies, mosquitoes, and fleas. Some arthropods act as disease vectors. That is, the animals transmit pathogenic microorganisms to humans. An arthropod may transmit a pathogen when biting and feeding on human blood. The *Anopheles* mosquito transmits

*Plasmodium* when it feeds on an infected human and carries the malaria parasite to another human. Some arthropods simply carry pathogens on their bodies. The housefly *Musca* can carry bacteria on its feet. In many cases, the arthropod is an essential part of the pathogen's life cycle. Humans will not get infected with the pathogen unless the appropriate arthropod vector is present. Therefore, it is very important to identify these arthropods and to understand their lives if the diseases they carry are to be controlled.

Other animals are also important for infectious diseases. Some animals act as reservoirs of infection, acting as sources of the pathogen and potential sources of disease. Certain hoofed animals and domestic cattle are reservoirs for African sleeping sickness. Deer and mice can carry the spirochete and harbor the tick that transmits Lyme disease. Still other animals are the only means by which a disease is transmitted. Rabies viruses are transmitted by the bite of infected raccoons, foxes, bats, and domestic dogs.

## ▶ Infection Prevention and Control

Effective prevention and control of infectious diseases requires knowledge of the nature of the pathogens and their means of transmission.

## Transmission and Epidemiology

Epidemiology is the study of the transmission, occurrence, distribution, and control of disease. Infectious diseases can be transmitted directly from an infected human to a susceptible human. This route is called horizontal transmission. Influenza, gonorrhea, measles, and many other diseases described elsewhere in this book are transmitted this way. Other infectious diseases are transmitted from one generation to the next, as when syphilis, HIV/AIDS, or ophthalmia neonatorum (an eye infection; see Chapter 12) are transmitted to newborns from infected mothers. This route is called vertical transmission.

Humans transmit pathogens in respiratory droplets, blood, semen, feces, urine, and through direct physical contact. Measles, pneumonia, tuberculosis, and influenza are well-known diseases transmitted in respiratory droplets generated by coughing and sneezing. HIV and hepatitis B and C are viruses transmitted in blood and blood products. Sexually transmitted diseases like gonorrhea, chlamydia, and HIV are transmitted in semen and vaginal secretions. Food poisoning, like salmonellosis, and dysentery are transmitted by consumption of fecal-contaminated food and water (see Chapter 10 for salmonella and dysentery).

In some cases, humans are not involved in direct transmission of a disease. For example, an effective campaign to control malaria would require control of the parasite's mosquito vector.

Study of the distribution and frequency of diseases can help predict and prevent disease. The number of new cases of a disease in a population is its incidence. The incidence of some diseases follows a pattern, as when influenza incidence increases in winter and subsides in summer, or when Lyme disease increases in summer and subsides in winter. The number of existing cases of a disease is known as its prevalence, and this information can tell how significant the disease is to a certain population When a disease always occurs at low levels in a population, it is said to be endemic. If a disease occurs in unusually large numbers over a specific area, it is said to be epidemic. Influenza occurs as epidemics. When an epidemic has spread to include several large areas worldwide, it is said to be pandemic. AIDS is considered to be pandemic. When a disease suddenly occurs in unexpected numbers in a limited area and then subsides, this is described as an outbreak.

Certain diseases are under constant surveillance in the United States. Such diseases are called notifiable diseases. Physicians are required to report the occurrence of these diseases to the Centers for Disease Control and Prevention. This ensures tracking and identification of disease occurrence and patterns. Chlamydia infections were not notifiable before 1998. After these infections were classified as notifiable, it was discovered that the number of chlamydial infections surpassed gonorrhea. Other notifiable infectious diseases include measles, mumps, polio, tuberculosis, Legionnares' disease, and tetanus.

Control of infectious diseases can be achieved by preventing transmission and by treating infected persons. Isolation of infected persons in hospitals and self-imposed isolation, such as when a person with influenza remains home in bed, can be effective. Quarantine is the separation of persons who may or may not be infected from healthy people until the period of infectious risk is passed. Disinfection of potentially infectious materials is necessary to prevent transmission. Medical and dental implements need disinfection to remove human pathogens after use. The Centers for Disease Control and Prevention recommends Standard Precautions be employed by all medical personnel during patient care. These precautions are used in all situations, whether a patient is infected or not, and include the use of gloves, correct disposal of bodily fluids, needles, and other waste. Sanitation techniques that remove infectious sewage from drinking and bathing water and prevent sewage from contaminating food can

## Prevention ➕ PLUS!

### Advice for Travelers

Traveling out of the country? Have you considered how you will protect yourself and your family from infectious diseases? In a different country, you will be faced with different infectious diseases to which you are unlikely to be immune. Will you need vaccinations or prophylactic medications? The Centers for Disease Control and Prevention in Atlanta, Georgia, maintains a Web site to advise travelers. Before you book your flight, go to www.cdc.gov for the latest information on infectious diseases at your destination.

dramatically reduce the incidence of cholera and dysentery. The treatment of infected persons is a critical component of prevention.

## Treatment of Infectious Disease

The effective treatment of an infectious disease depends on the type of causative pathogen. Bacterial infections can be treated with a variety of antibiotics. The target of some antibiotics is the unique bacterial cell wall. Penicillin and related drugs act on the cell wall, and they are especially useful in controlling gram-positive bacteria. Some antibiotics target the bacterial cell membrane, causing lysis. Other antibiotics target the protein synthesis machinery of the cell. This is effective because the ribosomes and enzymes involved in bacterial protein synthesis are sufficiently different from those in human cells. Other antibiotics interfere with bacterial metabolism or with DNA and RNA synthesis. Antibiotic resistance plays an important role in the increased incidence of bacterial infections.

Correct use of antibiotics can prevent the development of antibiotic resistance. Resistance arises when bacteria adapt to antibiotics and the adaptation becomes common in the bacterial population, soon rendering the antibiotics ineffective. An antibiotic should be used only for bacterial infections. A number of infections, like influenza and the common cold, are viral and are not treatable with antibiotics. Some viral ailments closely mimic bacterial infections. For example, it turns out that group A streptococci cause only 15% of pharyngitis cases, so only a small proportion of sore throats are really strep throat. Most sore throats are really caused by viral infections, some of which closely mimic strep throat because the symptoms include swelling and exudate. If antibiotics are used for many of these viral infections, bacterial populations will more likely evolve resistance to those antibiotics. The Centers for Disease Control and Prevention has asked physicians to take a throat swab and perform the rapid strep antigen test to confirm the presence of group A streptococci before prescribing antibiotics. If prescribed, the appropriate antibiotic must be selected. Guidelines are shared and updated for physicians so that the most effective types and dosages are used for certain infections. Patients need to follow through on the prescription. Patients should use the antibiotics for the entire time prescribed, should not end treatment early, and should not save antibiotics.

Viruses do not have the cell walls and cell membranes of bacteria, nor do they have metabolic or protein synthesis machinery. Viruses are not susceptible to antibiotics. Viruses need human cells to reproduce and decode their genetic material. Some antiviral drugs interfere with this process by acting as nucleic acid analogues, substances that mimic the correct DNA or RNA bases. These analogues are used to manufacture the viral genetic material but, in fact, do not function as the normal DNA or RNA bases. Viruses are not replicated correctly and are eventually reduced in number or eliminated. Other antiviral drugs interfere with the assembly of new virus particles inside cells or interfere with the attachment of viruses to host cells and thus prevent infection before disease begins.

Antifungal drugs target fungal walls and membranes but can affect human cells as well, leading to serious toxic side effects. Topical agents are effective for skin infections, such as infections of nails or ringworm, and pose fewer adverse effects. A systemic infection, however, requires systemic treatment, which entails the risk of serious side effects. Systemic treatment requires careful dosing and monitoring for side effects.

Protozoa are treated with drugs that interfere with protein synthesis and metabolism. Certain antibiotics may be used to treat protozoal infections.

Helminths are susceptible to drugs that paralyze their muscles or interfere with their carbohydrate metabolism.

Although effective treatments have been discovered and used for many important infections, certain problems remain. One complication is that resistant microorganisms can evolve, rendering existing treatments useless. Another difficulty is that some treatments are accompanied by unacceptable toxic side effects or allergies. For these reasons, preventive measures are the best choice for long-term control of certain diseases.

## Vaccination

Vaccination is the presentation of antigens from a microorganism to provoke an immune response in order to prevent future infection by that microorganism. Natural immunity occurs when a person is infected by or exposed to a microorganism. The individual's immune system responds and produces memory cells that are primed to protect the person from future encounters with that microorganism. The initial infection can cause a great deal of discomfort and major complications, including death. Preventive vaccination is recommended and practiced. Vaccines may contain dead bacteria, extracted antigens, inactivated toxins, virus particles, or genetically engineered proteins.

Because they are designed to prevent disease, vaccines have been used to help eliminate certain diseases. Smallpox was eliminated by thorough vaccination of susceptible populations. Polio will be the next major infectious disease to be eliminated through vaccination. Administration of a series of vaccines in infancy and childhood has controlled many serious childhood diseases. Diphtheria, whooping cough, measles, and other contagious and potentially serious infections are now much less common. Vaccines can protect health-care workers from hepatitis B and other pathogens. Table 3–3 describes the recommendations of the Centers for Disease Control and Prevention for vaccinations for various populations. Further details are discussed in Chapter 2.

## ▶ Emerging Infectious Diseases

Infections still account for a significant amount of morbidity and mortality in the United States. Recent data from the Centers for Disease Control and Prevention show that infectious disease mortality has increased significantly be-

| Table 3–3 Universally Recommended Vaccinations | |
|---|---|
| **Population** | **Vaccines** |
| All young children | Measles, mumps, and rubella |
| | Diphtheria-tetanus toxoid and pertussis |
| | Poliomyelitis |
| | *Haemophilus influenzae* type B |
| | Hepatitis B |
| | Varicella |
| Previously unvaccinated or partially vaccinated adolescents | Hepatitis B |
| | Varicella |
| | Measles, mumps, and rubella |
| | Tetanus-diphtheria toxoid |
| All adults | Tetanus-diphtheria toxoid |
| All adults aged >65 years | Influenza |
| | Pneumococcal |

tween 1980 and 1996 from about 42/100,000 to about 66/100,000. Moreover, certain infections that were once considered under control have re-emerged as important health threats.

The factors behind the re-emergence of tuberculosis are described in Chapter 9. One of the factors is increased antibiotic resistance of the tuberculosis pathogen. Antibiotic resistance plays an important role in the increased incidence of other bacterial infections. In addition to antibiotic resistance, changes in climate, urbanization, increased crowding, increased incidence of chronic disease, fast world travel, and disruption of social and governmental structure are responsible for the emergence of new pathology or re-emergence of old infectious diseases.

Climate changes can alter the breeding ranges of arthropod vectors like mosquitoes and flies. Malaria, Dengue fever, yellow fever—all mosquito-borne infections—show sensitivity to climate. Even in areas where malaria is endemic, it occurs with less frequency in higher and cooler elevations. In 1987, when the temperature averaged 1° higher than the previous year in Rwanda, the incidence of malaria increased 337% because higher, cooler, drier areas became favorable for the malarial mosquitoes.

After increased urbanization brought humans and deer in close proximity, Lyme disease became prominent in northeastern United States in recent years. Much of that area was cleared for farms, driving out deer and their predators. Forest and deer have reclaimed the farmland, but the predators have not returned. As urban centers grow, the human and deer populations inevitably come in contact with more frequency, giving the Lyme disease ticks ample opportunity to attach to humans and their pets.

The population of the world exceeds 6 billion people. Most of the growth has occurred and will continue to occur in the most densely populated and poorest cities. In the next few years, the World Health Organization projects that of the top 15 or so most populous cities, only Tokyo will be in a so-called industrialized nation. Crowding, chronic disease, malnutrition, and lack of medical resources will become critical. Infectious diseases thrive on these conditions.

Scientists must continue basic research into the cause, transmission, prevention, and treatment of infectious diseases for future generations.

## CHAPTER SUMMARY

Infectious diseases remain a significant cause of morbidity and mortality in the United States and throughout the world. The diseases are caused by a variety of pathogenic microorganisms, viruses, helminths, and arthropod vectors. The characteristics of each are important to understand to implement effective prevention and treatment. As human populations grow, pathogens will evolve, and infectious diseases likely will remain a threat to human life.

## RESOURCES

Biddle, W. 2002. *A Field Guide to the Germs,* 2nd ed.

Madigan, M.T., Martinko, J., & Parker, J. 2003. *Brock Biology of Microorganisms,* 10th ed.

American Society for Microbiology: www.asm.org

Centers for Disease Control and Prevention: www.cdc.gov

# Interactive Activities

## Cases for Critical Thinking

1. Based upon what you learned about transmission and control of infectious diseases, compare how one would approach the control of influenza with the control of malaria. Explain which methods would be useful for each disease.

2. Explain why antibiotics are ineffective against viral infections. What problems can arise when viral infections are treated with antibiotics?

3. Explain why vaccination is a particularly effective method for controlling infectious disease.

## Multiple Choice

1. A strain of cholera has appeared in unusual amounts in south Asia, South America, and even in North America. The occurrence of this cholera strain can be described as _____.

   a. endemic
   b. pandemic
   c. epidemic
   d. outbreak

2. Viruses are different from bacteria in that viruses _____.

   a. cannot grow on their own
   b. have have cell membranes
   c. have genetic material
   d. are single-celled organisms

3. Malaria is caused by _____.

   a. a mosquito
   b. *Plasmodium*
   c. *Trypanosoma*
   d. varicella virus

4. Penicillin disrupts bacterial _____.

   a. ribosomes
   b. cell membranes
   c. cell walls
   d. DNA synthesis

5. Which of these is not a contagious disease?

   a. influenza
   b. strep throat
   c. measles
   d. malaria

6. The gram stain is used to differentiate types of _____.

   a. bacteria
   b. viruses
   c. protozoa
   d fungi

7. _____ are long, whiplike appendages used for swimming.

   a. cilia
   b. endospores
   c. mycelia
   d. flagella

8. The protein coat of a virus is its _____.

   a. nucleus
   b. capsid
   c. core
   d. mycelia

9. Chitin is unique to _____ cell walls.

   a. bacterial
   b. protozoal
   c. fungal
   d. viral

10. Which is a fungal infection?

    a. measles
    b. rabies
    c. schistosomiasis
    d. ringworm

## True or False

_____ 1. Most microorganisms cause disease.

_____ 2. Viruses are not considered living organisms because they do not independently grow, metabolize, or reproduce.

_____ 3. When an infectious disease is transmitted directly from an infected human to a susceptible human, it is known as a horizontal transmission.

_____ 4. One of the factors behind the re-emergence of tuberculosis is increased antibiotic resistance of the tuberculosis pathogen.

_____ 5. *Ascaris* is a large flatworm that infects the blood vessels.

_____ 6. Food, water, and insects can all transmit infectious diseases.

_____ 7. Amoeboids move by using pseudopodia.

_____ 8. Pinworms and tapeworms infest human intestines.

_____ 9. Antibiotics are effective treatments for helminth infestations.

_____ 10. Fungi normally do not infect healthy tissues.

## Fill-Ins

1. Infectious diseases are those diseases caused by _____ _____.

2. _____ is the presentation of antigens from a microorganism to provoke an immune response and thus prevent future infection by that microorganism.

3. Animals with jointed legs and a hard exoskeleton are called _____.

4. _____ is the study of the transmission, occurrence, distribution, and control of disease.

5. Health-care workers must follow _____ _____ when handling patients.

6. Insects such as mosquitoes serve as _____ of infectious disease.

7. A source of pathogens in nature is called a _____.

8. Lyme disease is carried to humans by a species of _____.

9. The number of diseases occurring in a specific time frame is known as its _____.

10. The blood fluke _____ causes disease in south Asia, Africa, and South America.

# MedMedia
# Wrap-Up

**www.prenhall.com/mulvihill**
Remember to visit this website for extra study practice, including exercises, Internet links, news updates, and an audio glossary.

**Activity CD-ROM**
Check out the CD-ROM in the back of this book. You will find games, exercises, puzzles, and videos to help enhance your understanding of this chapter.

# Neoplasms

**CHAPTER**

# 4

## Learning Objectives

After studying this chapter, you should be able to

- Compare and contrast benign and malignant tumors
- Describe the biology of cancer and the process of malignant transformation
- Identify causes of cancer
- Discuss the warning signs and nonspecific signs and symptoms of cancer
- Describe diagnosis and treatment options for cancer

## Fact or Fiction?

Tobacco use is a major preventable cause of disease and premature death in the United States.

*Fact: Each year, a staggering 440,000 people die in the United States from tobacco use. Nearly 1 of every 5 deaths is related to smoking. Cigarettes kill more Americans than alcohol, car accidents, suicide, AIDS, homicide, and illegal drugs combined.*

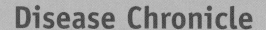

# Disease Chronicle

## Cancer

Nobody knows what the cause is, though some pretend they do; it is like some hidden assassin waiting to strike at you. Childless women get it, and men when they retire; it is as if there had to be some outlet for their foiled creative fire.

—W. H. Auden, 1907–1973, British-American Poet

## MedMedia
www.prenhall.com/mulvihill

Use the web address to the left to access the free, interactive Companion Website created for this textbook. It features chapter-specific exercises, Internet links, news links, and an audio glossary. Additionally, explore the CD-ROM that accompanies this book to discover Disease Focus videos and a rich array of activities that accompany this chapter.

# ▶ Introduction

Uncontrolled growth of cells, or neoplasia, can occur at any age and in any tissue of the body. A neoplasm, or tumor, is a mass of cells that grow more rapidly than normal cells. Neoplasms are divided into two classes: benign and malignant. A benign neoplasm is noncancerous and usually localized to a tissue or organ. Malignant tumors, or cancer, consist of rapidly dividing cells that accumulate uncontrollably, invade normal tissue, and have the ability to metastasize, or generate independent tumors at distant sites.

# ▶ Benign Tumors

Benign and malignant tumors are classified according to the tissue in which they develop. Benign growths are generally encapsulated with clearly defined edges, which makes their removal from surrounding tissues relatively easy. Benign tumors do not metastasize nor do they recur after surgical removal. A benign tumor differentiates in its development and resembles the tissue from which it grew.

Benign tumors may cause local tissues damage or affect the function of attached or adjacent organs. A benign tumor on the brain or spinal cord may cause pain by putting pressure on nerves. Any tumor can obstruct a passageway, such as the trachea or esophagus, and cause breathing or swallowing difficulties.

## Glandular

A benign tumor of a gland, or adenoma, can stimulate over secretion of hormone in the structure from which it develops. One form of high blood pressure is caused by a pheochromocytoma, a benign tumor on the adrenal glands that secretes epinephrine and norepinephrine.

## Fatty

A common benign fatty tumor, or lipoma, develops in adipose (fat) tissue. Lipomas occur more often in women than in men and are commonly found on the neck, back, or buttocks. Surgical removal is usually not required.

## Muscle

A myoma is a tumor of the muscle. These tumors are rare in voluntary muscle but do develop in smooth, involuntary muscles. Uterine myomas, or fibroids, are the most common pelvic neoplasms. Fibroids can cause excessive menstrual bleeding and pain, urinary or bowel complaints, recurrent spontaneous abortions, and infertility.

## Vascular

Angiomas are localized tumors that result from hyperplasia of blood or lymph tissue. Typical birthmarks (commonly called port-wine stains and strawberry marks) are benign tumors that frequently appear on the face and head. Port-wine stains are flat pink, red, or purplish lesions that are present at birth and usually do not fade. Strawberry marks develop shortly after birth and fade away spontaneously within 5 to 10 years.

## Epithelial

The common wart is an example of a papillary tumor, or papilloma. A papilloma originates from epithelial cells, projecting as a mass from the skin, or from squamous cells such as in the nasal cavity.

## Brain

Meningiomas are benign brain tumors that occur in the membranes that surround the brain. Meningiomas do not invade normal brain tissue, and may cause severe symptoms by compressing and putting pressure on adjacent parts of the brain. Although benign, meningiomas may need to be removed to prevent, restore, or maintain healthy neurological function.

# ▶ Cancer

Cancer is the second most common leading cause of death in the United States (American Cancer Society). According to the World Health

Organization, more than 10 million people are diagnosed with cancer every year. It is estimated that there will be 15 million new cases every year by 2020. Cancer causes 6 million deaths every year, or 12% of the deaths worldwide (Table 4–1). Lung, colorectal, and stomach cancer are among the five most common cancers in the world for both men and women. Among men, lung and stomach cancer are the most common cancers worldwide. Cervical and breast cancer are the most common cancers among women.

## Biology of Cancer

In normal tissues, cells are reproduced according to the need of the organism. Growth factors, growth inhibitors, cell cycle proteins called cyclins, and cell death, or apoptosis, regulate cell growth. In response to injury, cell growth is accelerated by growth factors. Once damaged tissue has been repaired, inhibitory growth factors decrease cell growth. Cell cycle proteins, or cyclins, regulate specific phases of cell division, allowing cells with normal DNA to complete cell division. If a cell has not completely and accurately replicated its DNA or does not have the full complement of substances required to complete cell division, the cell either is repaired or undergoes apoptosis, or cell death.

Unlike normal cells, cancer cells lose specialized structure and function of the cells from which they originated. Cell division proceeds indefinitely without regard for regulatory mechanisms. Cancer cells consume nutrients from the circulation, invade adjacent tissue, and may produce enzymes or proteins that further destroy healthy tissue. Abnormalities in cellular adhesion, and lymph node penetration, promote cancer metastasis and lead to advanced disease.

## Development of Cancer

Cancer cells develop from normal cells through a complex process called transformation. The first step in the process is initiation, in which a change in genetic material prepares the cell to become cancerous. Abnormal expression of tumor-promoting genes may initiate malignant transformation. Promotion is the second phase of malignant transformation whereby initiated cells proliferate and bear a resemblance to benign neoplasms. Benign neoplasms may regress to normal-appearing tissue through immune modulating mechanisms or by removal of the carcinogen. Several factors, such as the interaction between heredity, environmental carcinogens, and diet, are associated with progression, or transformation of precancerous cells to malignant cells.

## Causes of Cancer

**Heredity**   Hereditary causes of cancer have been linked to family history, inherited gene mutations, and inherited chromosomal disorders. Family history has been associated with childhood cancers such as retinoblastoma, or cancer of the retina, and Wilm's tumor, a childhood kidney tumor. Inherited mutations in tumor-suppressor genes and/or tumor-promoting genes, or oncogenes, have been identified in certain types of breast cancer, ovarian cancer, and bladder cancer. Inherited chromosome disorders may be associated with an increased risk for cancer. Fanconi's aplasia, Bloom's syndrome, and Down syndrome are chromosomal disorders that are associated with a high risk for leukemia.

**Environment**   At least one-third of all cancers can be attributed to living habits and carcinogens in the environment. Comprehensive prevention strategies for cancer prevention include bans on environmental carcinogens, such as tobacco smoking, toxic airborne chemicals, and asbestos.

**Tobacco**   Tobacco use is a major preventable cause of cancer and disease in the world today. It causes 80% to 90% of all lung cancer deaths in developing countries, including cancer of the oral cavity, larynx, esophagus, and the stomach. Tobacco smoking introduces mutagens into the lungs and oral cavity. These mutagens alter genetic expression and, through a multistep process, transform healthy cells into neoplastic cells or cancer cells.

**Chemicals**   Common chemical carcinogens include cancer medications or chemotherapy, asbestos, soot, mineral oil, arsenic, benzene, formaldehyde, and painting materials. Chemical carcinogens may promote the development of

## Table 4-1  Cancer Statistics and Risks: Ten Most Common Cancers

| Cancer | New Cases Annually | Risks |
|---|---|---|
| Lung | 1.2 million | Cigarette smoking |
| | | Chemical exposure: arsenic, organic chemicals, radon, asbestos |
| Breast | 1 million | Family history |
| | | Obesity |
| | | Alcohol |
| | | Increased breast density |
| | | Long menstrual history |
| Colorectal | 940,000 | Family history |
| | | Physical inactivity |
| | | Obesity |
| | | Red meat |
| | | Smoking |
| | | Excessive consumption of alcohol |
| Stomach | 870,000 | Nitrite consumption in diet |
| | | Bacterial infection |
| | | Diet lacking in fresh fruits and vegetables |
| Liver | 560,000 | Excessive alcohol consumption |
| | | Hepatitis |
| Cervical | 470,000 | Strains of the human papillomavirus |
| | | Genital herpes |
| | | Multiple sexual partners |
| | | Sexual activity at an early age |
| Esophageal | 410,000 | Cigarette smoking |
| | | Excessive consumption of alcohol |
| Head and neck | 390,000 | Cigar/cigarette smoking |
| | | Excessive consumption of alcohol |
| Bladder | 330,000 | Smoking |
| | | Workers in dye, rubber, or leather industries |
| Malignant non-Hodgkin's lymphoma | 290,000 | Human immunodeficiency virus |
| | | Occupational exposures to herbicides |

Source: World Health Organization, 2003

## Prevention ✚ PLUS!

### Cigarettes and Cancer

It is estimated that nearly one-third of all cancers can be prevented by lifestyle modification. Cigarette smoking accounts for at least 30% of all cancer deaths. It is a major cause of cancers of the lung, larynx (voice box), oral cavity, pharynx (throat), and esophagus, and is a contributing cause in the development of cancers of the bladder, pancreas, liver, uterine cervix, kidney, stomach, colon and rectum, and some leukemias. A lifestyle without smoking is a life with a significantly reduced risk of cancer.

Source: American Cancer Society

cancer by continuous exposure or by simultaneous exposure with another carcinogen or cancer risk factor, such as genetics or poor diet.

**Radiation** The carcinogenic effects of ultraviolet radiation or ionizing radiation are the result of direct damage that induces malignant changes to normal cells. The cancer risk from ionizing radiation appears to be higher if the radiation is accumulated over a short period of time, as was established by populations exposed to the atomic bomb. Solar ultraviolet radiation damages DNA and increases the risk for melanomas and squamous and basal cell carcinomas of the skin.

**Nutrition and Physical Activity** Dietary choices and physical activity can modify cancer risk. Overweight and obesity is linked to many types of cancers of the esophagus, colon and rectum, breast, endometrium, and kidney. Diets high in fruits, vegetables, and extra dietary fiber may have a protective effect against many cancers. Conversely, excess consumption of red and preserved meat is associated with breast, colon, and stomach cancers.

**Infections** Some cancers are associated with viral, bacterial, or parasitic infections. Viruses linked with human malignancies include human papillomavirus (cervical cancer), cytomegalovirus (Kaposi's sarcoma), and hepatitis B (liver cancer). Viruses invade healthy tissue and alter genetic material of the cell. The parasite *Schistosoma*

*haematobium* has been associated with bladder cancer, and the bacterium *Helicobacter pylori* is linked to stomach cancer. Bacteria and parasites induce inflammation and cause chronic tissue damage, giving rise to altered or mutagenic cells.

**Immune Disorders** Cancer is more likely to develop when the immune system is not functioning normally. Kaposi's sarcoma and lymphoma are associated with AIDS, or acquired immune deficiency syndrome. Kaposi's sarcoma commonly appears in the skin or the linings of the digestive tract or lung. High-grade lymphomas within the brain and spinal cord generally occur in late stages of AIDS.

## Classification of Cancer

Similar to benign tumors, malignant neoplasms are grouped by the tissue which they originate. Classifications of cancer include carcinoma, sarcoma, mixed cancers, and other types.

Carcinomas are the most common form of cancer, affecting epithelial cells that line body surfaces, including the skin and mucous membranes such as the breast, stomach, large intestine, prostate gland, and uterine cervix. Sarcomas are highly malignant connective tissue tumors that originate from muscle, fat, bone, and blood vessels. Mixed cancers originate in cells capable of differentiating into epithelial or connective tissue or when malignancies occur concurrently in adjacent tissue types. Other types of cancer may be classified as leukemias, lymphomas, or melanomas. Leukemia, or cancer of blood-forming tissue, is classified by cell type and disease duration. Lymphomas, or cancer of lymphoid tissue, are classified by cell type and degree of differentiation. Melanomas are malignant neoplasms derived from pigment producing cells called melanocytes, which may occur in the skin or any part of the body, eye, or, rarely, in mucous membranes.

## Signs and Symptoms of Cancer

Signs and symptoms of cancer vary with the site of the primary tumor and extent of metastasis. Because early-stage cancer symptoms tend to be subtle, they are often mistaken for signs of less-threatening diseases. For example, a persistent cough or sinusitis may be mistaken as symptoms of the common cold, although they are common symptoms in head and neck tumors (Table 4–2).

Pain and nutritional wasting (cancer cachexia) are signs of advanced disease. Cancer pain results from the effects of treatment or from the mechanical and pathological effects of cancer. Several metabolic abnormalities play a role in cachexia.

| Table 4–2   Some Nonspecific Warning Signs of Cancer |
| --- |
| Changes in bowel or bladder habits |
| A sore that does not heal |
| Unusual bleeding or discharge |
| Thickening or lump in the breast or any other part of the body |
| Indigestion or difficulty swallowing |
| An obvious change in a wart or mole |
| A nagging cough or hoarseness |
| Source: *American Cancer Society* |

## Head and Neck Cancer

Head and neck cancers are a heterogeneous group of tumors that arise from various sites and have distinct behavior patterns. Throat pain, mucosal ulcers, persistent nasal bleeding, hearing loss, and swallowing difficulties are common signs and symptoms of head and neck cancers.

## Lung Cancer

A new or changing cough, hoarseness, or bloody sputum (hemoptysis), shortness of breath, and chest pain are symptoms that usually inspire a smoker to quit just before the diagnosis of lung cancer. Common tumors of the lung include small cell carcinoma, squamous cell carcinoma, and adenocarcinoma. Adenocarcinoma is the most common type of lung cancer that occurs in nonsmokers.

## Gastric Cancer

Gastric cancer often progresses to an advanced stage before signs and symptoms develop. Symptoms of advanced disease include anorexia, loss of appetite, distaste for meat, weakness, and dysphagia, or swallowing difficulties.

## Colorectal Cancer

Intestinal polyps have the potential to evolve into colorectal cancer through a multistep process. Clinical signs and symptoms relate to the size and location of tumor. Right-sided tumors are often associated with dull abdominal pain, bleeding, weakness, and anemia. Changes in bowel habits, bleeding, gas, constipation, obstruction, and increased use of laxatives occur with cancerous lesions on the left side.

## Liver Cancer

Vague abdominal pain, fever, and anorexia can persist for up to two years before the diagnosis of liver carcinoma is made. Pain, fatigue, jaundice, ascites (accumulation of fluid in the abdomen), cachexia, and noticeable upper abdominal mass are ominous prognostic signs of liver cancer. The number, size, and location of liver tumors as well as portal vein involvement determine prognosis for liver cancer. Survival rates for liver cancer are also affected by the extent and type of liver resection and available hepatic reserve following treatment.

## Breast Cancer

Breast lumps and spontaneous nipple discharge are the most common signs of breast cancer. Milky and purulent discharges are usually due to infection, whereas serous, bloody, or watery discharges are highly suspicious of breast cancer. Signs of life-threatening disease include extensive lymph node involvement and metastasis to the lungs and liver. Breast cancer is discussed further in Chapter 12.

## Cancer of the Uterine Cervix

Symptoms of early-stage invasive cervical cancer include vaginal discharge, bleeding, and postcoital spotting. Physical findings on pelvic exam include the appearance of gray discolored areas and appearance of obvious masses. Invasive cervical cancer may spread into other pelvic structures and along lymph node chains.

## Ovarian Cancer

Ovarian cancer is the most lethal of all gynecological cancers. Early ovarian carcinoma is asymptomatic. Any pelvic mass in a woman who is more than one year postmenopausal is suspicious for ovarian cancer. Symptoms are often nonspecific and include irregular menstruation in postmenopausal women, urinary frequency, constipation, abnormal vaginal bleeding, and abdominal bloating and discomfort.

## Prostate Cancer

The symptoms of prostate cancer are similar to benign prostatic hypertrophy that commonly occurs in middle adulthood. Difficulties passing urine, blood in the urine, pain in the lower abdomen, and the presence of tumor markers in blood tests are highly suggestive of prostate cancer. Prostate-specific antigen (PSA) is a tumor marker measured in blood, which is significantly elevated in men with prostate cancer. Prostate cancer is discussed further in Chapter 12.

## Testicular Cancer

The most common symptom of testicular cancer is a painless enlargement; however, painful tumors are usually the result of bleeding in the tumor. Nearly all cancers of the testes that occur in younger age groups originate from germ cells. The risk for developing testicular cancer is higher in cases where the testes are retained in the abdomen. Tumor markers commonly detected in blood tests for testicular cancer are alpha-feto-protein (AFP) and beta human chorionic gonadotropin (βHCG). The presence of AFP and βHCG in the blood is used to monitor the amount of cancer present following surgical removal of the tumor.

## Renal Cancer

The kidney is a frequent metastatic landing site for a number of malignancies, including cancers of the lung, ovary, colon, and breast. Hematuria, or blood in the urine; steady, dull, flank pain; and weight loss are common presenting symptoms of renal cancer. Leg edema, which causes obstruction of the veins or lymphatic tissue, is suggestive of advanced disease.

## Lymphoma and Leukemia

**Lymphoma**  Lymphomas are cancer of the lymphocytes and may be either confined to a single lymph node or dispersed throughout the body. The most common complaint of patients with Hodgkin's lymphoma and non-Hodgkin's lymphoma is lymphadenopathy, or enlargement of the superficial lymph nodes. Fevers, night sweats, and weight loss are symptoms of advanced stages of Hodgkin's lymphoma and aggressive non-Hodgkin's lymphoma. Pain in the abdomen may be due to splenomegaly, or enlargement of the spleen, and bone pain may reflect localized areas of bone destruction or diffuse bone marrow infiltration.

**Leukemia**  Leukemia is cancer of white blood cells and can originate in the bone marrow or

lymph nodes or both. Chronic fatigue and reduced exercise tolerance are the first symptoms
to develop in acute leukemia. Severe fatigue, anemia, bruising, weight loss, and bleeding are signs
of advanced disease.

## Skin Cancer

Basal cell carcinomas and squamous cell carcinomas
may cause a sore on the skin. Pearly lesions with
visible blood vessels and an ulcer with a rolled up
edge are common warning signs for basal cell

carcinomas. Squamous cell carcinomas appear
on skin that is visibly damaged as rough, flaky,
red scales, with or without ulceration. Malignant
melanoma, or cancer of pigment-producing cells,
may appear spontaneously or from a pigmented
mole that has been present for years. The majority of moles on the skin are benign. The sudden
appearance of a new lesion, with irregular borders and patchy brown, black, or blue color are
among the warning signs of a melanoma. Sudden
changes to an existing mole, such as an increase
in size, or bleeding, or development of satellite le-

| Table 4–3 | Summary of American Cancer Society Recommendations for Early Detection of Cancer in Asymptomatic People |
|---|---|
| **Site** | **Recommendation** |
| Breast | Annual mammography for women over 40 |
|  | Annual breast exam |
|  | Monthly self-breast examination |
| Colon and rectum | Beginning at age 50: |
|  | Fecal occult blood test every year or |
|  | Flexible sigmoidoscopy every 5 years or |
|  | Annual fecal occult blood test and flexible sigmoidoscopy every 5 years |
|  | A double contrast barium enema every 5 to 10 years |
|  | A colonoscopy every 10 years |
|  | Combined testing is preferred over annual tests every 5 years; people at moderate or high risk should talk with doctor about a different testing schedule |
| Prostate | Prostate-specific antigen test and digital rectal exam should be offered annually beginning at age 50; men at risk should start testing at age 45 |
| Uterus | Cervix: All women who are sexually active or who are 18 and older should have an annual Pap test and pelvic exam |
|  | Endometrium: all women should be informed about the risks and symptoms of endometrial cancer |
| Cancer-related checkup | A cancer-related check up is recommended every 3 years for people aged 20 to 39 years and every year for people 40 and older; exam should include health counseling and, depending on a person's age, examinations for cancers of the thyroid, oral cavity, skin, lymph nodes, testes, ovaries, as well as for some nonmalignant diseases |

Source: American Cancer Society

sions, are important danger signs of skin cancer. Skin cancer is further discussed in Chapter 17.

## Diagnosis of Cancer

Evaluation of cancer begins with a careful history and physical exam. Cancer-screening tests can help identify cancer before it causes symptoms (Table 4–3). Two of the most widely used screening tests in women are the Papanicolaou (Pap) test to detect cervical cancer and mammography to detect breast cancer. Measuring blood levels or urine levels of certain substances, or tumor markers, may uncover the likelihood that a cancer is present. X-ray techniques, particularly those using contrast dyes, are used to show location, size, and mass of the tumor. CT scans provide a cross sectional view of a tumor, whereas MRI, and ultrasound provide a detailed view inside the body. Direct visualization techniques, or endoscopy, are used to assess specific locations and to obtain a tissue biopsy. Tissue biopsy, the surgical removal and examination under a microscope, is required to

### Table 4–4  Breast Cancer Staging

**Stage 0**

Noninvasive breast cancer. No evidence of cancer cells breaking through to or invading neighboring normal tissue.

**Stage I**

Invasive breast cancer (cancer cells are breaking through to or invading neighboring normal tissue) in which the tumor measures up to 2 centimeters, and No lymph nodes are involved.

**Stage II**

This stage describes invasive breast cancer in which:

The tumor measures at least 2 centimeters, but not more than 5 centimeters, or

Cancer has spread to the lymph nodes under the arm on the same side as the breast cancer.

Affected lymph nodes have not yet stuck to one another or to the surrounding tissues, a sign that the cancer has not yet advanced to stage III. (The tumor in the breast can be any size.)

**Stage IIIA**

This stage describes invasive breast cancer in which:

The tumor measures larger than 5 centimeters, or

The tumor has spread to lymph nodes, and nodes are clumping or sticking to one another or surrounding tissue.

**Stage IIIB**

This stage describes invasive breast cancer in which a tumor of any size has spread to the breast skin, chest wall, or internal mammary lymph nodes (located beneath the breast inside the chest) and includes inflammatory breast cancer.

**Stage IV**

This stage includes invasive breast cancer in which a tumor has spread beyond the breast, underarm, and internal mammary lymph nodes. The tumor may have spread to the supraclavicular lymph nodes (nodes located at the base of the neck, above the collarbone), lungs, liver, bone, or brain.

Source: American Cancer Society

confirm a diagnosis and assess prognosis, or potential course of the disease.

Once cancer is diagnosed, staging tests are used to define the extent of disease and the prognosis and treatment. Staging systems generally include the following factors: origin of the tumor; histology or microanatomy; size; invasion of adjacent tissues; involvement of nerves, blood vessels or lymphatic system; sites of metastasis; and functional status of the patient.

A number of staging systems are used to classify tumors. The TNM staging system assesses tumors in three ways: extent of primary tumor (T); absence or presence of regional lymph node involvement (N); and absence or presence of distant metastasis (M). Once the T, N, and M, are determined, a stage of I, II, III, or IV is assigned, with stage I being early stage and IV being advanced. If cancer cells are present only in the layers of cells where they developed and they have not spread, the stage is in situ. If cancer cells have spread beyond the original layer of tissue, the cancer is invasive. Table 4–4 gives examples of staging for breast cancer.

## Cancer Treatment

Cancer treatment begins with primary prevention and early detection. Once an environmental cause of cancer has been determined, the major approach to cancer prevention is avoidance of the precipitating agent. Chemoprevention is the use of nutrients or compounds to decrease the incidence of malignancy developing. A striking example of effective chemoprevention is the use of cis-retinoic acid in patients with oral leukoplakia, lesions that have a high propensity for neoplastic progression, to reduce the incidence of head and neck cancers in a population of smokers. The American Cancer Society publishes cancer prevention guidelines that are assessed annually (Tables 4–5 and 4–6).

---

### Table 4–5  Guidelines on Nutrition and Physical Activity for Cancer Prevention

**Eat a variety of healthful foods, with an emphasis on plant sources**

- Eat five or more servings of vegetables and fruit each day
- Choose whole grains in preference to processed (refined) grains and sugars
- Limit consumption of red meats, especially high fat and process meats
- Choose foods that help maintain a healthful weight

**Adopt a physically active lifestyle**

- Adults: Engage in at least moderate activity for 30 minutes or more on 5 or more days of the week; 45 minutes or more of moderate to rigorous activity on 5 or more days per week may further enhance reductions in the risk of breast and colon cancer
- Children and adolescents: Engage in at least 60 minutes per day of moderate to vigorous physical activity at least 5 days per week

**Maintain a healthful weight throughout life**

- Balance caloric intake with physical activity
- Lose weight if currently overweight or obese

**If you drink alcoholic beverages, limit consumption**

Source: American Cancer Society

**Table 4–6    Prevention Measures for Melanoma and Other Skin Cancers**

Avoid exposure to the sun between the hours of 10 a.m. and 4 p.m., when ultraviolet rays are the most intense

Wear hats with a brim wide enough to shade face, ears, and neck, as well as clothing that covers as much as possible of the arms, legs, and torso

Cover exposed skin with a sunscreen lotion with a sun protection factor (SPF) of 15 or higher

Avoid tanning beds and sun lamps, which provide an additional source of UV radiation.

Source: American Cancer Society

Optimal treatment of advanced disease requires an interdisciplinary approach, including surgery, medication or chemotherapy, and radiation. Surgery is one of the oldest treatments for cancer and is used to diagnose, stage, treat, and prevent cancer. Curative surgery is most promising when a tumor is confined to one area. Chemotherapy is the systemic administration of medications to kill tumor cells. Frequent administration of chemotherapy is used to decrease the tumor burden and must be continued after the tumor is no longer clinically evident to achieve a cure. Many cancer cells develop drug resistance and require treatment with combinations of medications with different mechanisms of action. Radiation therapy may be used alone or in combination with surgery and chemotherapy. The curative goal of radiation therapy is to halt tumor growth while producing reversible and tolerable toxicity to surrounding normal tissues.

## CHAPTER SUMMARY

Neoplasms, or tumors, are divided into two classes: benign and malignant. Benign tumors are generally encapsulated, and they neither metastasize nor recur after surgical removal.

Uncontrolled growth and metastasis are hallmark features of malignant neoplasms that develop from complex cellular mutations. Causes of cancer have been linked to heredity, environment, lifestyle, infections, and immune compromise. The symptoms of cancer are usually nonspecific and often mistaken for less serious diseases. A careful history, physical exam, x-ray techniques, and a biopsy is required to confirm a diagnosis of cancer. Cancer treatment begins with prevention and early detection. Optimal treatment of advanced disease requires an interdisciplinary approach, including surgery, chemotherapy, and radiation therapy.

## RESOURCES

*The Merck Manual,* 17th ed.

American Cancer Society, Cancer Facts and Figures, 2002.

*Current Medical Diagnosis and Treatment,* 42nd ed., 2003.

www.breastcancer.org: A nonprofit organization for breast cancer education

# Interactive Activities

## Cases for Critical Thinking

1. J. W. is a 52-year-old female who recently read an article stating that cancer may be genetically determined. Concerned with this finding, J. W. decides to make an appointment with her general practitioner for a "cancer exam."

   What are some of the signs and symptoms of cancer? In addition to genetics, what are some other likely causes of cancer?

2. D. A. is a 33-year-old mother of four children, ages 8, 7, 4, and 1. After giving birth to her fourth child, D. A. reports "not feeling" as strong as before. She has had a number of recent infections, with weight loss, and a cough that does not seem to go away. Upon examination, D. A.'s doctor recommended the following tests: Complete blood count, Papanicolaou smear, chest x-ray, abdominal ultrasound, and mammography. Describe the value of diagnostic tests for cancer screening.

   How often are cancer-screening tests recommended? Are there specific diagnostics tests that should be performed on men versus women?

3. G. W. is a 57-year-old male who presents to his physician with lower abdominal back pain, fever, loss of appetite, and weight loss. He is a recovering alcoholic and a chronic smoker. Despite recent weight loss, G. W. complains of "feeling bloated," and he is constipated. The nurse practitioner orders a complete blood count, including a prostate-specific antigen, evaluation of liver function, and an abdominal ultrasound. G. W.'s complete blood count shows evidence of anemia. G. W. is discouraged because he was told that losing weight would be beneficial to his overall health. What are his risk factors for cancer? What type of information is needed to accurately diagnose cancer? If G. W. does have cancer, how would his doctors determine his prognosis?

## Multiple Choice

1. A noncancerous growth on a gland is called a _____.

   a. lipoma     c. myoma
   b. adenoma     d. angioma

2. Rapidly dividing cells with metastasis are characteristic of _____.

   a. apoptosis     c. intestinal polyps
   b. carcinoma in situ     d. melanoma

3. The spread of cancer to a distant site is called _____.

   a. lymphadenopathy     c. metastasis
   b. papilloma     d. transformation

4. The causes of cancer include all of the following except _____.

   a. DNA     c. mutagens
   b. genetic mutations     d. oncogenes

5. _____ is nutritional wasting and is characteristic of advanced cancer.

   a. Neoplasia     c. Apoptosis
   b. Cachexia     d. Progression

6. A woman should do a breast self exam _____.

   a. daily     c. once a month
   b. once a week     d. once a year

7. The TNM staging system assesses tumors for all of the following except _____.

   a. cyclins     c. lymph node involvement
   b. size of the tumor     d. metastasis

8. The systemic administration of medications to kill tumor cells is _____.

   a. radiation therapy     c. chemotherapy
   b. surgery     d. prevention

## True or False

_____ 1. Benign tumors do not metastasize.

_____ 2. Squamous cell carcinomas are tumors of pigment-producing cells.

_____ 3. Apoptosis regulates cell growth.

_____ 4. Bladder cancer may be caused by smoking tobacco.

_____ 5. Sarcomas are highly malignant tumors of epithelial cells.

_____ 6. Carcinomas are the most common form of cancer.

_____ 7. All women who are sexually active or who are 18 years and older should have an annual PAP test and pelvic exam.

_____ 8. Optimal treatment requires surgery, chemotherapy, and radiation.

## Fill-Ins

1. A sunscreen with a sun protective factor of _____ _____ is recommended to prevent skin cancer.

2. Tumor markers commonly measured to monitor testicular cancer include _____ and _____.

3. Localized tumors of blood or lymph tissue are _____.

4. The _____ staging system assesses tumors by size, lymph node involvement, and metastasis.

5. A direct visualization technique called _____ is used to assess the location of the tumor and to obtain a sample of the tumor.

6. Surgical removal and microscopic examination of a tumor, or a _____, is required to confirm a diagnosis of cancer.

7. Cell cycle proteins also know as _____ regulate specific phases of cell division.

8. _____ is the first step of malignant transformation.

# MedMedia Wrap-Up

**www.prenhall.com/mulvihill**
Remember to visit this website for extra study practice, including exercises, Internet links, news updates, and an audio glossary.

**Activity CD-ROM**
Check out the CD-ROM in the back of this book. You will find games, exercises, puzzles, and videos to help enhance your understanding of this chapter.

**CHAPTER**

# 5

# Heredity and Disease

## Learning Objectives

After studying this chapter, you should be able to

- Understand DNA's role in heredity
- Describe mechanisms of transmission of hereditary diseases and give examples
- Discuss abnormal chromosome diseases
- Describe genetic diseases involving the sex chromosomes
- Describe congenital diseases

## Fact or Fiction?

Familial hypercholesterolemia, a disorder in which a person has very high blood cholesterol, can be inherited.

*Fact: Five types of hypercholesterolemia are known and all can be inherited; a common form is an autosomal dominant disorder.*

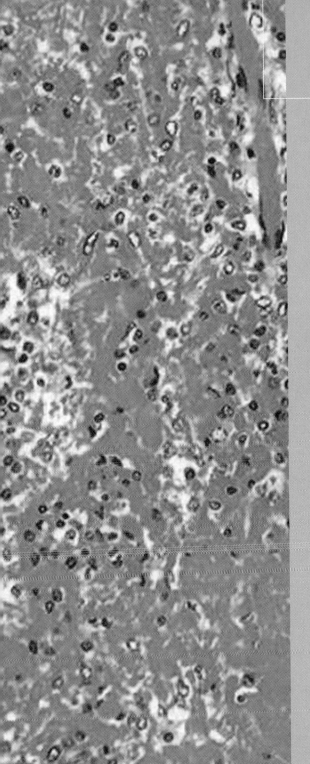

# Disease Chronicle

## President Lincoln and Marfan Syndrome

Some say that President Abraham Lincoln had a hereditary disease called Marfan syndrome, which today affects 1 in 10,000 people. President Lincoln exhibited key traits associated with Marfan, including a tall stature with a slender skeleton, long fingers, and long, narrow face. Marfan also causes an abnormally shaped chest, loose joints, and weak ligaments, which results in curvature of the spine. Weakened connective tissue in the walls of large arteries leads to aortic aneurysms. With aging, the heart and other organs fail.

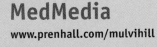

## MedMedia
www.prenhall.com/mulvihill

Use the web address to the left to access the free, interactive Companion Website created for this textbook. It features chapter-specific exercises, Internet links, news links, and an audio glossary. Additionally, explore the CD-ROM that accompanies this book to discover Disease Focus videos and a rich array of activities that accompany this chapter.

# ▶ Introduction to Heredity

DNA, which stands for deoxyribonucleic acid, is the blueprint for protein synthesis within the cell. DNA is a double helix (spiral staircase) made of four chemical bases, pairs of which form the "steps" of the DNA molecule. All genes are made of these four bases, arranged in different orders and in different lengths.

Within the nucleus of cells the DNA is assembled into units called chromosomes, which must be copied during cell division and distributed to the resulting daughter cells. Sex cells contain 46 chromosomes and divide by a process called meiosis (Figure 5–1) and produce gametes (egg and sperm) that contain 23 chromosomes each. Egg and sperm unite during fertilization; therefore, each human cell contains 46 chromosomes in 23 pairs.

The chromosomes contain thousands of genes, each of which is responsible for the synthesis of one protein. Forty-four of the chromosomes are called autosomes, and two are called the X and Y (or sex) chromosomes. A male has a combination of one X and one Y chromosome and a female has two X chromosomes. The chromosomal composition of the nucleus is called the karyotype of the cell. The karyotype can be visualized by extracting the chromosomes from the nucleus and photographing them under a microscope. In this way, abnormalities in number or structure of the chromosomes can be detected (Figure 5–2).

Begun in 1990, the U.S. Human Genome Project (HGP) was a 13-year effort coordinated by the U.S. Department of Energy and the National Institutes of Health. The project originally was planned to last 15 years, but rapid technological advances accelerated the completion date to 2003. Project goals were to identify all of the approximate 30,000 genes in human DNA, determine the sequences of the 3 billion chemical base pairs that make up human DNA, and store this information in databases.

The full DNA sequence was completed and published in April 2003. Upon publication of the majority of the genome in February 2001, Francis Collins, the director of the National Human Genome Research Institute, noted that the genome could be thought of in terms of a book with multiple uses. "It's a history book—a narrative of the journey of our species through time. It's a shop manual, with an incredibly detailed blueprint for building every human cell. And it's a transformative textbook of medicine, with insights that will give health-care providers immense new powers to treat, prevent, and cure diseases." Genes for some hereditary diseases have been located and are listed in Table 5–1; a complete list can be found at www.ncbi.nlm.nih.gov.

The genes for a particular trait, such as eye color, hair color, and hair type, occupy a particular site on a chromosome. Alleles are alternative forms of a gene. If the pair of alleles is similar, the person is homozygous for that trait. If the alleles are different, one for dark and one for

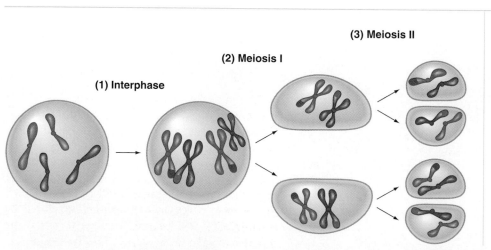

**(1) Interphase**  **(2) Meiosis I**  **(3) Meiosis II**

Figure 5–1
Meiosis.

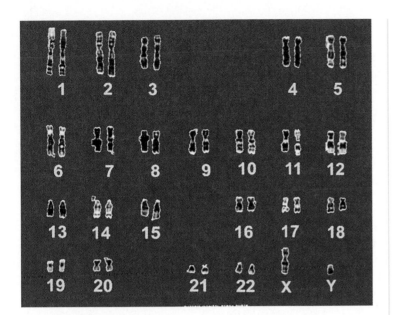

Figure 5–2
Human karyotype. (©Custom Medical Stock Photo.)

light hair, for example, the person is heterozygous. Some alleles always produce their trait when inherited and are said to be dominant. The result of the dominant allele is the same whether a person is homozygous or heterozygous. The allele for brown eyes, for example, is dominant to that for blue eyes. Other alleles are recessive and only manifest themselves when the person is homozygous for the trait. This is significant in many hereditary diseases.

Certain factors may cause a deviation from the basic principles of inheritance that have been described. Some alleles are codominant, so that when both are inherited, both traits are expressed. An example of codominant alleles is found in blood type AB. The allele for the A factor is inherited from one parent and that for the B factor from the other, but both alleles are expressed. At times, a dominant allele is not fully expressed, a condition known as *reduced penetrance*. Various factors modify the expression of genes, including other genes, environmental conditions, and gender.

### ▶ Transmission of Hereditary Diseases

Many of the diseases described throughout this book are called *hereditary* or *familial diseases.* In this chapter, the mechanism of transmission is explained. Some diseases are caused by inheriting a single autosomal dominant allele. One such defective gene causes Huntington's chorea, a disease described in Chapter 14, and another causes polydactyly, explained later in this chapter. Other diseases are caused by inherited autosomal recessive alleles. In this case,

| Table 5–1 Hereditary Disease Locations | |
|---|---|
| **Disease** | **Location** |
| Huntington Disease | Chromosome 4 |
| Achondroplasia | Chromosome 4 |
| Parkinson's Disease | Chromosome 4 |
| Cystic Fibrosis | Chromosome 7 |
| Sickle Cell Anemia | Chromosome 11 |
| Phenylketonuria | Chromosome 12 |
| Tay-Sachs Disease | Chromosome 15 |
| Marfan Syndrome | Chromosome 15 |

expression of the disease occurs only when one defective allele is inherited from each parent, making the person homozygous for that trait. Cystic fibrosis, described in Chapter 9, is such a disease. A third type of inheritance is sex-linked, in which the defective allele is located on the X chromosome. Red-green color blindness and hemophilia are examples of sex-linked inherited diseases and are explained later in this chapter.

## Autosomal Dominant

A defective dominant allele is usually transmitted from a parent who is heterozygous for the trait. If the other parent is normal for the particular condition, each child has a 50% chance of being affected and manifesting the genetic defect. This is illustrated in Figure 5–3. The disease appears in every generation, with males and females being equally affected. Exceptions to the rule are minimal.

Polydactyly, extra fingers or toes, is an example of an autosomal dominant disorder. A boy or girl inheriting the defective allele from either parent will have the abnormality.

Achondroplasia is another disorder resulting from one defective dominant allele (Figure 5–4).

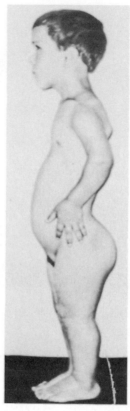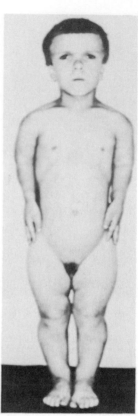

**Figure 5–4** A 12-year-old achondroplastic dwarf. (Note the disproportion of the limbs to the trunk, the curvature of the spine, and the prominent buttocks.)

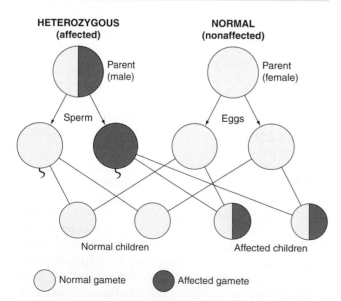

**Figure 5–3** Transmission of autosomal dominant disorders (50% chance for an affected child).

In this disease, cartilage formation in the fetus is defective. Normally, the fetal skeleton first forms as cartilage and is gradually replaced by bone. In achondroplasia, the defective cartilage formation results in improper bone development and achondroplastic dwarfism. The long bones of the arms and legs are short, the trunk of the body is normal in size, the head is large, and the forehead is very prominent. The person develops sexually, has normal intelligence, and is muscular and agile.

Marfan syndrome results from the dysfunction of the gene that codes for the connective tissue protein fibrillin. Fibrillin is essential for the maintenance of connective tissue in various organs, including tendons, heart valves, and blood vessels. Tendons and blood vessel walls with abnormal connective tissue become loose and cannot support normal body functions.

Because connective tissue is widespread in the body, Marfan syndrome is a multisystemic disease. Lack of fibrillin causes skeletal changes, dilatation of the aorta, floppy heart valves, and ocular changes, including lens displacement, retinal detachment, and blindness. Death is most often caused by heart failure or aortic aneurysm.

Familial hypercholesterolemia affects 1 in 500 Americans and is a common cause of cardiovascular disease in this country. A common form of familial hypercholesterolemia is caused by a mutation in the gene encoding the receptor for low-density lipoprotein (LDL). LDLs transport approximately 70% of the total blood cholesterol and are the principal carriers for the removal of cholesterol from the blood. The receptor deficiency in patients with familial hypercholesterolemia causes LDL cholesterol to be removed by a less efficient receptor-independent mechanism. Inefficient cholesterol removal results in hypercholesterolemia and the deposition of lipids in the arteries. This results in accelerated atherosclerosis and increased incidence of coronary heart disease. The progression of familial hypercholesterolemia can be slowed by a low-fat diet and drugs that block uptake of cholesterol in blood vessels.

## Autosomal Recessive

Autosomal recessive diseases manifest themselves only when a person is homozygous for the defective allele. Two parents who are both carriers of the recessive allele are themselves heterozygous for the trait but do not have the disease. Each of their children has a 25% chance of inheriting two recessive alleles and the disease. This is shown in Figure 5–5. The chance for inheriting two recessive alleles increases in close intermarriage. Cystic fibrosis is an autosomal recessive disease affecting the respiratory and digestive systems, and is discussed in Chapter 9.

Phenylketonuria (PKU) is caused by an autosomal recessive allele. Persons with PKU lack a specific enzyme that converts one amino acid, phenylalanine, to another, tyrosine. This mechanism is illustrated in Figure 5–6. As a result, high levels of phenylalanine and its derivatives

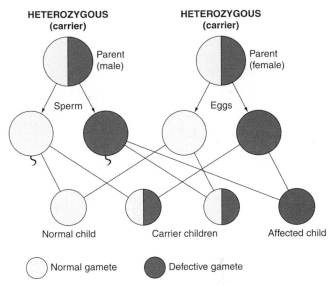

**Figure 5–5** Transmission of recessive disorders (25% chance for an affected child).

build up in the blood and are toxic to the brain, interfering with normal brain development. If the condition is not diagnosed and treated early, severe mental retardation results. Physical development proceeds normally, but the child is very light in color. Production of the pigment melanin is impeded because of inadequate tyrosine, a result of the missing enzyme. The child may manifest disorders of the nervous system, such as a lack of balance, and may suffer convulsions.

To prevent the serious mental retardation that accompanies PKU, newborn babies are routinely screened for the defective gene. If the gene is found, a synthetic diet is prescribed that eliminates phenylalanine. Good results have been achieved with this treatment. The diet is unpleasant, and controversy exists as to the length of time the diet must be maintained. Beginning treatment immediately and continuing during the earliest years of life seems to be the most critical factor in preventing mental retardation.

Galactosemia is another example of an inborn error of metabolism resulting from autosomal recessive inheritance. The person with this disease lacks the enzyme necessary to convert

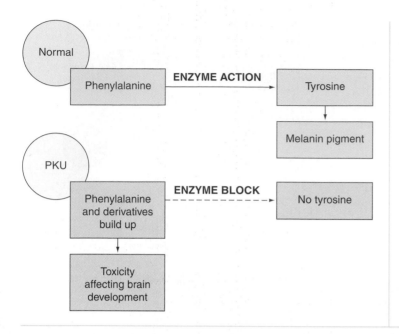

**Figure 5–6**
Enzyme block in phenylketonuria (PKU).

galactose, a sugar derived from lactose in milk, to glucose. Galactose accumulates in the blood and interferes with development of the brain, liver, and eyes. If untreated, mental retardation develops. The liver becomes enlarged and cirrhotic, and ascites fluid (see Chapter 10) accumulates in the abdominal cavity. Intestinal distress results in vomiting and diarrhea. Early diagnosis and treatment of galactosemia can prevent these problems, allowing development to proceed normally. The treatment consists of eliminating lactose from the diet.

Sickle cell anemia, a severe anemia generally confined to blacks, is described in Chapter 8. Sickle cell anemia is an autosomal recessive disorder in which the hemoglobin is abnormal, resulting in deformed red blood cells. The improperly formed cells become lodged in capillar-

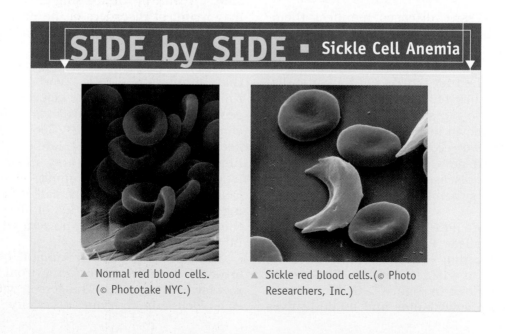

▲ Normal red blood cells. (© Phototake NYC.)

▲ Sickle red blood cells. (© Photo Researchers, Inc.)

ies and block circulation, causing necrosis and infarcts, death of tissues. The sickle-shaped red blood cells rupture easily, and they are removed from the circulation by the spleen. The depletion of red blood cells results in severe anemia.

The person with sickle cell anemia is homozygous, having inherited one defective allele from each parent. A person who is heterozygous has both normal and abnormal hemoglobin and possesses the sickle cell trait. The person is mildly anemic, but the one defective allele provides an advantage because sickle cell trait confers increased resistance to malaria.

Tay-Sachs is an autosomal recessive condition that primarily affects families of Eastern Jewish origin. Tay-Sachs is caused by the absence of the enzyme Hexosaminodase A (Hex-A). Without Hex-A, a lipid called GM2 ganglioside accumulates in cells, especially nerve cells of the brain. The result is progressive mental and physical retardation. Symptoms appear by 6 months of age when no new skills are learned, convulsions occur, and blindness develops. A cherry-red spot may be seen on each retina. Children usually die between 2 and 4 years of age. No cure exists, and treatment is aimed at relieving symptoms.

There are two tests available to determine if someone is a carrier of Tay-Sachs. An enzyme assay measures the level of Hex-A in blood. Carriers have less Hex-A than noncarriers. DNA-based carrier-testing looks for specific mutations in the gene that codes for Hex-A. Some carriers may not be identified by DNA analysis alone because not all known mutations in the Hex-A gene are detected by the test. Other mutations responsible for the disease have yet to be identified.

Albinism is an autosomal recessive disorder that is easily recognized. The skin and hair color are very white and do not darken with age. People with albinism have an increased risk for skin cancer and exhibit visual problems such as nearsightedness and abnormal sensitivity to light.

## Sex-Linked Inheritance

Diseases of sex-linked inheritance generally result from defective genes on the X chromosome, because the Y chromosome is small and carries very few genes. Because a male has only one X chromosome, if he inherits a defective recessive gene, the trait is expressed. A female may be heterozygous for the gene, having a defective recessive allele on one X chromosome but a normal allele on the other X. In that case, the female carries the disease, and she has a 50% chance of transmitting the allele to her sons and daughters. A male transmits the disease only to his daughters. His sons are unaffected, because the Y chromosome is normal. This is illustrated in Figure 5–7. Thus, the abnormalities of sex-linked inheritance tend to occur more frequently in males, but are transmitted by females. It is far less common for a female to inherit a sex-linked disease because she must inherit two defective X chromosomes. Duchenne's muscular dystrophy is an X-linked recessive disease that is discussed in Chapter 16.

## Color Blindness

Red-green color blindness, the inability to distinguish between certain colors, is a disorder of sex-linked inheritance. The defect that causes color blindness is apparently in certain specialized receptors of the retina called *cones*. Three types of receptors are stimulated by wavelengths of the primary colors: red, green, and blue. Impulses are then sent to the brain and interpreted. The color-blind person is most frequently unable to distinguish reds and greens. Corrective lenses are available that may offer some treatment for red-green color blindness.

## Hemophilia

People with hemophilia do not bleed more profusely or bleed faster than normal; they bleed for a longer period of time. There have been significant advances in treating hemophilia in the last decade. A new genetically engineered clotting protein is now used for treatment of some types of hemophilia. Research is also underway to develop gene therapy for the disease. The therapy will replace the missing or deficient gene with one that has the instructions for producing the clotting factor. Gene therapy has been successful in treating mice with hemophilia B.

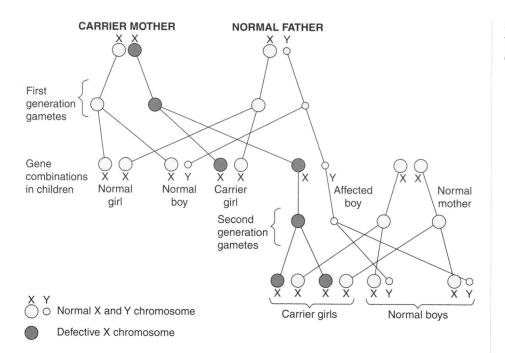

**CARRIER MOTHER** **NORMAL FATHER**

First generation gametes

Gene combinations in children

Normal girl  Normal boy  Carrier girl

Second generation gametes

Affected boy  Normal mother

Carrier girls  Normal boys

X Y ◯ ○ Normal X and Y chromosome

● Defective X chromosome

**Figure 5–7**
Transmission of sex-linked disorders.

## Fragile X Syndrome

Fragile X syndrome is a genetic condition associated with mental retardation. It is identified by a break, or weakness, on the long arm of the X chromosome. Because this is an abnormality of a sex chromosome, it is often referred to as X-linked. Mothers are the carriers, and their sons are at risk of being affected, whereas daughters are at risk of being carriers and sometimes are mildly affected. The prevalence of Fragile X is approximately 1 in 1,000 males, and the prevalence of carriers in the population is 1 in 600. Fragile X is the most common inherited cause of mental retardation known, accounting for up to 10% of cases. The gene responsible for Fragile X has been identified (FMR-1), and Fragile X is diagnosed by DNA testing.

About 80% of boys with Fragile X have mental impairment ranging from severe retardation to low-normal intelligence. The majority are mildly to moderately retarded. Men and boys with Fragile X are usually socially engaging, but they have an unusual style of interacting with other people. They tend to avoid direct eye contact during conversation, and hand-flapping or hand-biting is common. They may have an un-

usual speech pattern characterized by a fast and fluctuating rate of repetitions of sound, words, or phrases. They also may have a decreased attention span, hyperactivity, and motor delays. Girls are much less affected, with estimates that about 30% with the condition have some degree of mental retardation. The physical features are often more subtle in females.

There is no cure for Fragile X syndrome, but medical intervention can improve the problems in attention and hyperactivity. A variety of medications can treat attention span, hyperactivity, and other behavior problems. In addition, speech and physical therapy as well as vocational training can be beneficial.

## Familial Diseases

Some diseases appear in families, but the means of inheritance is not understood. Examples of diseases with a higher incidence in certain families are epilepsy, diabetes, cardiovascular problems, allergies, and familial polyposis. The cause of these diseases does not seem to be a single gene but the effect of several genes working together. In fact, some familial diseases may not be inherited at all, but instead result from unique environmental conditions or behaviors that are shared by family members.

## ▶ Abnormal Chromosome Diseases

The hereditary diseases described to this point result from a defective gene. Abnormalities in the chromosomes, either in their number or structure, also cause disorders. At times, chromosomes fail to separate properly during cell division, causing one daughter cell to be deficient and one to have an extra chromosome. The loss of an autosomal chromosome is usually incompatible with life because each autosome contains a large number of essential genes. A fetus affected by this condition is generally spontaneously aborted. The loss of a sex chromosome or the presence of an extra one is less serious, but many abnormalities accompany the condition.

### Down Syndrome

Down syndrome is an example of a disorder caused by the presence of an extra autosomal chromosome. Chromosome 21 is inherited in triplicate, a condition called trisomy 21. The extra chromosome results from nondisjunction, the failure of two chromosomes to separate as the gametes, either the egg or the sperm, are being formed. The incidence of Down syndrome is higher among children born to mothers over age 35.

The Down syndrome child is always mentally retarded. The excessive enzyme production from the extra genes may have a toxic effect on the brain. The child can be taught simple tasks and is generally very affectionate.

The life expectancy of a child with Down syndrome is relatively short because of complications that accompany the condition, including congenital heart diseases, greater susceptibility to respiratory tract infections, including pneumonia, and a higher incidence of leukemia than in a normal child.

The Down syndrome child has a characteristic appearance. The eyes appear slanted be-

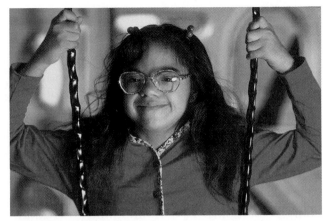

**Figure 5–8** Girl with Down syndrome. (© Beebe/Custom Medical Stock Photo.)

cause of an extra fold of skin at the upper, medial corner of the eye; the tongue is coarse and often protrudes; and the nose is short and flat. The child is usually of short stature, and the sex organs are underdeveloped. A straight crease extends across the palm of the hand, and the little finger is often shorter than normal (Figure 5–8).

### Cri Du Chat Syndrome

Cri du chat syndrome, or cat cry syndrome, is caused by a deletion of part of the short arm of chromosome 5. Infants with cri du chat syndrome have an abnormally small head with a deficiency in cerebral brain tissue, eyes that are spaced far apart, and mental retardation. Those who are born alive have a weak, catlike cry. Treatment is supportive until the infant dies.

## ▶ Sex Anomalies

### Turner's Syndrome

One of the sex chromosomes is missing in Turner's syndrome, resulting in a karyotype of 45, XO, indicating the presence of 45 chromosomes, with only one X chromosome. The person appears to be female, but the ovaries do not develop; thus, there is no ovulation or menstruation, and the person is sterile. The nipples are widely spaced, the breasts do not develop, and the person is short of stature and has a stocky build. Congenital heart disease, particularly coarctation of the aorta (described in Chapter 7), frequently accompanies Turner's syndrome. Facial deformities are often present. Figure 5–9 shows a patient with Turner's syndrome.

## Klinefelter's Syndrome

An extra sex chromosome is present in Klinefelter's syndrome, resulting in a karyotype of 47, XXY, indicating the presence of 47 chromosomes, including two X and one Y chromosomes. This person appears to be a male but has small testes that fail to mature and that produce no sperm. At puberty, with the development of secondary sex characteristics, the breasts enlarge and female distribution of hair develops. There is little facial hair, and the gen-

eral appearance is that of a eunuch. The person is tall (with abnormally long legs), is mentally deficient, and is sterile (Figure 5–10).

## Hermaphrodites

The number of true hermaphrodites who have both testes and ovaries is small. Pseudo-hermaphrodites do develop, and they have either testes or ovaries, usually nonfunctional, but the remainder of the anatomy is mixed. This condition is referred to as *sex reversal*, in which the chromosomal sex is different from the anatomic sex. Sex reversal occurs during fetal life. The sex glands are neutral during the first few weeks after conception, until the male gonads differentiate at about the sixth week under the influence of masculinizing hormone. In the absence of an adequate amount of this hormone, ovaries develop, and the individual devel-

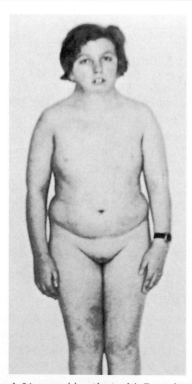

**Figure 5–9** A 21-year-old patient with Turner's syndrome. The chest is broad, and the nipples are small and pale. Pubic hair is totally lacking.

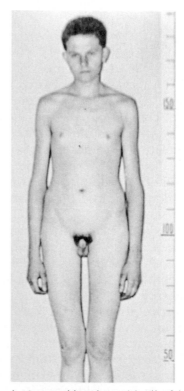

**Figure 5–10** A 19-year-old patient with Klinefelter's syndrome. Extremities are excessively long, pubic hair is scanty, and genitals are undeveloped. Body proportions resemble those of a eunuch.

ops anatomically female but chromosomally male (XY).

Some cases of pseudohermaphroditism result from excessive production of sex hormones from the adrenal cortex. An affected female develops male secondary sexual characteristics at a very early age. The external genitalia of pseudohermaphrodites are ambiguous, resembling that of both males and females. A pseudohermaphrodite is shown in Figure 5–11.

## ▶ Genetic Counseling

A genetic counselor usually begins with a complete family history of both prospective parents. A complete, detailed family history is called a *pedigree.* Pedigrees are used to determine the

pattern of inheritance of a genetic disease within a family. When the pedigree is complete, the genetic counselor can inform prospective parents of the possibility of having genetically abnormal offspring. Once armed with this information, the couple can make an informed decision on whether to have children.

### Diagnosis of Genetic Diseases

Early diagnosis is critical to prevention and treatment of genetic diseases. During amniocentesis, a small amount of amniotic fluid is withdrawn after the 14th week of pregnancy. Fetal cells in the amniotic fluid are removed, the chromosomes are examined, and the amniotic fluid is analyzed for biochemical abnormalities. Test results in amniocentesis are available approximately 2 weeks after the procedure. Amniocentesis can detect approximately 200 genetic diseases before birth.

Chorionic villi are projections of the membrane that surrounds the embryo in early pregnancy. Chorionic villus sampling involves removing cells from the villi through the cervix. Samples may be taken between 8 and 10 weeks of pregnancy. The chromosomes of the cells obtained can be analyzed immediately.

In addition to fetal testing, DNA testing is available for some hereditary diseases.

## ▶ Congenital Diseases

Congenital diseases are those appearing at birth or shortly after, but they are not caused by genetic or chromosomal abnormalities. Congenital defects usually result from some failure in development during the embryonic stage, or in the first 2 months of pregnancy. Congenital diseases cannot be transmitted to offspring.

Various factors—inadequate oxygen, maternal infection, drugs, malnutrition, and radiation—can interfere with normal development. Rubella, or German measles, contracted by the mother during the first trimester of pregnancy, can produce serious birth defects. The rubella virus can cross the placental barrier and affect the central nervous system of the embryo, caus-

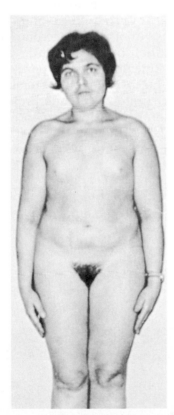

**Figure 5–11** A 22-year-old patient with pseudohermaphroditism, reared as a girl because of ambiguous genitalia. Surgery and tissue studies showed the gonads to be testes.

ing mental retardation, blindness, and deafness. Cerebral palsy and hydrocephalus can develop as a result of the viral infection.

Syphilis can be transmitted to a developing fetus and cause multiple anomalies: structural deformities, blindness, deafness, and paralysis. Children with congenital syphilis may become insane. Syphilitic infection of a fetus frequently results in spontaneous abortion or a stillbirth. A mother with syphilis should be treated for it before the fifth month of pregnancy to prevent fetal infection. A child born with syphilis should be treated immediately with penicillin, but considerable irreversible damage may have already occurred. Syphilis is discussed further in Chapter 12.

The tragic effect of the drug thalidomide, introduced in the 1950s and used during pregnancy until 1962, alerted the public to the danger of drugs to the developing embryo. Babies who had been exposed to thalidomide before birth were born without limbs or had flipper-like appendages.

Many congenital defects result from improper development, such as the failure of organ walls to form or close, or the failure of two parts to unite and fuse. The chambers and vessels of the heart are sites of such abnormalities, and congenital heart diseases are discussed in Chapter 7. Spina bifida, an improper union of parts of the vertebral column, is an example of a neural tube defect (NTD). Although the cause of NTD is unknown, folic acid intake prior to and through the first few weeks of pregnancy decreases the incidence of NTD. Since neural tube closure occurs at 28 days after conception and prior to the recognition of pregnancy by many women, NTD prevention is best achieved by adequate folic acid (0.4 mg per day) intake throughout the reproductive years. Spina bifida is further explained in Chapter 14.

Cleft lip and cleft palate comprise the fourth most common birth defect in the United States. One of 700 newborns is affected by cleft lip and/or cleft palate, which is a gap between the left and right halves of the lip or upper palate (roof of the mouth). The defects are due to failure of the two sides to fuse during gestation, and affect speech, respiration, feeding, and physical appearance. Clefts can be corrected with surgery.

A variety of types of congenital defects occur in the alimentary tract. The absence of a normal opening in an organ is called atresia. The lack of an opening from the esophagus to the stomach is esophageal atresia; it is frequently accompanied by an abnormal opening between the esophagus and the trachea.

Intestinal atresia is a complete obstruction of the intestine, resulting in vomiting, dehydration, scanty stool production, and distention of the abdomen. Another congenital obstruction of the intestinal tract is pyloric stenosis, in which the pyloric sphincter hypertrophies, closing the opening between the stomach and the duodenum. Symptoms include projectile vomiting, dehydration, constipation, and weight loss. Corrective surgery has been very effective in removing these congenital obstructions of the intestinal tract, just as it has been for congenital heart disease.

The bile ducts are blocked in biliary atresia, causing severe jaundice to develop. In biliary atresia, the liver and spleen become greatly enlarged.

## Prevention ✚ PLUS!

### Rubella and Pregnancy

Rubella infection during pregnancy can harm the fetus. The best way to prevent rubella during pregnancy is to get vaccinated before even thinking about getting pregnant. However, because the vaccine itself can harm the fetus, pregnant women must not get the rubella vaccine, and women should wait 3 months after vaccination before becoming pregnant.

## CHAPTER SUMMARY

Genetic information is encoded in the DNA molecule, which duplicates in preparation for cell division. DNA comprises the genes that are arranged on the chromosomes and provides a blueprint for protein synthesis in the daughter cells. Some genes are dominant and are always expressed when inherited, whereas others are recessive and require the inheritance of two copies for the expression of a trait. One pair of chromosomes, the X and Y chromosomes, determine the gender of the fetus. The other 44 chromosomes are called autosomes.

Some diseases develop if a single dominant autosomal gene is received. An example of this is familial hypercholesterolemia. Other diseases develop if a recessive gene is received from each parent, as is the case in phenylketonuria. Other diseases are sex-linked, which primarily affect males and are usually transmitted by females. Sex-linked disorders and diseases include color blindness, hemophilia, and Fragile X syndrome. Some diseases, such as epilepsy, diabetes, and allergies, occur within families but are not attributable to one particular gene, and may instead be caused by the action of several genes.

Gross chromosomal abnormalities cause other disorders. Down's syndrome is caused by chromosome 21 being in triplicate (trisomy 21). A missing or extra sex chromosome produces sex anomalies and usually mental retardation.

Certain conditions are apparent at birth or soon after, but they are not the result of genetic or chromosomal abnormalities. These are congenital diseases caused by various factors during early development. Certain heart malformations, absence of a natural body opening, or failure of a structure to close are examples of congenital diseases. Congenital diseases are not passed on to offspring.

## RESOURCES

The National Center for Biotechnology Information: www .ncbi.nlm.nih.gov

The National Library of Medicine: www.nlm.nih.gov

The National Marfan Foundation: www.marfan.org

National Human Genome Research Institute: www.nhgri .nih.gov

# Interactive Activities

## Cases for Critical Thinking

1. What is the reason that Turner's and Klinefelter's syndromes can occur as a result of nondisjunction in either the sperm or the egg, but XYY can occur only as a result of nondisjunction in the sperm?

2. Marfan syndrome is an autosomal dominant disease. What is the probability that a child with a parent with Marfan syndrome will have Marfan syndrome?

3. If a mother is a carrier for the X-linked disease hemophilia A, what is the probability that her male child will have hemophilia A? Her female child?

## Multiple Choice

1. The sex chromosomes of a normal male are
   _____.
   a. XX                    c. YY
   b. XY                    d. XXY

2. Except for sperm and ova, human cells each have
   _____ chromosomes.
   a. 23                    c. 96
   b. 46                    d. 21

3. _____ alleles manifest themselves only when
   the person is homozygous for the trait.
   a. Recessive             c. Homozygous
   b. Dominant              d. Heterozygous

4. Sex-linked diseases affect men more than women because
   _____.
   a. men have two X chromosomes
   b. men have two Y chromosomes
   c. men have one X chromosomes
   d. men have no Y chromosome

5. Color-blind people most frequently can't distinguish
   _____.
   a. red and yellow        c. red and green
   b. green and blue        d. blue and yellow

6. Galactosemia is a(n) _____ disorder.
   a. autosomal dominant    c. sex-linked
   b. autosomal recessive   d. congenital

7. If a female is a carrier of a sex-linked disease, she has a
   _____% chance of transmitting the allele to
   her children.
   a. 25                    c. 75
   b. 50                    d. 100

8. If both parents are carriers of an autosomal recessive disease, each child has a _____% chance of getting the disease.
   a. 0                     c. 50
   b. 25                    d. 100

9. If alleles are different, the person is _____ for
   that trait.
   a. homozygous            c. heterozygous
   b. recessive             d. dominant

10. Forty-four of our chromosomes are called
    _____.
    a. sex chromosomes       c. autosomes
    b. genes                 d. alleles

## True or False

_____ 1. DNA contains genetic information.

_____ 2. The incidence of Down's syndrome increases with the mother's age.

_____ 3. Fragile X syndrome is found equally in men and women.

_____ 4. A patient with Turner's syndrome has an extra sex chromosome.

_____ 5. Tay Sach's is an autosomal dominant disease.

_____ 6. Down's syndrome is caused by an extra sex chromosome

_____ 7. Albinism is a sex-linked disease.

_____ 8. If allele pairs are similar, the person is homozygous for that trait.

_____ 9. If one parent is heterozygous for an autosomal dominant disease and the other parent is normal, a child has a 50% chance for getting the disease.

_____ 10. DNA is the blueprint for protein synthesis within the cell.

## Fill-Ins

1. _____ diseases are those appearing at birth or shortly after, but they are not caused by genetic or chromosomal abnormalities.

2. _____ have both functional testes and ovaries.

3. _____ alleles only manifest themselves when the person is homozygous for that trait.

4. _____ encode information for the synthesis of proteins.

5. _____ are alternative forms of a gene.

6. _____ is the condition of extra fingers or toes.

7. _____ is the failure of two chromosomes to separate as the gametes are being formed.

8. Sex cells contain _____ chromosomes.

9. The chromosomal composition of the nucleus is called the _____ of the cell.

10. Sex cells are produced by a type of cell division called _____.

**MedMedia
Wrap-Up**

**www.prenhall.com/mulvihill**
Remember to visit this website for extra study practice, including exercises, Internet links, news updates, and an audio glossary.

**Activity CD-ROM**
Check out the CD-ROM in the back of this book. You will find games, exercises, puzzles, and videos to help enhance your understanding of this chapter.

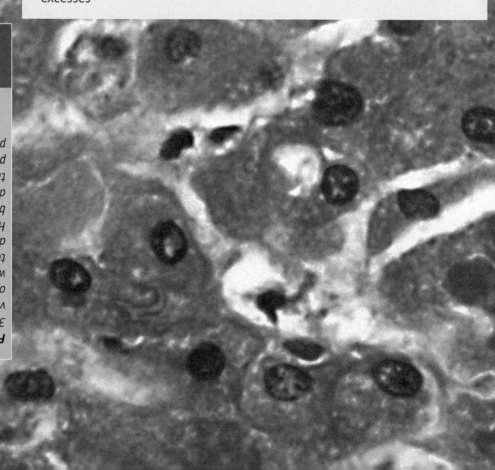

# Nutrition and Disease

**CHAPTER**

**6**

## Learning Objectives

After studying this chapter, you should be able to

- Describe the role of nutrition in health promotion
- Describe the consequences of overnutrition and undernutrition
- Identify appropriate treatment for obesity and protein-calorie malnutrition
- Define the biological role of carbohydrates, fats, proteins, vitamins, and minerals
- Identify the consequences of vitamin and mineral deficiencies and excesses

## Fact or Fiction?

Large doses of vitamin C prevent the common cold.

*Fiction:* Systematic analysis of 30 clinical trials concluded that vitamin C in doses as high as one gram daily over several winter months had no consistent beneficial effect on incidence of the common cold. High doses of vitamin C may be beneficial in reducing the duration of the cold. However, the relation of dose to therapeutic benefit needs further exploration.

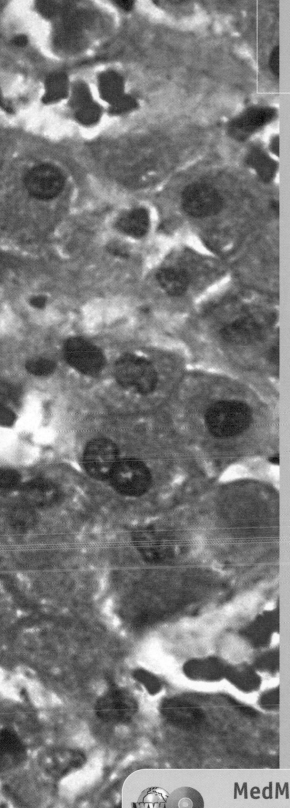

# Disease Chronicle

## James Lind: A Treatise of the Scurvy

In 1747, as the HMS *Salisbury* sailed from England to America, the ship's physician, James Lind, performed a simple experiment to determine what might be an effective cure for scurvy.

On the 20th May, 1747, I took twelve patients in the scurvy on board the *Salisbury* at sea. They all in general had putrid gums, the spots and lassitude, with weakness of their knees. They lay together in one place, being a proper apartment for the sick in the fore-hold; and had one diet in common to all, viz., water gruel sweetened with sugar in the morning; fresh mutton broth often times for dinner; at other times puddings, boiled biscuit with sugar etc.; and for supper barley, raisins, rice and currants, sago and wine, or the like. Two of these were ordered each a quart of cyder a day. Two others took twenty five gutts of elixir vitriol three times a day upon an empty stomach, using a gargle strongly acidulated with it for their mouths. Two others took two spoonfuls of vinegar three times a day upon an empty stomach, having their gruels and their other food well acidulated with it, as also the gargle for the mouth. Two of the worst patients, with the tendons in the ham rigid (a symptom none the rest had) were put under a course of sea water. Of this they drank half a pint every day and sometimes more or less as it operated by way of gentle physic. Two others had each two oranges and one lemon given them every day. They continued but six days under this course, having consumed the quantity that could be spared. The two remaining patients took the bigness of a nutmeg three times a day of an electuary recommended by an hospital surgeon made of garlic, mustard seed, *rad. raphan.*, balsam of Peru and gum myrrh, using for common drink barley water well acidulated with tamarinds, by a decoction of which, with the addition of *cremor tartar,* they were gently purged three or four times during the course.

The consequence was that the most sudden and visible good effects were perceived from the use of the oranges and lemons; one of

those who had taken them being at the end of six days fit four [sic.] duty.

I shall here only observe that the result of all my experiments was that oranges and lemons were the most effectual remedies for this distemper at sea.

## ▶ Nutrition

Nutrients are chemical compounds consumed in food that are required for vital cellular processes that ensure growth and development, recovery from illness, and prevention of chronic disease. The human body requires approximately 40 nutrients. Essential nutrients include vitamins, minerals, certain amino acids and fatty acids, and some carbohydrates that cannot be synthesized by the human body. Nonessential nutrients are those that the body can synthesize from compounds that are derived from the diet. The body also requires a continuous supply of energy in the form of carbohydrates and fat, indigestible carbohydrate (fiber) to aid in proper digestion, additional nitrogen for growth and recovery from illness, and water to maintain hydration.

Recommended Dietary allowances (RDAs) describe quantitative and qualitative nutritional requirements for most healthy people. Diets that meet the RDA of food choices ensure intake of enough nutrients to maintain health and physical activity. The food guide pyramid translates the RDA into food choices that are important for a healthy diet (Figure 6–1). The goal for a proper diet is to achieve optimal body composition necessary for physical and mental activity. The daily dietary requirements for essential nutrients vary with age, sex, height, weight, and metabolic and physical activity.

### Diet, Health, and Disease

The importance of nutrition in health promotion and disease prevention is evident with growing scientific information and health outcomes observed among different cultures. Malnutrition, including overnutrition and undernutrition, are major causes of morbidity and mortality in developing and industrialized countries. Dietary choices are shaped by cultural, social, and religious traditions. Accessibility of various food choices is at times limited by economic, ecologic, and social conditions that may or may not meet nutritional requirements.

Nutrition is often compromised in persons with chronic physical and mental illnesses, and malnutrition may occur as a complication of certain medical and surgical procedures. Starvation, overeating, substance abuse, endocrine diseases, fever and infections, gastrointestinal disease, liver disease, and kidney disease are among many conditions that compromise nutrition and health. Furthermore, nutritional factors play a role in the causation of many chronic degenerative diseases such as cancer, cardiovascular disease, and diabetes.

## ▶ Malnutrition

The concept of malnutrition is generally associated with inadequate availability of food, but one can suffer nutritional deficiencies in the midst of plenty. Malnutrition results from imbalance between the body's needs and the intake of nutrients. Malnutrition includes both disorders in which nutrients are oversupplied and undernutrition in which nutrient intake fails to meet physiological needs. Overnutrition results from overeating, insufficient exercise, overuse of fad or prescription diets, or excess intake of certain vitamins and minerals. Undernutrition can result from inadequate intake, or starvation; malabsorption; abnormal systemic loss of nutrients

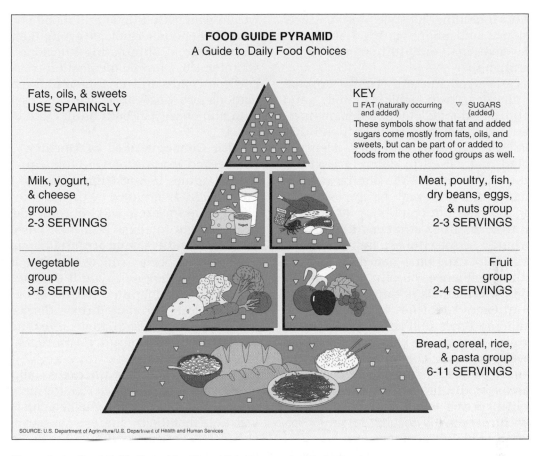

**Figure 6-1** Food Guide Pyramid. (*Source:* U.S. Department of Agriculture.)

due to vomiting, diarrhea, hemorrhage, renal failure, or excessive sweating; infection; or addiction to drugs or alcohol.

## Overnutrition

**Obesity** Obesity is one of the most common health problems in the United States and among the most frustrating and difficult to manage. Nearly one-third of adult Americans are overweight or obese despite published recommendations for healthy eating and healthy lifestyles. Health-care costs associated with obesity amount to nearly $100 billion annually within the United States. Despite access to health care, approximately 300,000 deaths per year in the United States result from the ill effects of obesity.

Overweight and obesity customarily has been defined in terms of body weight, but current measures and risks for obesity are based on assessment of body mass index (BMI). The BMI is a calculated measure that is obtained by dividing measured body weight in kilograms by height in meters squared. The National Institutes of Health define a normal BMI as 18.5 to 24.9. Overweight is defined as a BMI of 25 to 29.9. Class I obesity is 30 to 34.9; class II obesity is 35 to 39.9; and class III (extreme) obesity is a BMI of 40 or greater.

**Causes of Obesity** Obesity is most simply understood as overindulgence. The regulation of body weight, however, is a complex and precise behavioral and metabolic process that is shaped by genetic, biological, psychological, and environmental factors. Genes and biology regulate human development, including body size, shape, metabolism, behavior, and emotions.

Environment, including lifestyle and cultural traits, influence and shape eating habits and preferences, emotions, and attitudes relating to body size and shape.

Genetic causes of human obesity are assessed by identical twin, sibling, family, and adoption studies. Adopted children demonstrate a close relationship between their BMI and that of their biologic parents. Similarly, identical twins adopted and raised in different environments from birth, develop BMIs similar to each other. Genetic influences may be important in determining the distribution of body fat and the metabolic abnormalities that contribute to greater morbidity in select obese individuals.

More than 300 candidate genes have been identified that influence obesity in humans. Genetic studies in animals account for relationships between candidate genes as well as mutations in candidate genes that result in obesity. A mutation in the *ob* gene, for example, results in massive obesity in mice. The ob gene codes the protein leptin, which is produced in fat cells, and regulates areas of the brain that direct energy and metabolism as well as influence body weight.

Sedentary lifestyle with chronic intake of excess calories, availability of certain types of high-calorie food, as well as cultural and social traditions are among many environmental explanations for obesity. Children raised in families with one overweight parent have a 40% chance of becoming overweight as an adult. This risk increases to 80% for children raised in families in which both parents are overweight.

Obese and nonobese individuals eat in response to emotional cues such as feelings of anxiety, depression, loneliness, boredom, and anger. Emotional patterns of overeating are commonly reported among severely obese individuals with binge eating problems. Binge eaters eat large amounts of food in response to depression, anxiety, and self-contempt. The use of food as comfort, as a substitute for feeling loved, and as a way to avoid conflict plays a role in both the development and maintenance of obesity.

Secondary causes of obesity include endocrine disorders, such as Cushing's syndrome and hypothyroid disease, and long-term pharmacotherapy with certain medications. Unexplained weight gain with fatigue and mood changes warrant further endocrinologic evaluation, including serum–thyroid stimulating hormone levels (see Chapter 13). Chronic medication treatment with corticosteroids and certain antipsychotic medications are associated with excessive weight gain and obesity in both adults and children.

**Health Consequences of Obesity** Obesity is the second leading preventable cause of death among adults in the United States. Excess fat and weight is coupled with adverse metabolic changes associated with chronic degenerative diseases that increase both morbidity and mortality. The most significant and common health problems in obese and overweight individuals include hypertension, type II diabetes mellitus, hyperlipidemia (elevated plasma cholesterol and triglycerides), coronary artery disease, peripheral vascular disease, gastrointestinal disease, osteoarthritis, respiratory disorders, and certain types of cancer.

Obese individuals with excess abdominal or visceral fat have a higher risk for metabolic syndrome. Metabolic syndrome is a cluster of physical and metabolic changes associated with a significant risk for peripheral vascular disease, cardiovascular disease, stroke, and diabetes. Individuals with abdominal obesity are more likely to have high blood pressure, elevated plasma triglycerides and cholesterol, and resistance to insulin. Both insulin resistance with hyperglycemia and hyperlipidemia contribute to atherosclerotic changes that result in peripheral vascular disease, hypertension, coronary artery disease, and strokes.

Respiratory complications in obese individuals include obstructive sleep apnea syndrome (OSAS) and obesity-hypoventilation syndrome (pickwickian syndrome). OSAS is defined as recurrent episodes of apnea during sleep caused by occlusion of the upper airway. Increased fat surrounding the structures of the upper airway limits expansion of airways causing hypoventilation and accumulation of carbon dioxide. Hypoventilation with accumulation of carbon dioxide, or pickwickian syndrome, increases risks for premature death from pulmonary and cardiac disorders.

Obesity may lead to orthopedic disturbances of weight-bearing and non-weight-bearing muscles and joints. Excess weight stresses joints, leading to inflammation and erosion of cartilage, muscle strain, degenerative joint disease, and osteoarthritis. Chronic orthopedic pain limits activity and contributes to physical and social disability.

Skin disorders are particularly common in obese individuals. Persistent inflammation of the skin, immobility, and veno-occlusive disease often result in skin ulcers and infections. Sweat and skin secretions, trapped in thick folds of skin, produce a culture conducive to fungal and bacterial growth that is often difficult to identify until serious infections result.

Prejudice and social discrimination relating to size, self-control, and social image are often cited psychosocial stresses in obese individuals. Obese children and adolescents experience psychological pain from isolation and social rejection that may continue through adulthood. Obese children and adults have difficulty participating in sports and are often teased and ridiculed by their peers. Obese women report problems with disparagement of body image, in which they feel that their body is grotesque and as a result feel others view them with hostility. Depression, anxiety, loneliness, and guilt perpetuate a cycle of withdrawal, inactivity, and persistent health problems.

**Treatment of Obesity** Obese individuals who achieve and maintain a 10% reduction in body weight, regardless of BMI, are likely to lower their blood pressure, serum glucose, cholesterol, triglycerides, and resultant morbidity from diabetes or cardiovascular disease. The most successful diet programs for obesity integrate a multidisciplinary approach to weight loss, including calorie restrictions, behavior modification, aerobic exercise, and social support.

Behavior modification techniques include education that encourages changes in eating behavior, such as lifestyle changes that includes time for meal planning, awareness of dietary choices, and exercise. Continued contact with health-care providers is important for long-term maintenance of weight loss.

Pharmacological agents for weight loss include medications that enhance satiety, decrease appetite, and decrease fat absorption. Similar to behavior modification, medication therapy requires close monitoring of weight, blood pressure, and adherence to healthy dietary choices. Vitamin and mineral supplementation is recommended with agents that decrease fat absorption.

Surgical treatment for obesity includes vertical-banded gastroplasty and gastric bypass. Both procedures result in significant weight loss that is maintained. Nutritional side effects include undernutrition, nutrient malabsorption, and dumping syndrome. Vitamin and mineral supplementation should be encouraged with both surgical procedures.

Exercise offers a number of advantages to patients trying to lose weight and keep it off. Aerobic exercise directly increases the daily energy expenditure and is particularly useful for long-term weight control, healthy cardiovascular function, and good mental health.

## Undernutrition

Undernutrition, or suboptimal supply of nutrients, results in decreased tissue mass and energy stores needed for proper growth and development. Undernutrition affects all age groups across the life span, from conception to older adults, and impedes homeostatic responses such as immune function to fight illness and inflammatory responses to promote healing. Health consequences of undernutrition range from intrauterine growth retardation and brain damage to reduced physical and mental capacity in childhood to diet-related chronic diseases in adulthood and later in life. Poverty, poor dentition, gastrointestinal disease, abdominal pain, anorexia (decreased appetite), dysphagia (difficulty swallowing), depression, social isolation, and pain from eating are some of the many causes of poor nutrition.

**Digestion and Malnutrition** A healthy and intact gastrointestinal tract is needed for adequate digestion and absorption of nutrients. Gastrointestinal disorders may prevent solubilization of nutrients, mechanical and chemical breakdown, and absorption of nutrients. Secretion of enzymes, coenzymes, gastric acid, hormones, and neurotransmitters are also needed to facilitate chemical and physical processes of digestion. Physical conditions that impair digestion contribute to several types of malnutrition, including vitamin and mineral deficiencies, protein-calorie malnutrition, and essential fatty acid and amino acid deficiency.

Bowel disorders, including inflammatory bowel disease and Crohn's disease, discussed in Chapter 10, result in malabsorption of essential nutrients. Protein and energy undernutrition is prevalent among individuals with inflammatory bowel disease. Crohn's disease, on the other hand, tends to result in extensive nutritional problems. Bacterial overgrowth or surgical removal of the bowel can decrease the absorptive surface area of both the small and large bowel. Resections of the ileum can cause bile salt deficiency, resulting in fat malabsorption and subsequent deficiency of the fat-soluble vitamins (A, D, E, and K). Vitamin $B_{12}$ intrinsic-factor complex is absorbed in the ileum, and complete ileal resection produces a vitamin $B_{12}$ deficiency. Excess fluid losses in either inflammatory bowel disease or Crohn's disease can cause depletion of electrolytes (sodium, potassium, chloride, magnesium, phosphate), minerals such as iron, and trace elements such as zinc.

Fat malabsorption and severe abdominal pain common in pancreatitis impair both intake of nutrients and utilization of nutrients. Bile secretion, essential for the absorption of lipids, including the fat-soluble vitamins A, D, E, and K, may be compromised by liver or gallbladder disease, or other conditions that obstruct the bile ducts. Severe abdominal pain following meals in acute and chronic pancreatitis results in reduced food intake for symptom control.

The liver is involved in many of the body's metabolic processes, including regulation of protein, fat, and carbohydrate metabolism, vitamin storage and activation, and detoxification and excretion of waste products. Impaired liver function can lead to vitamin deficiencies, protein and energy deficiency, fatty acid deficiency, and impaired storage of nutrients within the liver. Conversely, undernutrition from other causes, such as alcoholism, anorexia nervosa, poverty, or mental illness, can impair liver function by affecting the liver's structural integrity.

**Protein Energy Malnutrition**   Protein energy malnutrition (PEM) is caused by inadequate intake of carbohydrates, fats, proteins, minerals, and water. When consumed in adequate quantities, carbohydrates and fats spare the use of tissue protein as a source of energy. Furthermore, unless sufficient nonprotein calories are available from either dietary sources or tissue stores (particularly of fat), protein cannot be used efficiently for tissue maintenance, replacement, or growth. Although infants and children of some developing nations dramatically exemplify this type of malnutrition, it can occur in persons of any age in any country.

The balance of nonprotein and protein sources of energy and resultant physical changes determines differential diagnoses of PEM. Marasmus is referred to as the "dry form" of PEM and results from starvation with deficiency of protein and nonprotein nutrients. The marasmic child appears very thin from the loss of muscle and body fat. Kwashiorkor, or the "wet form" of PEM, occurs in children who are weaned too quickly from breast milk and are fed a thin gruel with poor nutritional quality. Protein deficiency is greater relative to the energy deficiency in the child with kwashiorkor. The combined form of PEM is termed marasmic kwashiorkor and is characterized by edema or accumulation of an excessive amount of watery fluid and more body fat than those with marasmus (Table 6–1).

Marasmus and kwashiorkor are associated with growth failure, impaired immune function, weakness, and decline in functional status with difficulties associated with daily care and living. Infections with a wide variety of bacteria-producing pneumonia, diarrhea, otitis media, genitourinary infections, and sepsis often result from poor hygiene and impaired immunity. Electrolyte abnormalities with decreases in plasma potassium, calcium, phosphorus, and magnesium exacerbate muscle weakness.

Death within the first days of treatment is usually due to electrolyte imbalance, infections, hypothermia, or heart failure. The first step for

| Table 6–1 Marasmus and Kwashiorkor | | |
|---|---|---|
| | **Marasmus** | **Kwashiorkor** |
| **Description** | Dry | Wet |
| **Cause** | Near starvation | Early weaning from breast milk |
| **Nonprotein/protein sources of energy** | Deficiency in both protein and nonprotein nutrients | Protein deficiency greater than energy deficiency |
| **Age** | Younger than 5 years | Older than 5 years |
| **Appearance** | Growth retardation with wasting of subcutaneous fat and muscle | Generalized edema (fluid accumulation); flaky dermatitis; thin, discolored hair |

treatment of PEM begins with assessment and treatment of fluid and electrolyte disorders, current infections, and diarrhea. Fluid and electrolyte replacement is initiated first along with antimicrobial medications to treat existing infections. Once diarrhea subsides, re-feeding is introduced with fortified milk-based formulas. Some children recover completely with adequate treatment, while others suffer lifelong immune function impairment, mental retardation, and permanent organ damage.

## ▶ Vitamin Deficiency, Excess, and Dependency

Vitamins are organic compounds that have important functions in metabolic reactions that result in the release or storage of energy from carbohydrates, fats, and proteins. Minerals are inorganic elements that do not provide energy but are needed for a number of anabolic and catabolic biochemical reactions within the body. Vitamins and minerals are crucial throughout life for proper growth, development, and metabolism. Physical vitamin requirements vary throughout the life cycle. In general, cellular requirements for vitamins and minerals are greater in infancy, adolescence, pregnancy, and lactation.

The Food and Nutrition Board of the National Research Council established recommended dietary allowances for most vitamins and minerals based on extensive review of published scientific data. Dietary reference intakes, or DRIs, established by the Institute of Medicine and the National Academy of Sciences, provide a range of safe and appropriate amounts of vitamins and minerals that are needed to prevent chronic disease.

Despite the relative ease of meeting RDA with a well-balanced diet, many adults in the United States consume vitamin and mineral supplements. Deficiencies in the western world are most often associated with malabsorption, alcoholism, kidney disease, liver disease, food faddism, or inborn errors of metabolism. In parts of the world where food supply is inadequate, multiple vitamin and mineral deficiencies are encountered more often than deficiencies of single vitamins. Disorders caused by vitamin deficiency and excesses are listed in Table 6–2.

Individual vitamins differ in chemical composition and are categorized as either fat-soluble or water-soluble. Fat-soluble vitamins include vitamin A ( retinol, carotenoids), D (cholecalciferol), E (tocopherols), and K (phylloquinone, menaquinone, and menadione). Water-soluble vitamins include vitamin C (ascorbic acid), and the B complex vitamins; $B_1$ (thiamine), $B_2$ (riboflavin), $B_3$ (niacin), $B_5$ (pantothenic acid), $B_6$ (pyridoxine), $B_{12}$ (cobalamin), folic acid, and biotin. Fat-soluble vitamins require some dietary fat for absorption and are stored in fat tissue.

## Table 6–2  Vitamin Deficiencies and Excesses

| Nutrient | Principal Sources | Functions | Effects of Deficiency and Toxicity |
|---|---|---|---|
| **Vitamin A** (retinol) | Fish liver oils, liver, egg yolk, butter, cream, vitamin A-fortified margarine; ascarotenoids: dark green, leafy vegetables; yellow fruits; red palm oil | Photoreceptor mechanism of retina, integrity of skin | **Deficiency:** night blindness, keratomalacia, increased morbidity and mortality in young children<br>**Toxicity:** headache, peeling of skin |
| **Vitamin D** (cholecalciferol, ergocalciferol) | Ultraviolet irradiation of the skin (main source); fortified milk (main dietary source); fish liver oils, butter, egg yolk, liver | Calcium and phosphorus absorption; resorption, mineralization, and maturation of bone | **Deficiency:** rickets (sometimes with tetany), osteomalacia<br>**Toxicity:** anorexia, renal failure, |
| **Vitamin E group** (α-tocopherol and other tocopherols) | Vegetable oil, wheat germ, leafy vegetables, egg yolk, margarine, legumes | Intracellular antioxidant, scavenger of free radicals in biologic membranes | **Deficiency:** RBC hemolysis or rupture of red blood cells, neurologic damage,<br>**Toxicity:** interference with enzymes |
| **Vitamin K group** (phylloquinone and menaquinones) | Leafy vegetables, pork, liver, vegetable oils, intestinal flora after newborn period | Formation of coagulation factors, and bone proteins | **Deficiency:** Hemorrhage from deficiency of coagulation factors |
| **Thiamine** (vitamin B$_1$) | Dried yeast, whole grains, meat (especially pork, liver), enriched cereal products, nuts, legumes, potatoes | Carbohydrate metabolism, central and peripheral nerve cell function, heart function | **Deficiency:** beriberi (peripheral nerve degeneration, heart failure, Wernicke-Korsakoff syndrome |
| **Riboflavin** (vitamin B$_2$) | Milk, cheese, liver, meat, eggs, enriched cereal products | Many aspects of energy and protein metabolism, integrity of mucous membranes | **Deficiency:** dry lips, mouth sores, dermatitis. |
| **Niacin** (nicotinic acid, niacinamide) | Dried yeast, liver, meat, fish, legumes, whole-grain enriched cereal products | Carbohydrate metabolism | **Deficiency:** pellagra (Dermatitis, swelling of the tongue, gastrointestinal and nervous system disturbance) |
| **Vitamin B$_6$ group** (pyridoxine, pyridoxal, pyridoxamine) | Dried yeast, liver, organ meats, whole-grain cereals, fish, legumes | Many aspects of protein metabolism | **Deficiency:** convulsions, nervous system disturbance,<br>**Toxicity:** peripheral degeneration of nervous tissue |
| **Folic acid** | Fresh green leafy vegetables, fruits, organ meats, liver, dried yeast | Maturation of red blood cells | **Deficiency:** anemia, neural tube defects |
| **Vitamin B$_{12}$** (cobalamins) | Liver, meats (especially beef, pork, organ meats), eggs, milk and milk products | Maturation of red blood cells, neural function, DNA synthesis | **Deficiency:** pernicious anemia, megaloblastic anemia |

| Nutrient | Sources | Functions | Deficiency/Toxicity |
|---|---|---|---|
| Biotin | Liver, kidney, egg yolk, yeast, cauliflower, nuts, legumes | Amino acid and fatty acid metabolism | **Deficiency:** dermatitis, swelling of the tongue |
| Vitamin C (ascorbic acid) | Citrus fruits, tomatoes, potatoes, cabbage, green peppers | Essential to bone tissue, collagen formation, vascular function, tissue oxygenation, and wound healing | **Deficiency:** scurvy (hemorrhages, loose teeth, gingivitis, bone disease) |
| Sodium | Wide distribution—beef, pork, sardines, cheese, green olives, corn bread, potato chips, sauerkraut | Acid-base balance, fluid balance, blood acidity, muscle contractility, nerve transmission | **Deficiency:** confusion, coma  **Toxicity:** confusion, coma |
| Chloride | Wide distribution—mainly animal products but some vegetables, similar to sodium | Acid-base balance, fluid balance, blood acidity, kidney function | **Deficiency:** failure to thrive in infants  **Toxicity:** increase in extracellular volume, hypertension |
| Potassium | Wide distribution—whole and skim milk, bananas, prunes, raisins, meats | Muscle activity, nerve transmission, intracellular acid-base balance and water retention | **Deficiency:** paralysis, cardiac disturbances  **Toxicity:** paralysis, cardiac disturbances |
| Calcium | Milk and milk products, meat, fish, eggs, cereal products, beans, fruits, vegetables | Bone and tooth formation, blood coagulation, neuro-muscular irritability, muscle contractility, myocardial conduction | **Deficiency:** long term: osteoporosis, tetany, neuromuscular hyperexcitability  **Toxicity:** gastrointestinal paralysis, kidney failure, psychosis |
| Phosphorus | Milk, cheese, meat, poultry, fish, cereals, nuts, legumes | Bone and tooth formation, acid-base balance, component of nucleic acids, energy production | **Deficiency:** irritability, weakness, blood cell disorders, gastrointestinal tract and kidney dysfunction  **Toxicity:** accumulation in kidney disease |
| Magnesium | Green leaves, nuts, cereal grains, seafood | Bone and tooth formation, nerve conduction, muscle contraction, enzyme activation | **Deficiency:** neuromuscular irritability  **Toxicity:** hypotension, respiratory failure, cardiac disturbances |
| Iron | Wide distribution (except dairy products)—soybean flour, beef, kidney, liver, beans, clams, peaches. Heme iron in meat well absorbed (10–30%); nonheme iron in vegetables poorly absorbed (1–10%) | Hemoglobin and myoglobin formation, cytochrome enzymes, iron-sulfur proteins | **Deficiency:** anemia, decreased work performance, impaired learning ability  **Toxicity:** nausea, vomiting, diarrhea, gastrointestinal damage; fatal in children |

(continued)

## Table 6-2 Vitamin Deficiencies and Excesses (continued)

| Nutrient | Principal Sources | Functions | Effects of Deficiency and Toxicity |
|---|---|---|---|
| Iodine | Seafood, iodized salt, eggs, dairy products, drinking water in varying amounts | Synthesis of thyroid hormones | **Deficiency:** hypothyroid, impaired fetal growth and brain development<br>**Toxicity:** hyperthyroidism |
| Fluorine | Seafood, vegetables, grains, tea, coffee, fluoridated water (sodium fluoride 1.0–2.0 ppm) | Bone and tooth formation | **Deficiency:** predisposition to dental caries, osteoporosis<br>**Toxicity:** mottling and pitting of permanent teeth |
| Zinc | Meat, liver, eggs, oysters, peanuts, whole grains | Component of enzymes; skin integrity, wound healing, growth | **Deficiency:** growth retardation, small reproductive gland (testes) acrodermatitis enteropathica cause zinc deficiency |
| Copper | Organ meats, oysters, nuts, dried legumes, whole-grain cereals | Enzyme component, red blood cell synthesis, bone formation | **Deficiency:** anemia in malnourished children<br>**Toxicity:** nausea, vomiting, diarrhea, brain damage |
| Chromium | Brewer's yeast, liver, processed meats, whole-grain cereals, spices | Promotion of glucose tolerance | **Deficiency:** impaired glucose tolerance in malnourished children, some diabetics, and some elderly persons |
| Selenium | Wide distribution—meats and other animal products | Functions as an antioxidant with vitamin E | **Deficiency:** rare; muscle weakness<br>**Toxicity:** loss of hair and nails, nausea, dermatitis, polyneuritis |
| Manganese | Whole-grain cereals, green leafy vegetables, nuts, tea | Component of enzymes | **Primary Deficiency:** rare<br>**Toxicity:** Rare due to occupational exposure |
| Molybdenum | Milk, beans, breads, cereals | Component of coenzyme | **Deficiency:** tachycardia, headache, nausea, disorientation |

*Source:* Modified from Merck Manual, 1999

Water-soluble vitamins are more easily absorbed and, when consumed in excess, are excreted in the urine. Acute and chronic toxicities occur with fat- and water-soluble vitamins. However, very large doses of fat-soluble vitamins are categorically more toxic.

## Fat-Soluble Vitamins

Fat-soluble vitamins include the following:

Vitamin A (retinol, carotenoids)

Vitamin D (cholecalciferol)

Vitamin E (tocopherols)

Vitamin K (phylloquinone, menaquinone, menadione)

### Vitamin A (Retinol and Carotenoids)

Vitamin A is available from fish-liver oils, liver, egg yolks, butter, and cream. Most of the body's vitamin A is stored in the liver. Vitamin A combines with opsin to form rhodopsin, a pigment receptor that absorbs light in the rods of the retina in the eye. Vitamin A also combines with receptors on DNA to regulate differentiation of epithelial tissue that line the respiratory, gastrointestinal, and urogenital tracts.

Primary vitamin A deficiency is usually caused by prolonged dietary deprivation. It is endemic in areas such as southern and eastern Asia, where rice, devoid of carotene, is the main source of nutrition. Secondary vitamin A deficiency may be due to inadequate conversion of carotene to vitamin A, or interference with absorption, storage, or transport of vitamin A. Interference with absorption or storage is likely in celiac disease, cystic fibrosis, pancreatic disease, duodenal bypass, congenital obstruction of the jejunum, obstruction of the bile ducts, parasitic infections such as giardiasis, and cirrhosis of the liver.

Vitamin A deficiency results in night blindness or the inability to see in dim light, dryness of the mucous membranes, impaired immunity, and increased susceptibility for infections. Dryness of the mucous membranes is most notable within the cornea of the eye. With persistent, untreated vitamin A deficiency, dryness of the mucous membranes may lead to perforation and ulceration of the cornea of the eye, and drying of mucous membranes throughout the body.

High doses of vitamin A are especially toxic in children. Signs of toxicity include drowsiness, irritability, headaches, vomiting, and drying and peeling of the skin. Symptoms of toxicity resolve within one to four weeks after elimination of vitamin A from the diet.

### Vitamin D (Ergocalciferol and Cholecalciferol)

Vitamin D occurs in two forms: ergocalciferol and cholecalciferol. Ergocalciferol is found in irradiated yeast, and cholecalciferol is formed in human skin by exposure to sunlight. Milk is fortified with both forms of vitamin D, but synthesis in the skin is the major source of vitamin D. Vitamin D is required for absorption of calcium and phosphorus from the gastrointestinal tract and for mineralization of bone.

Inadequate exposure to sunlight and low dietary intake are usually responsible for the development of vitamin D deficiency. Metabolic bone disease resulting from vitamin D deficiency is called rickets in children and osteomalacia in adults. Disturbances in growth with skeletal growth deformities, muscle weakness, delayed walking and crawling, and bone pain are symptoms of rickets in infants, children, and adolescents. Osteomalacia in adults is characterized by demineralization and softening of bone and vertical shortening of the vertebrae. Rickets and osteomalacia are further described in Chapter 16.

Type I vitamin D dependency (pseudovitamin D deficiency) is an autosomal recessive syndrome characterized by severe rickets with low or normal concentrations of plasma calcium and low plasma phosphate levels. Type II vitamin D dependency is due to mutations in a transcription factor that results in production of an ineffective form of vitamin D. Type I vitamin D dependency responds to physiologic replacement of vitamin D, whereas type II vitamin D dependency may or may not respond to vitamin D replacement.

Vitamin D in doses beyond the upper limits of the DRI produces toxicity within one to four months in infants. Vitamin D may accumulate for many years, causing toxicity in adulthood. Symptoms of toxicity include loss of appetite, nausea, and vomiting, followed by weakness, nervousness, severe itching of the skin, increased thirst, and excessive urination.

**Vitamin E (Tocopherols)**   The role of vitamin E as nature's antioxidant is shaped by the physiological role of vitamin E in cell membranes and the implications of free radicals in a variety of disease processes. Cardiovascular disease and carcinogenesis are hypothesized to result from uninhibited oxygen free radicals that damage cellular constituents such as DNA, lipids, and proteins. By preventing propagation of oxygen free radicals, vitamin E is thought to be the first line of defense against cellular damage and disease.

Food sources for vitamin E include salad oil, shortening, margarine, whole grains, legumes, and dark green leafy vegetables. The most prominent form of vitamin E with antioxidant activity is alpha tocopherol.

Vitamin E deficiency from poor food intake is uncommon in adults and children. Premature infants and some full-term infants are born with a relative vitamin E deficiency that resolves as the digestive system matures. Limited placental transport, intestinal malabsorption, and rapid growth control integration of vitamin E in newborns. Children with chronic hepatobiliary disease or cystic fibrosis develop vitamin E deficiency from fat malabsorption.

The primary manifestation of vitamin E deficiency is hemolytic anemia. Neurological signs of vitamin E deficiency, though not common, include muscle weakness and loss of deep tendon reflexes.

Vitamin E toxicity is rare, though documented cases of weakness, nausea, and vomiting have been reported with persistent administration of doses beyond the DRI. The most significant toxic effect of vitamin E is inhibition of synthesis of vitamin K–dependent clotting factors resulting in hemorrhage.

**Vitamin K (Phylloquinone, Menaquinone, and Menadione)**   Vitamin K is required for synthesis of coagulation factors within the liver. Vitamin K is widely distributed in plant and animal tissues and is reasonably conserved by the human body. Green, leafy vegetables are rich in vitamin K, and resident gut microbiological flora produce vitamin K.

Vitamin K deficiency is uncommon in adults. Prolonged marginal intake, extended treatment with antimicrobial medication, and malabsorption syndromes can bring about a vitamin K deficiency. Without sufficient bodily stores, defective coagulation results in easy bruising, mucosal bleeds, and hemorrhage.

Newborns are at risk for vitamin K deficiency during the first week of life. Placental transfer of vitamin K is poor, and the immature liver of the newborn cannot adequately synthesize vitamin K–dependent clotting factors. Breast milk contains small amounts of vitamin K, and the newborn gut is sterile from bacteria needed to synthesize vitamin K. Untreated vitamin K deficiency of the newborn may result in hemorrhagic disease with severe intracranial bleeding. Newborns are routinely administered vitamin K to prevent bleeding from birth trauma.

Vitamin K toxicity is rare and occurs with ingestion of large amounts of vitamin K precursors. Ironically, vitamin K toxicity may result in hemolytic anemia and elevated plasma bilirubin in newborns.

### Water-Soluble Vitamins

Water-soluble vitamins include the following:

Vitamin $B_1$ (thiamine)
Vitamin $B_2$ (riboflavin)
Vitamin $B_3$ (niacin, nicotinic acid, niacinamide)
Vitamin $B_5$ (pantothenic acid)
Vitamin $B_6$ (pyridoxine)
Vitamin $B_{12}$ (cobalamin)
Vitamin C (ascorbic acid)
Folic acid
Biotin

**Vitamin $B_1$ (Thiamine)**   Thiamine, or vitamin $B_1$, is activated within the human body to a coenzyme required for carbohydrate metabolism. Thiamine also plays a role in neural transmission and is required for a healthy nervous system. Sources of thiamine include dried yeast, whole grains, liver and pork, enriched cereal, nuts, legumes, and potatoes.

Thiamine deficiency, also known as beriberi, may result from inadequate intake, impaired absorption and utilization, and in association with physiological conditions that increase carbohydrate metabolism. Thiamine requirements are greater during pregnancy and lactation, and in people with hyperthyroid disorders where physical metabolism is increased. Alcohol interferes with absorption of thiamine, and it is routinely prescribed to alcoholics.

Early signs of thiamine deficiency include fatigue, irritation, poor memory, sleep disturbances, loss of appetite, abdominal discomfort, and constipation. Dry beriberi is a syndrome of thiamine deficiency characterized by peripheral and bilateral paresthesia, or numbness and tingling of the toes, feet, and calves. Wet beriberi is thiamine deficiency with high-output heart failure that can result in pulmonary and peripheral edema or shock if left untreated. Cerebral beriberi, also known as Wernicke-Korsakoff syndrome, is a complication of chronic alcoholism characterized by severe brain disturbances causing mental confusion and memory loss. Cerebral beriberi may progress to Wernicke's encephalopathy, in which further thiamine deficiency and altered metabolism progress to coma and death.

### Vitamin B₂ (Riboflavin)

Riboflavin, similar to thiamine, is an essential coenzyme required for carbohydrate and protein metabolism. Physiological and epidemiological studies link riboflavin supplementation to prevention of cardiovascular diseases, cancer, and development of corneal cataracts.

Riboflavin is available in a variety of foods, although milk and milk products (cheese) make a particularly important contribution to the riboflavin intake of populations in Western countries. Other dietary sources of riboflavin include green vegetables, liver, wheat germ, eggs, and fish.

Physiological requirements for riboflavin are greater during pregnancy and lactation and in those taking oral contraceptives or the prescription medication probenecid. Riboflavin deficiency is endemic in regions where intake of milk products and meat is limited. A decline in consumption of milk and milk products in Western countries may contribute to poor riboflavin status reported among young individuals and the elderly.

Signs of riboflavin deficiency include appearance of magenta colored mucosa; fissures around the angles of the mouth; and scaly lesions on the skin under the nose, around the ears and eyelids, and in the genital area. Riboflavin deficiency is most common in those with chronic diarrhea, liver disease, and alcoholism.

Current scientific studies in humans and animals have not identified disorders associated with excess dietary riboflavin.

### Vitamin B₃ (Niacin)

Unlike most other vitamins, niacin can be synthesized from the amino acid tryptophan, which is readily available from dietary meat; fish; poultry; green, leafy vegetables; whole grains; and enriched breads and cereals. Niacin is an essential component of coenzymes involved in carbohydrate, lipid, and protein metabolism. Organ systems vulnerable to niacin deficiency or excess involve gastrointestinal tract, skin, and central nervous system.

Severe primary deficiencies in niacin usually occur in areas where maize or Indian corn is a major part of the diet. The intestinal tract does not absorb niacin bound to maize unless it is chemically altered, as in the preparation of tortillas. Niacin deficiency may also occur secondary to diarrhea, cirrhosis of the liver, and alcoholism.

Niacin deficiency, commonly known as pellagra, produces symptoms easily attributed to other illnesses with similar symptoms. Common complaints include loss of appetite, heartburn, weakness, irritability, soreness of the mouth, and weight loss. With advanced deficiency, inflammatory changes progress to severe mental confusion; delirium; hallucinations; memory loss; and a scaly, symmetrical, hyperpigmented dermatitis on sun-exposed areas of the skin.

Niacin is used therapeutically in high doses to treat hyperlipidemia. Side effects, including stomach pain, nausea, intestinal gas, and facial flushing, are commonly reported with niacin excess.

### Vitamin B₅ (Pantothenic Acid)

Pantothenic acid is widely distributed in dietary sources and is an essential component of coenzyme A, which is an essential cofactor for protein metabolism. Food sources of pantothenic acid include chicken, beef, potatoes, oats, tomatos, liver, yeast, egg yolk, grains, and green, leafy vegetables.

Pantothenic acid deficiency usually occurs in conjunction with deficiency of other B vitamins. Symptoms of pantothenic acid deficiency include fatigue, abdominal discomfort, muscle cramping, and burning and numbness in the feet.

Pantothenic acid is usually nontoxic, even in large doses. Isolated cases of itching, numbness, difficulty breathing, and dermatitis have been reported, though a causal relationship to pantothenic acid has not been established.

**Vitamin B$_6$ (Pyridoxine)** Pyridoxine includes a group of related vitamins involved in amino acid metabolism and the synthesis of heme, the oxygen-carrying group in red blood cells. Food sources of pyridoxine include meat; whole-grain cereals; dark green, leafy vegetables; and potatoes.

Pyridoxine deficiency is a common adverse event associated with medication treatment with immune suppressants, oral contraceptives, and certain antibiotics. Vitamin B$_6$ deficiency is also a nutritional consequence of alcoholism, heart failure, and malabsorption.

Vitamin B$_6$ deficiency results in a clinical syndrome similar to that seen with deficiencies of other B vitamins, including mouth soreness, inflammation of the tongue, dry chapped lips, weakness, and irritability. Severe deficiency can result in anemia, numbness of the extremities, and seizures.

Although pyridoxine has generally been considered relatively nontoxic, chronic administration of large doses can result in sensory neurological pain and numbness. Peripheral nerves appear to be most vulnerable to excessive dosing or high doses pyridoxine.

**Vitamin B$_{12}$ (Cyanocobalamin)** Dietary sources of vitamin B$_{12}$ are required for carbohydrate, protein, and lipid metabolism; cell reproduction; and synthesis of red blood cells. Animal foods, including milk, eggs, meat, poultry, and fish, are sources of vitamin B$_{12}$.

Vitamin B$_{12}$ deficiency results in megaloblastic anemia and neurological degeneration of neurons. It occurs in strict vegetarians who do not consume animal products and in gastrointestinal disorders with malabsorption. Increased requirements with pregnancy, hyperthyroid, liver disease, and renal disease may also result in a vitamin B$_{12}$ deficiency.

Vitamin B$_{12}$ is usually nontoxic in large doses; however, mild diarrhea, peripheral vascular clots, itching, and bodily swelling have been reported with intravenous doses. Pulmonary edema and congestive heart failure have also been reported, possibly because of increased blood volume induced by vitamin B$_{12}$.

**Vitamin C (Ascorbic Acid)** Vitamin C, as an antioxidant, protects tissues against free radicals. Vitamin C is also needed for the synthesis of collagen, wound healing, and the absorption of iron. Major food sources of vitamin C are fresh fruits and vegetables.

Dietary vitamin C is required to prevent and treat scurvy. Scurvy is a disease marked by anemia, bleeding of the mucous membranes, and ulceration of the gums; hemorrhages into the skin; and poor wound healing. Most cases of vitamin C deficiency are due to poor dietary intake, chronic alcoholism, cancer, and chronic kidney failure.

Large doses of vitamin C have been advocated for lessening the severity of and for the prevention of the common cold. Most large, controlled research studies fail to demonstrate the value of vitamin C in the treatment or prevention of the common cold. Very large doses of vitamin C can increase oxalate crystal accumulation in kidney stones and cause gastrointestinal irritation, with gas and diarrhea.

**Folic Acid (Folate)** Folic acid, along with vitamin B$_{12}$, serves as a component in protein, lipid, and carbohydrate metabolism and for red blood cell synthesis. Dietary sources of folic acid include whole-grain breads and cereals, orange juice, lentils, beans, yeast, liver, and green, leafy vegetables.

Folic acid deficiency results in macrocytic anemia due to impaired red blood cell synthesis and is associated with coronary atherosclerosis, stroke, and thromboembolism. Deficiency of folic acid in pregnancy is associated with an increased risk of neural tube defects such as spina bifida as well as an increased risk for preterm delivery and low birth weight.

Folic acid is rarely associated with toxic effects. Chronic supplementation with high doses has been associated with loss of appetite, nausea, mental confusion, irritability, and difficulties concentrating.

**Biotin** Biotin functions as a coenzyme in gas exchange and in fat and carbohydrate metabolism. Biotin is widely distributed in a variety of foods.

Prolonged consumption of raw egg whites, which contain a biotin antagonist, results in dermatitis and tongue swelling that respond to supplementation of biotin. Retarded physical and mental development, hair loss, and impaired immunity have been reported in children with deficiencies in enzymes that depend on biotin for metabolic reactions.

## ▶ Minerals

Minerals are inorganic metals that do not furnish energy but play a vital role in a number of physiologic functions. Macrominerals are required in gram quantities daily and include sodium, potassium, chloride, calcium, magnesium and phosphorus. Essential trace minerals, or microminerals, include iron, iodine, fluorine, zinc, chromium, selenium, manganese, molybdenum, and copper.

### Macrominerals

#### Electrolytes (Sodium, Potassium, and Chloride)
Requirements for sodium, potassium, and chloride vary widely based on age, gastrointestinal status, cardiovascular status, kidney disease, and endocrine disease. Sodium, potassium, and chloride are widely available in animal products, fruits, and vegetables, and are vital for neurotransmission, muscle contractility, and regulation of fluid balance and blood pH.

Acid balance in the blood, muscle contractility, neural transmission, and body-fluid regulation depend on a delicate balance of sodium and chloride in the blood and within cells. Sodium concentrations are higher in the blood and, as such, regulate blood volume and extracellular metabolic processes. Excess sodium along with

excess chloride within extracellular space increase blood volume and blood pressure. Sodium and chloride deficiencies usually occur with diseases that commonly cause dehydration. Signs of sodium deficiency or sodium excess are nonspecific and include confusion and dizziness with progression to coma and death. Isolated chloride deficiencies in infants are associated with failure to thrive.

Potassium is an important regulator for muscle activity and transmission of nerve impulses. Potassium concentrations are higher within cells and, as such, regulate intracellular acid and fluid balance. Potassium deficiency or excess can cause severe cardiac conduction abnormalities and paralysis that can result in death. Depletion of potassium occurs with excess vomiting, diarrhea, and disorders that impair absorption of nutrients.

#### Electrolytes (Calcium, Magnesium, and Phosphorus)
Most of the body's calcium, phosphorus, and magnesium are deposited in bones and teeth. Bones also store and release calcium, phosphorus, and magnesium when needed for cellular metabolism.

Calcium is vital for bone and tooth formation, blood coagulation, neurotransmission, muscle contractility, and myocardial function. Table 6–3 lists the recommended calcium intake for people of different ages. Physical requirements for calcium are higher for adolescents and pregnant or lactating females. Chronic calcium deficiency, especially in postmenopausal women, is associated with osteoporosis (see Chapter 16). Calcium deficiencies in children result in improper bone and tooth formation. Acute calcium deficiencies manifest as neuromuscular irritability, impaired muscle contractility, and myocardial conduction. Severe calcium deficiency can result in muscle tetany and death. Calcium toxicity can result in kidney failure, paralysis of the gut, and psychosis.

In addition to bone and tooth formation, phosphorus regulates acid balance and energy production, and is a vital component of DNA and RNA. Phosphorus deficiencies result in irritability, weakness, blood cell disorders, gastrointestinal dysfunction, and kidney dysfunc-

| Table 6–3 | Recommended Calcium Intakes |
|---|---|
| **Age** | **Amount (mg/day)** |
| Birth–6 months | 210 |
| 6 months–1 year | 270 |
| 1–3 years | 500 |
| 4–8 years | 800 |
| 9–13 years | 1300 |
| 14–18 years | 1300 |
| 19–30 years | 1000 |
| 31–50 years | 1000 |
| 51–70 years | 1200 |
| 70 or older | 1200 |
| Pregnant or lactating | |
| 14–18 years | 1300 |
| 19–50 years | 1000 |

*Source:* Dietary Reference Intakes for Calcium, National Academy

tion. Kidney disease results in accumulation of phosphorus. Chronic treatment with phosphate binders is necessary to prevent toxicity from phosphate overload in kidney disease.

Magnesium works with calcium to support bone and tooth formation, nerve conduction, and muscle contractions. Magnesium alone is an important regulator for enzyme activation. Muscular irritability is the primary manifestation of magnesium deficiency. Excess magne-sium is toxic and associated with low blood pressure or hypotension, respiratory failure, and cardiac conduction disturbances.

## ▶ Microminerals

Except for fluorine and chromium, essential trace elements are incorporated into enzymes or hormones required for metabolism. Fluoride forms a compound with calcium ($CaF_2$), which stabilizes the mineral matrix in bones and teeth and prevents tooth decay. Except for iron and zinc, micromineral deficiencies are uncommon in industrialized countries. Infants and children are particularly vulnerable to mineral deficiencies because of their rapid growth and variation in intake. Microminerals can be toxic if consumed in excess.

### Iron

Iron is a component of hemoglobin (blood protein), myoglobin (muscle protein), and many enzymes in the body. Heme iron, found mainly in animal products, is the most absorbable form of iron. The absorption of nonheme iron found in vitamins is enhanced when it is consumed with vitamin C.

Iron deficiency anemia is the most common nutritional deficiency in the world. Iron deficiency results from inadequate consumption, especially in infants, adolescent females, and pregnant women. Blood loss can produce an iron deficiency in both males and females of all ages. Supplementation is usually adequate-to replace iron deficiency.

Iron may accumulate in the body from overdoses or from repeated blood transfusions. Symptoms of iron toxicity include vomiting, di-

## Prevention ➕ PLUS!

### Bone Loss

All humans gain bone early in life, during growth. Following a plateau in bone formation, a gradual loss of the bone matrix occurs during adulthood. Accelerated bone loss may lead to osteoporosis. Recommended intake of calcium may help prevent or slow the progress of osteoporosis.

arrhea, and intestinal irritation and damage. Iron overload can be potentially fatal, especially in young children.

## Iodine

Iodine is an important element for the synthesis of thyroid hormones necessary for normal growth and development. The thyroid gland stores about 80% of the iodine that is ingested. Iodine occurs in soil and seawater, which is vaporized into the air, where much of the iodine is lost. The usual intake of iodine comes from table salt fortified with iodine.

Severe iodine deficiency results in reduced synthesis of thyroid hormone and hyperthyroid disease. Metabolic disturbances in thyroid hormone synthesis can cause growth retardation, especially in children, and reduced metabolism, as well as fatigue, depression, and weight gain in adults. See Chapter 13 for more on the role of iodine in the synthesis of thyroid hormone and the effects of iodine deficiency.

Ironically, iodine toxicity may lead to inhibition of thyroid hormone synthesis or increases in thyroid hormone synthesis. Changes in taste, increased salivation, gastric irritation, and acne-like lesions have been associated with high doses of iodine.

## Fluorine

Fluorine, though not an essential mineral, is necessary for the prevention of dental caries. Fluoridation, the addition of fluorine compounds called fluorides to water, has significantly reduced the incidence of dental caries.

Excess accumulation of fluoride occurs in communities where excess fluoride is available in drinking water. Excess fluoride is most evident in permanent teeth. Irregular, chalky white patches occur in the surface of tooth enamel with acute fluoride toxicity. Severe and prolonged toxicity weakens the enamel, resulting in characteristic yellow-brown staining with a pitted, bony appearance to the teeth.

## Zinc

Zinc is found mainly in bones, teeth, hair, skin, liver, muscles, white blood cells, and the testes. Zinc is a constituent of various enzymes involved in DNA and RNA synthesis. Food sources of zinc include meat, liver, eggs, and seafood.

Signs of zinc deficiency include loss of appetite, growth retardation, delayed sexual maturation, hair loss, immune disorders, dermatitis, night blindness, and impaired taste and wound healing. Zinc deficiency develops from protein-calorie malnutrition and liver disease. Acrodermatitis enteropathica is a rare autosomal recessive disorder that results from malabsorption of zinc. The defect involves the failure to generate a transport protein that enables zinc to be absorbed in the intestine. Symptoms usually begin after an infant is weaned from breast milk. This disorder is characterized by dermatitis, hair loss, growth retardation, and diarrhea.

Ingesting zinc in large quantities occurs with consumption of acidic food or drink from a galvanized container and can cause vomiting and diarrhea. Excess doses of zinc may interfere with copper metabolism and cause neutropenia (a decrease in white blood cells).

## Chromium

The role of chromium (Cr) in human nutrition is currently debatable, as physiologic evidence currently is only available from animal studies. Chromium supplementation in animals enhances insulin's activity. Apparent chromium deficiency in humans, characterized by glucose intolerance, may respond to chromium supplementation.

## Selenium

Selenium (Se), along with vitamin E, functions as an antioxidant in fatty acid metabolism. Selenium is also a constituent of enzymes involved in thyroid hormone regulation. Selenium deficiency is rare in humans. However, toxicity produces a syndrome of dermatitis, hair loss, and peripheral nerve numbness.

## Manganese

Manganese (Mn) is a component of several enzyme systems essential for normal bone structure. Intake varies greatly, depending mainly on the consumption of rich sources, such as unrefined cereals; green, leafy vegetables; and tea. Cases of manganese deficiency are rare, and toxicity has been reported in people who refine ore. Prolonged exposure to manganese results in symptoms that resemble Parkinson's disease, such as body rigidity and tremors.

## Molybdenum

Molybdenum (Mo) is a transition metal that is a component of coenzymes. Molybdenum is derived from organ meats, whole-grain cereals, and legumes. Molybdenum deficiency or toxicity is rare. Deficiencies of molybdenum may be characterized by tachycardia or rapid heartbeat, headaches, nausea, and dizziness.

## Copper

Copper (Cu) is a heavy metal whose unbound ions are toxic. Almost all of the copper in the body is present as a component of copper proteins. Excess copper is excreted through the bile produced by the liver. Copper deficiencies are rare, with cases occurring most commonly in those with protein-calorie malnutrition. Copper toxicity causes symptoms of nausea, vomiting, and diarrhea. Continued copper toxicity can result in brain damage.

## CHAPTER SUMMARY

A well-balanced diet is necessary to obtain essential nutrients required for cellular processes that ensure growth and development, recovery from illness, and prevention of chronic disease. Fats and carbohydrates provide energy necessary for synthesis and storage of proteins. Proteins are essential building blocks for cellular growth, energy, repair, and synthesis of substances needed for metabolism as well as products of metabolism. Vitamins and minerals have important metabolic utility in biochemical reactions involving energy storage and energy release.

Malnutrition results from imbalance between the body's needs and the intake of nutrients. Malnutrition in-

cludes disorders in which nutrients are oversupplied, as in obesity, and undernutrition in which nutrient intake fails to meet physiological needs, as in protein-calorie malnutrition. Obesity and undernutrition result in metabolic changes that increase risks for associated diseases and death.

Vitamins are organic compounds, and minerals are inorganic compounds. Individual vitamin and mineral requirements vary throughout the life cycle, and deficiencies are most commonly caused by malabsorption, protein-calorie malnutrition, alcoholism, food faddism, liver disease, or inborn errors of metabolism. Acute and chronic toxicities can occur with both vitamins and minerals; however, fat-soluble vitamins are categorically most toxic if consumed in excess.

## RESOURCES

Douglas, R. M., E. B. Chalker, & B. Treacy. Vitamin C for preventing and treating the common cold (Cochrane Review). In *The Cochrane Library*, Issue 2, 2004. Chichester, UK: John Wiley & Sons, Ltd.

Lind, James. *A Treatise of the Scurvy in Three Parts. Containing an Inquiry into the Nature, Causes and Cure of that Disease, together with a Critical and Chronological View of what has been published on the subject.* A. Millar, London, 1753.

Baron, Robert B. (2004). Nutrition. In L.M. Turney, Jr., S.J. McPhee, M.A. Papadakis, *Current medical diagnosis and treatment, 43rd ed.* New York: Lange Medical Books/McGraw-Hill.

*The Merck Manual of Diagnosis and Therapy,* 17th ed. (1999), Centennial Edition, Section 1, Nutritional Disorders.

Centers for Disease Control and Prevention (CDC). Third Report of the National Cholesterol Education Program (NCEP), Expert Panel on Detection, Evaluation, and Treatment of High Blood Cholesterol in Adults (ATPIII), released May 15, 2001.

U.S. Department of Agriculture created a powerful and enduring icon, the Food Guide Pyramid.

# Interactive Activities

## Cases for Critical Thinking

1. A middle-aged car salesman presents to his family physician for his yearly physical exam. He complains of fatigue, burning in his feet, decreased memory, and heartburn. Over the years, he gained an excess of 20 pounds, mainly around the waist. He drinks alcohol socially and exercises modestly. What additional information is important to obtain from this patient? What are some possible metabolic changes associated with this patient's symptoms?

2. A. M., a 15-year old girl who is on the school's varsity cross-country team, presents to her physician for a fainting episode. She reports feeling dizzy at times, with shortness of breath and muscle cramping. A. M. recently received a referral from the physician for visual difficulties. On examination, the following are reported: BMI = 17; dermatitis; bruising below the knees; normal blood pressure and heart rate. What clues might suggest that A. M. has nutritional deficiencies? What are some of the possible causes of her fainting and muscle cramping? What nutrient deficiencies is she at risk for developing?

## Multiple Choice

1. Deficiencies in the which of the following vitamins are associated with anemia?
   a. vitamin C
   b. folic acid
   c. vitamin $B_5$
   d. vitamin $B_6$

2. Which of the following disorders produces signs and symptoms of thiamine deficiency?
   a. pellagra
   b. rickets
   c. beriberi
   d. marasmus

3. Metabolic syndrome is associated with obesity and _____.
   a. hypoglycemia, hypertension, and vitamin toxicity
   b. obstructive sleep apnea syndrome
   c. coronary artery disease
   d. osteoarthritis

4. Secondary causes of obesity include
   a. Cushing's syndrome
   b. diabetes
   c. gastrointestinal disease
   d. none of the above

5. Which of the following measures most accurately distinguishes between excess fat and muscle?
   a. lean body weight
   b. dietary reference intake
   c. abdominal fat
   d. body mass index

6. Which of the following provides the vitamin that combines with opsin to form the pigment receptor in the retina of the eye?
   a. biotin
   b. pantothenic acid
   c. carotene
   d. cobalamin

7. The major source of vitamin D is _____.
   a. the skin
   b. milk products
   c. meat products
   d. the water supply

8. Which of the following vitamins is needed for the synthesis of coagulation factors?
   a. vitamin C
   b. vitamin $B_{12}$
   c. vitamin K
   d. vitamin E

9. Cardiac arrest occurs with either a deficiency or toxicity in _____.
   a. calcium
   b. potassium
   c. sodium
   d. chloride

10. Failure to thrive may result in infants with a deficiency in _____.
    a. chloride
    b. magnesium
    c. potassium
    d. phosphorus

## True or False

_____ 1. Iodine is important for the synthesis of thyroid hormones.

_____ 2. Copper is an essential component of myoglobin.

_____ 3. Acrodermatitis enterpathica is a condition that results from zinc deficiency.

_____ 4. The ob gene is a candidate gene that codes for brain regulation of energy and metabolism.

_____ 5. The risk for obesity is greater for children with one obese parent.

_____ 6. Marasmus is due to early weaning from breast milk.

_____ 7. Vitamin D deficiency results in metabolic bone disease in adults.

_____ 8. Vitamin E along with vitamin A are naturally occurring antioxidants.

_____ 9. Vitamin E toxicity may result in hemorrhage.

_____ 10. Alcoholism is associated with thiamin deficiency.

## Fill-Ins

1. Fat-soluble vitamins include vitamins _____.

2. The _____ describe quantitative nutrient requirements.

3. Dietary choices are shaped by _____ traditions.

4. Oral health problems occur from inadequate supply of _____ in drinking water.

5. _____ exhibit antioxidant properties.

6. Pharmacologic doses of _____ are used to treat hyperlipidemia.

7. Most of the body's _____ is stored in bones and teeth.

8. _____ result in malabsorption of nutrients.

9. _____ is essential for the absorption of fat-soluble vitamins.

10. Chromium supplementation may enhance _____ sensitivity and reduce _____ intolerance.

# MedMedia Wrap-Up

**www.prenhall.com/mulvihill**

Remember to visit this website for extra study practice, including exercises, Internet links, news updates, and an audio glossary.

**Activity CD-ROM**

Check out the CD-ROM in the back of this book. You will find games, exercises, puzzles, and videos to help enhance your understanding of this chapter.

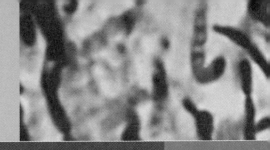

# Part II

# Diseases of the Systems

Part II presents diseases of the body's systems. Each chapter reviews the normal structure and function of a body system, and then discusses diseases associated with that system. Signs, symptoms, etiology, diagnosis, treatment, and prevention are described for each disease.

## Chapters

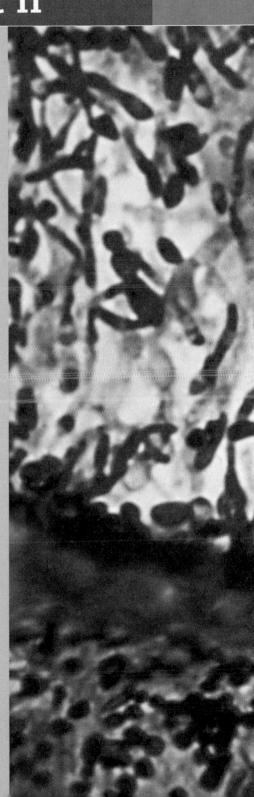

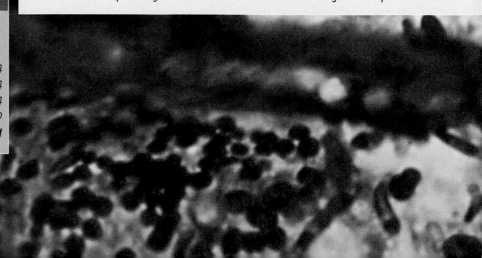

This photomicrograph reveals histopathologic changes indicative of endocarditis caused by the fungus *Candida albicans*. (Courtesy of the CDC/Sherry Brinkman, 1963.)

# 7

# Diseases of the Cardiovascular System

## Learning Objectives

After studying this chapter, you should be able to

- Describe the normal structure and function of the cardiovascular system
- Describe the key characteristics of major diseases of the heart
- Describe common forms of heart disease
- Know the causes and treatment for coronary artery disease
- Explain the causes and symptoms of cardiovascular disease
- Name the diagnostic procedures for cardiovascular disease
- Describe treatment options for cardiovascular disease
- Describe infectious diseases that attack the heart valves, muscle, and lining
- Distinguish between valve insufficiency and stenosis
- Discuss the pathogenesis of atherosclerosis
- Describe the relationship between hypertension and kidney disease
- Discuss the causes of and treatment for hypertension
- Define shock and describe its causes and treatment
- Describe the primary causes and treatment for Raynaud's phenomenon

## Fact or Fiction?

Aspirin therapy reduces the risk of myocardial infarction.

*Fact: By minimizing platelet aggregation and clot formation, aspirin therapy reduces the risk of a myocardial infarction.*

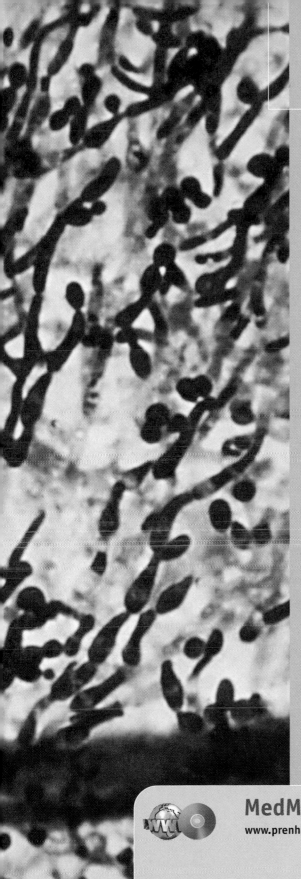

# Disease Chronicle

## Dr. Christiaan Barnard

Dr. Christiaan Barnard performed the first human heart transplant in 1967. In the Union of South Africa, Dr. Barnard performed this famous surgery on a 53-year-old dentist named Louis Washkansky. The dentist received the donated heart of a 25-year-old auto accident victim named Denise Davall. Although the surgery was a technical triumph and a beacon of hope for many with terminal heart disease, Washkansky died 18 days later from infection. Still risky today, heart transplants owe their successes to the generosity of Denise Davall, the courage of Louis Washkansky, and the brilliance of Dr. Barnard, who died of an apparent heart attack in 2001.

## ▶ Introduction to the Cardiovascular System

The cardiovascular system supplies blood to the body's tissues, ensuring a continual flow of oxygen and nutrients to every cell. The cardiovascular system consists of the heart, a muscular pump that propels the blood, and blood vessels that convey the blood throughout the body. This chapter briefly reviews the normal structure and function of the cardiovascular system, then discusses the diseases of the system. Diseases involving the cardiovascular system may be classified into one of five categories:

1. congenital heart disease
2. inflammatory heart disease
3. ischemic vascular disease
4. hypertensive disease
5. metabolic disease

## ▶ Structure and Function of the Heart

The heart is a hollow muscular organ located in the center of the chest. The heart consists of four chambers: a right and left atrium and a right and left ventricle. The chamber walls consist of cardiac muscle, known as myocardium, and their internal lining consists of a smooth, delicate membrane called the endocardium, which is continuous with the lining of the blood vessels. The pericardium, a double-layered membrane, encloses the heart. Figure 7–1 shows the tissues of the heart.

The right and left sides of the heart have an upper atrium that collects blood from the body and the lungs and a lower ventricle that ejects blood throughout the body and the lungs.

Valves between the atria and the ventricles, the atrioventricular (AV) valves, permit one-way bloodflow from atria to ventricles. The mitral valve between the left atrium and left ventricle has two flaps called cusps that meet when the valve is closed. The tricuspid valve between the right atrium and right ventricle is named for its

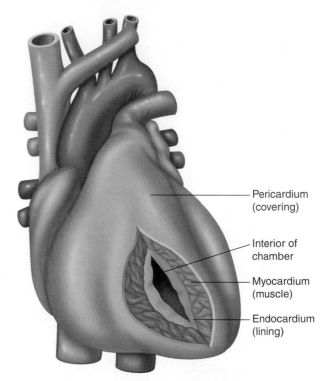

**Figure 7–1**   Heart covering and layers of the heart.

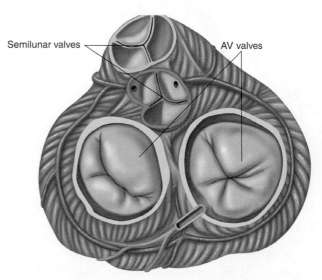

**Figure 7–2**   Heart valves in closed position viewed from the top.

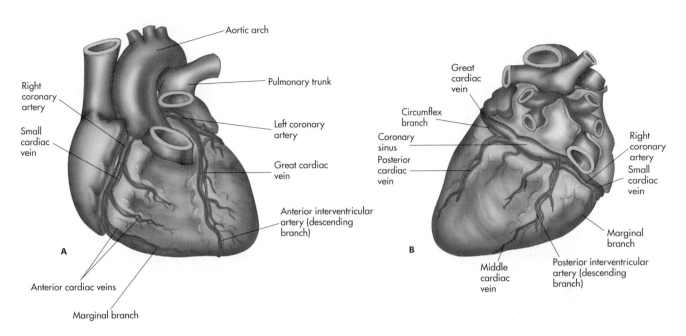

**Figure 7-3** Coronary arteries and major blood vessels.

three cusps. Figure 7–2 shows these valves in the closed position.

The pulmonary semilunar valve permits one way bloodflow from the right ventricle to the pulmonary artery, while the aortic semilunar valve controls bloodflow from the left ventricle to the aorta.

During every heart cycle, each heart chamber relaxes as it fills, and then contracts as it pumps blood. This filling period is the diastole, or the diastolic phase, while the contracting phase of each chamber is the systole, or systolic phase. The alternate contraction and relaxation of atria and ventricles comprises the cardiac cycle, which takes about 0.8 of a second. The flow of blood through the heart chambers, vessels, and lungs is reviewed in Figures 7–3 and 7–4.

Coronary arteries provide the heart muscle with a reliable blood supply. The left coronary artery begins at the aorta on the front of the heart and divides within an inch into the anterior interventricular coronary artery and the circumflex artery, which continues left around the back of the heart. The right coronary artery also branches from the front of the aorta and sends

divisions to the right side and back of the heart (Figure 7–5).

Unlike skeletal muscle, cardiac muscle contracts continuously and rhythmically without conscious effort. A small patch of tissue, the sinoatrial node (SA node), acts as the pacemaker of the heart. The impulse for contraction initiates at the SA node, spreads over the atria, and passes to the ventricles via conductive tissue called the atrioventricular (AV) node. The impulse continues along left and right bundle branches, and terminates in the Purkinje fibers, which further branch throughout the ventricle walls. This conduction system is illustrated in Figure 7–6.

Heart muscle does not depend on nerve stimulation for contraction, but it is influenced by the autonomic nervous system and hormones such as epinephrine. Two sets of nerves work antagonistically, one slowing the heart and the other accelerating it. The vagus nerve slows heart rate during rest and sleep by means of a chemical it secretes, acetylcholine. The excitatory portion of the autonomic nervous system increases heart rate during periods of stress, strenuous physical activity, and excitement. This excitation is brought about by the release of epinephrine and its cousin norepinephrine, which stimulate the heart's pacemaker.

Blood flows through two circulatory routes: the systemic circulation and the pulmonary circulation. The systemic circulation distributes oxygenated blood from the left ventricle, beginning at the aorta and continuing through arteries to all parts of the body, and returns deoxygenated blood by veins to the right atrium. The pulmonary circulation carries deoxygenated blood from the right ventricle, beginning at the pulmonary trunk and continuing through smaller arteries to the lungs to be oxygenated,

and returns the blood through pulmonary veins to the left atrium (Figure 7–7). Partitions called the interatrial septum and interventricular septum separate oxygenated from deoxygenated blood in the atria and ventricles respectively.

Branches of the aorta carry blood to the head, upper extremities, chest, abdomen, pelvis, and lower extremities. These arteries continue to divide into smaller and smaller arteries, and eventually into vessels called arterioles, the smallest arteries. Arterioles lead into capillaries, the connecting links between arteries and veins. Capillaries deliver oxygen and nutrients to tissues. Blood continues into venules, the smallest veins, and then into larger veins. Veins from the

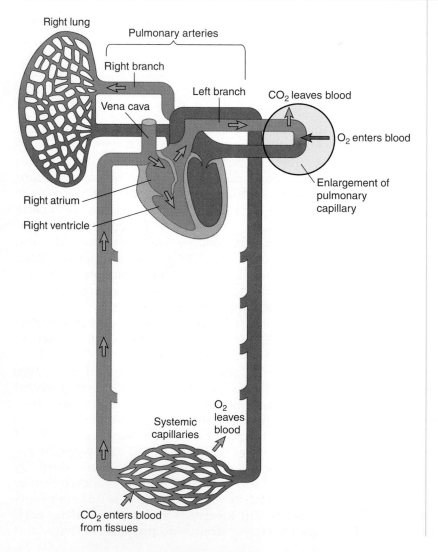

**Figure 7–4**
Venous return to the heart and bloodflow to the lungs.

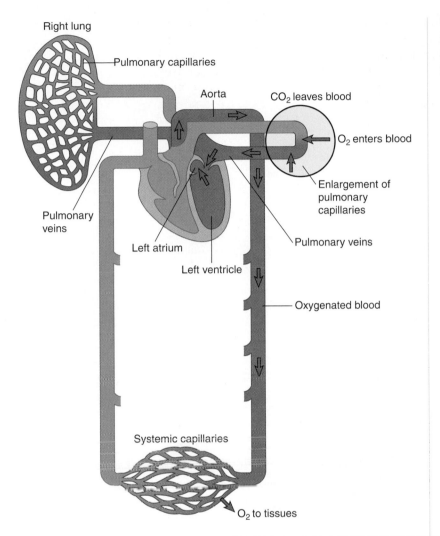

**Figure 7–5**
Return of oxygenated blood to heart and entry into aorta (red = oxygenated blood, blue = deoxygenated blood).

upper body empty blood into the superior vena cava, and veins of the lower body carry blood to the inferior vena cava. The superior and inferior venae cavae deliver systemic blood to the right atrium.

## ▶ Structure and Function of the Blood Vessels

The walls of arteries are muscular, thick, and strong, with considerable elastic tissue, and are lined with endothelium. Arterioles have a smaller diameter than arteries, with thinner walls consisting mostly of smooth muscle fibers arranged circularly, and a lining consisting of endothelium. Arterioles can change their diameter by constricting or dilating, which alters bloodflow to the tissues. Capillaries are minute vessels about 1/2 to 1 mm long with a lumen as wide as a red blood cell. Their wall consists only of a layer of endothelium. Vein walls are much thinner than companion arteries, but their lumens are considerably larger. With less muscle and elasticity in their walls, veins tend to collapse when empty. Veins, particularly those of the legs, contain valves that help return blood upward to the heart against gravity.

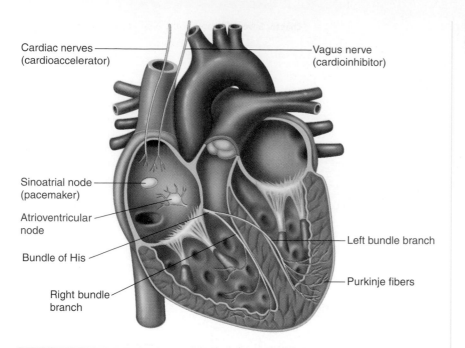

Cardiac nerves (cardioaccelerator)

Vagus nerve (cardioinhibitor)

Sinoatrial node (pacemaker)

Atrioventricular node

Bundle of His

Right bundle branch

Left bundle branch

Purkinje fibers

**Figure 7–6**
Conducting system of the heart.

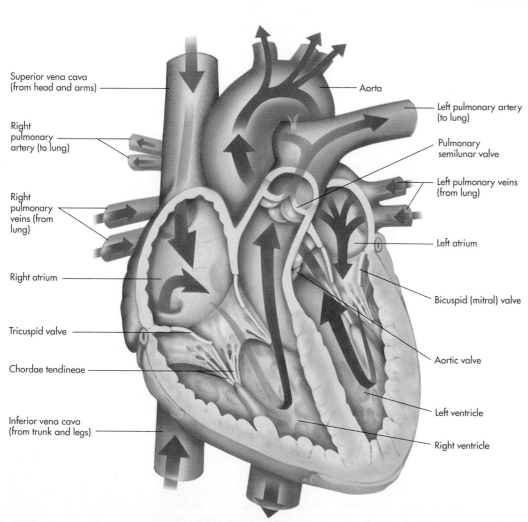

Superior vena cava (from head and arms)

Right pulmonary artery (to lung)

Right pulmonary veins (from lung)

Right atrium

Tricuspid valve

Chordae tendineae

Inferior vena cava (from trunk and legs)

Aorta

Left pulmonary artery (to lung)

Pulmonary semilunar valve

Left pulmonary veins (from lung)

Left atrium

Bicuspid (mitral) valve

Aortic valve

Left ventricle

Right ventricle

**Figure 7–7**
The bloodflow through the heart.

## ▶ Arteriosclerosis

Arteriosclerosis and atherosclerosis are diseases of the arteries. Because these diseases significantly contribute to the development of many other diseases in the cardiovascular system, most notably heart disease, they are discussed first.

In arteriosclerosis, artery walls thicken and become hard and inflexible, partly due to calcium deposition. "Hardening of the arteries" aptly describes this condition, because affected arteries are unable to stretch and rebound in response to the pressure of blood as it is forced through them by contraction of the heart. As a result, arteriosclerosis leads to hypertension. The most common cause of arteriosclerosis is atherosclerosis (discussed next) in which fatty material accumulates within the walls of the artery (Figure 7–8).

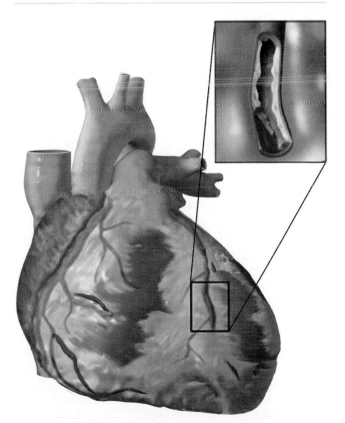

**Figure 7–8** An atherosclerotic artery.

## ▶ Atherosclerosis

Atherosclerosis is characterized by deposition of fatty material within artery walls. The artery walls thicken, narrowing the lumen and reducing bloodflow. In some instances, the lumen becomes completely blocked (occluded).

Atherosclerosis begins with inflammation in the artery wall, which might be triggered by a tear, infection, or chronic damage from hypertension. In response, monocytes accumulate under the inner lining of the arterial wall, forming an atheroma (Figure 7–8). The cells begin accumulating fat and form fatty deposits called plaques. This fatty material consists mostly of cholesterol and may also contain complex carbohydrates, blood clots, fibrous tissue, and calcium deposits. Although all arteries may be affected, typically atherosclerosis develops in the aorta and its branches as well as smaller coronary and cerebral arteries (Figure 7–9). If occluded, bloodflow to an organ is interrupted, a condition called ischemia, which is especially dangerous for heart and brain tissue. Ischemia is the basis for heart attacks and strokes, among other diseases.

Heredity plays a role in atherosclerosis, and it is a common complication of diabetes. Atherosclerosis is also associated with a sedentary lifestyle, a diet high in fat and cholesterol, and obesity. A low-cholesterol diet and regular exercise reduces the risk of developing atherosclerosis. The role of atherosclerosis and arteriosclerosis in heart disease is discussed later in this chapter. Table 7–1 summarizes the interplay between artery disease, various risk factors, and heart disease.

## ▶ Diseases of the Heart

### Coronary Artery Disease

Cardiac muscle receives a fraction (about 5%) of the blood flowing through the atria and the ventricles. Coronary arteries arising from the aorta supply the heart with oxygen-rich blood, and cardiac veins return oxygen-depleted blood to the right atrium. Unfortunately, these small

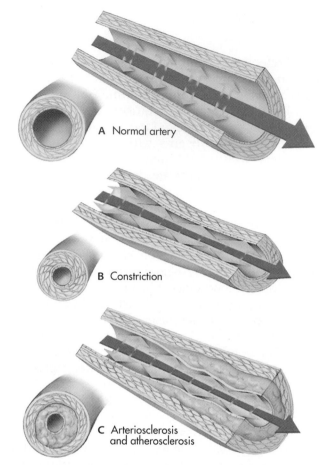

**Figure 7–9** Blood vessels: (A) normal artery; (B) constriction; (C) arteriosclerosis and atherosclerosis.

vessels can become occluded by blood clots or by the narrowing of the lumen caused by atherosclerosis. Figure 7–10 illustrates the sequence of events leading to artery occlusion.

Ischemia to cardiac muscle can result in a heart attack. Lack of oxygen and nutrients quickly kills cardiac muscle, and because this dead tissue is called an infarct, a heart attack is known as a myocardial infarction. Heart attacks and other heart diseases are the leading cause of death in the United States. Although treatment for acute myocardial infarction has improved, heart attacks continue to take their toll. Survival rates for MI are shown in Figure 7–11.

Angina pectoris is temporary chest pain caused by transient oxygen insufficiency. Angina is characterized by pain and a sensation of pressure below the breastbone, which may radiate to the neck, jaw, and arms, and a feeling of tightness and suffocation. Angina is triggered by physical activity, lasts no more than a few minutes, and subsides with rest. Angina may also be triggered by heavy meals, exposure to cold, or emotional stress. Recurrent angina is described as chronic unstable angina. Treatment includes nitroglycerin administered in tablet form under the tongue, which dilates coronary arteries, restoring adequate blood flow. Physical activity and stress should be monitored closely to prevent angina attacks. Transdermal nitroglycerin patches may reduce the frequency of episodes.

Angina is a sign that cardiac muscle is not receiving sufficient blood, but it should not be confused with a heart attack. Although severe chest pains generally accompany a heart attack, the pain may be sensed in the neck or left arm and may be accompanied by nausea, restlessness, cold sweats, vomiting, lightheadedness, and clammy skin. Like angina, heartburn may be confused with a heart attack, so it is important to recognize the signs and symptoms associated with these conditions (Table 7–2).

The prognosis for a myocardial infarction depends on many factors, including the speed with which medical attention is provided. Cardiopulmonary resuscitation (CPR) can maintain bloodflow and the oxygen supply to the brain and heart until emergency care is available. Among those who survive a heart attack, the prognosis varies, depending on the amount of cardiac muscle damage. Prognosis and survival rates are presented in Figure 7–11.

The extent of cardiac muscle damage in a heart attack depends on the number and size of the coronary vessels that are occluded. This can be determined by a diagnostic angiogram (discussed at end of this chapter). Because the dead cardiac cells release their contents into the blood, the severity of a heart attack can be determined by identifying the type and level of certain enzymes found in the blood (Figure 7–12).

The damaged cardiac muscle repairs itself with scar tissue. The damaged myocardium is susceptible to rupture, which is a dangerous complication, so rest is required for adequate

## Table 7–1 Risk Factors for Heart Disease

| Risk Factor | Indicators of High Risk | Role in Heart Disease |
| --- | --- | --- |
| Blood pressure | >140/90 mm Hg | Stresses heart muscle and damages arteries |
| Cholesterol | 0.240 mg/100mls blood | Forms plaque in coronary artery walls |
| Diabetes | Insulin insensitivity | Hypertension damages vessels |
| Smoking | Current or past heavy cigarette use | Inflames, narrows arteries |
| Calcium deposits | Deposits detected by CT scans | Hardens coronary arteries |
| C-reactive protein(CRP) | >3.0mg/L blood | Indicator of inflammation |
| Fibrinogen | Elevated concentration in blood | Promotes abnormal clotting |
| Homocysteine | Elevated concentration in blood | Linked to artery damage |
| Lipoprotein(a) | Increased blood clots | Induces atherosclerosis |

*Source:* Modified from *Science News* 31, January 2003, Heart Health Indicators

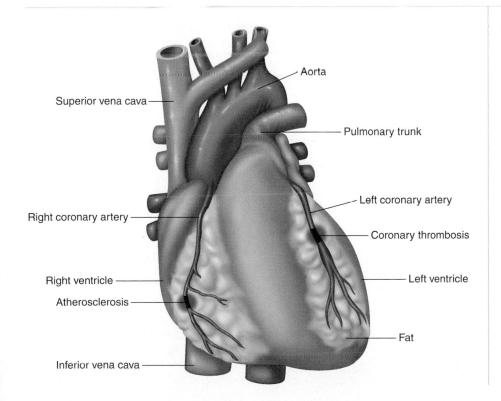

**Figure 7–10**
Blockage of coronary arteries.

Aorta

Superior vena cava

Pulmonary trunk

Left coronary artery

Right coronary artery

Coronary thrombosis

Right ventricle

Left ventricle

Atherosclerosis

Fat

Inferior vena cava

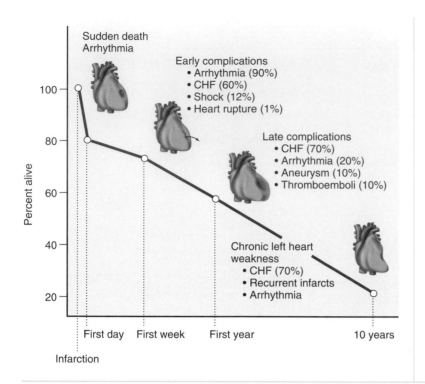

Sudden death
Arrhythmia

Early complications
• Arrhythmia (90%)
• CHF (60%)
• Shock (12%)
• Heart rupture (1%)

Late complications
• CHF (70%)
• Arrhythmia (20%)
• Aneurysm (10%)
• Thromboemboli (10%)

Chronic left heart
weakness
• CHF (70%)
• Recurrent infarcts
• Arrhythmia

Percent alive

First day  First week  First year  10 years

Infarction

**Figure 7–11**
Outcome of myocardial infarction. Forty percent of one-week survivors have late complications resulting in death. Ten-year survival is about 25%.

healing. After healing, controlled exercise is advised to maintain circulation.

Advances in the treatment of heart attacks have increased survival and recovery rates. Severe damage to heart muscle has been reduced by early administration of thrombolytic (blood clot-dissolving) drugs, including TPA (tissue plasminogen activator) and streptokinase. Anticoagulants such as aspirin and coumadin may reduce the risk of a second heart attack.

Angioplasty can also open a partly occluded artery. The procedure involves inserting a balloon-tipped catheter into the femoral artery, guiding it to the heart and into the narrowed

## Table 7–2   Signs and Symptoms of Heartburn and Heart Attack

| Heartburn | Heart Attack |
| --- | --- |
| Burning, irritation below breastbone | Crushing pressure and pain on chest in men, but not common in women |
| Central chest pain | Pain sensed in shoulders, neck, arm, jaw, especially in women |
| Usually occurs after meals | Irregular heartbeat |
| Gets worse when lying down | Shortness of breath, fatigue |
| Antacids help reduce or stop pain | Cold sweats |
| Rarely causes dizziness or shortness of breath | Nausea and paleness, especially in women; vomiting, lightheadedness, weakness, dizziness |

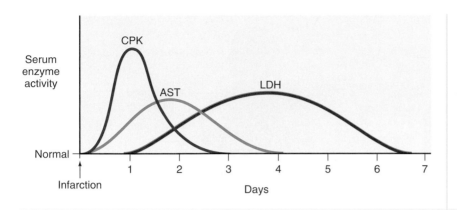

**Figure 7–12**
Serum enzyme level patterns used to diagnose myocardial infarction. AST = aspartate aminotransferase, CPK = creatine phosphokinase, and LDH = lactate dehydrogenase.

coronary artery. The balloon is expanded to press against the vessel walls and open the lumen. A stent, which is a cylindrical wire mesh of stainless steel or other alloy, surrounds the balloon. Expansion of the balloon forces the mesh into the lining of the vessel, which physically holds the lumen open. Because the vessels commonly become occluded again (restenosis) within months or a year, stents are coated with drugs that prevent restenosis. Treatment of a heart attack may require coronary bypass surgery in which a portion of the saphenous vein of the leg is removed and surgically attached to route blood around the occluded section of a coronary artery.

## Cor Pulmonale

Cor pulmonale is a life-threatening condition characterized by right-side heart failure. Cor pulmonale follows chronic lung disease and respiratory failure and results from increased pressure in the blood vessels, a condition called pulmonary hypertension. As hypertension stresses the right ventricle, the ventricle dilates, enlarges, and eventually fails. Treatment is aimed at the underlying lung disease.

## Congestive Heart Disease

Congestive heart disease is a progressive decrease in the ability of the heart to contract. Congestive heart disease can be caused by many diseases that damage the heart and interfere with circulation, including coronary heart disease, infection, heart valve disorders, and hypertension.

Congestive heart disease may involve the right or left side of the heart. Right-sided heart disease results in a build-up of blood flowing into the right side of the heart, causing edema of the ankles, distention of the neck veins, and enlargement of the spleen. Left-sided heart failure leads to a build-up of fluid in the lungs, a serious condition called pulmonary edema, which causes shortness of breath. Figure 7–13 shows the effect of each type of congestive heart failure.

## Congenital Heart Disease

Most congenital heart abnormalities occur in the septum that separates the right and left sides of the heart. An opening in this septum allows a mixing of deoxygenated and oxygenated

## Prevention ✚ PLUS!

### Coronary Heart Disease
Women can reduce their risk of coronary heart disease by 30 to 40% by walking briskly for three or more hours each week.

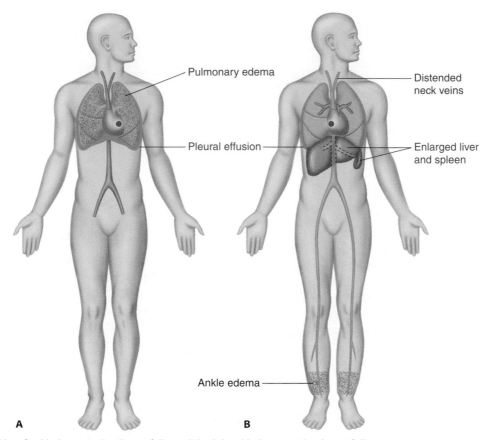

**Figure 7–13** (A) Left-sided congestive heart failure. (B) Right-sided congestive heart failure.

blood, which stresses the heart as it attempts to compensate for lower oxygen levels.

Septal defects may be large or small, with the smaller defects causing virtually no problem. An example of a small septal defect is failure of the foramen ovale to close after birth. The **foramen ovale** is a small, natural opening that allows blood from the right side of the heart to enter the left directly, bypassing the nonfunctional fetal lungs. Failure of this opening to close at birth

is the most common but least serious septal defect.

Septal defects may occur between the two atria, an atrial septal defect (ASD), or between the ventricles, a ventricular septal defect (VSD), which may be large. Because blood pressure is higher on the left side than on the right side of the heart, blood is generally shunted through the opening in a left-to-right direction. This shift increases the workload of the right ventricle,

**Prevention ✚ PLUS!**

**Dietary Salt and Congestive Heart Disease**

A low-salt diet can decrease blood volume and fluid accumulation in congestive heart failure. Dietary sodium can easily be reduced to 2 to 4 g per day by eliminating cooking salt.

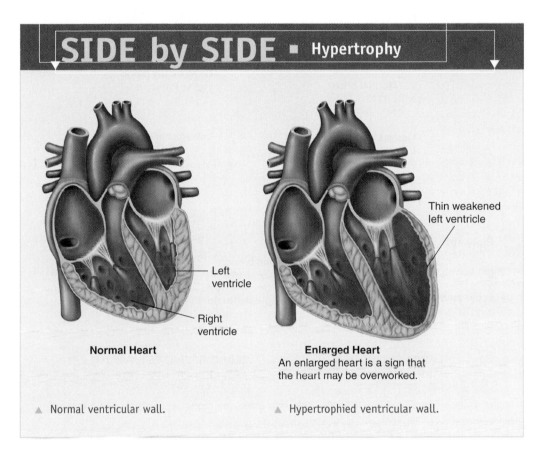

## SIDE by SIDE ■ Hypertrophy

Left ventricle

Right ventricle

Thin weakened left ventricle

**Normal Heart**

**Enlarged Heart**
An enlarged heart is a sign that the heart may be overworked.

▲ Normal ventricular wall.

▲ Hypertrophied ventricular wall.

which already receives blood from the venae cavae. To accommodate the increased blood volume, the right ventricle enlarges (hypertrophies).

Cyanosis, a blue color in the tissues, does not occur if the shunt of blood through the septal defect remains left to right. If the pressure becomes greater in the right ventricle than in the left, the shunt reverses and cyanosis occurs. The deoxygenated blood from the right side of the heart then enters the general circulation, causing cyanosis (Figure 7–14).

Tetralogy of Fallot is one of the most serious of the congenital defects and consists of four abnormalities. The baby with this condition is born cyanotic, with all the tissues a definite blue. The first abnormality is pulmonary stenosis, a narrowed pulmonary artery, which prevents blood from reaching the lungs to be oxygenated. The second abnormality is a large ventricular septal defect. The third defect is right ventricle hypertrophy that results from the pulmonary stenosis. The fourth abnormality is a misplaced aorta that crosses the interventricular septum. Normally,

only oxygenated blood from the left ventricle enters the aorta, but in this case, the right ventricle also feeds into the aorta, permitting the mixing of oxygenated and deoxygenated blood.

Other abnormalities develop as a result of these heart defects, including secondary polycythemia, a disease described in Chapter 8, which occurs to compensate for the low oxygen level. Clubbed fingers and curled fingernails develop because of poor oxygen supply to tissues at the fingertips. As a result, a child may experience dyspnea, difficulty breathing, after any exertion, even crying.

Surgical repair consists of patching the ventricular septal defect, opening the narrowed pulmonary valve, and closing any abnormal connection made between the aorta and the pulmonary artery. Figure 7–15 shows the four abnormalities in the tetralogy of Fallot.

Patent ductus arteriosus (PDA) is a common congenital disease in which a fetal blood vessel that connects the pulmonary artery and the aorta persists after birth. In a fetus, this vessel

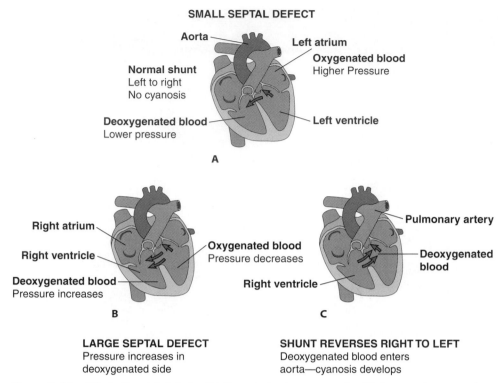

**SMALL SEPTAL DEFECT**

Aorta

**Normal shunt**
Left to right
No cyanosis

**Deoxygenated blood**
Lower pressure

Left atrium

**Oxygenated blood**
Higher Pressure

**Left ventricle**

**A**

Right atrium

Right ventricle

**Deoxygenated blood**
Pressure increases

**Oxygenated blood**
Pressure decreases

**B**

**Pulmonary artery**

**Deoxygenated blood**

Right ventricle

**C**

**LARGE SEPTAL DEFECT**
Pressure increases in
deoxygenated side

**SHUNT REVERSES RIGHT TO LEFT**
Deoxygenated blood enters
aorta—cyanosis develops

**Figure 7–14** Effect of septal defects. (A) Normal shunt: no cyanosis. (B) Increased pressure in right ventricle. (C) Shunt reversal: cyanosis develops.

shunts blood away from the nonfunctional fetal lungs (Figure 7–16), but after birth, it normally closes. If it remains open, blood intended for the body flows from the aorta to the lungs, overloading the pulmonary artery. Because this blood is oxygenated, there is no cyanosis. PDA is associated with a risk of heart failure and infection at the site of the lesion. The PDA may be closed surgically.

Coarctation of the aorta is a narrowing, or stricture, of the artery that provides blood to the entire body. The stricture occurs beyond the arterial branches to the head and arms, so the blood supply to the upper part of the body is adequate. Bloodflow is reduced, however, to the abdomen and legs, resulting in significantly lower blood pressure in the legs. Blood pressure remains high in the arms. Many collateral blood vessels develop to compensate for the poor blood supply to the legs. The coarctation can be corrected surgically by cutting out the narrowed segment of the aorta and rejoining the healthy ends.

## Valve Disorders

Valves maintain unidirectional flow of blood through the heart. Valve disorders include stenosis and valvular insufficiency. Because valve disorders affect bloodflow, valve defects cause heart murmurs with characteristic sounds that indicate the nature of the defect.

In mitral stenosis, the mitral valve opening is narrow, and the cusps that form the valve, normally flexible flaps, become rigid and fuse together. A deep funnel shape develops, increasing resistance to bloodflow from the left atrium to the left ventricle. As back-pressure develops in the left atrium, it becomes hypertrophied. The right side of the heart is also affected (Figure 7–17). Pressure within the heart makes it difficult for the pulmonary veins to deliver blood to the right atrium, leading to increased pressure within veins. As the congestion builds in the veins, fluid from the blood leaks out into the tissue spaces, causing edema. Poor circula-

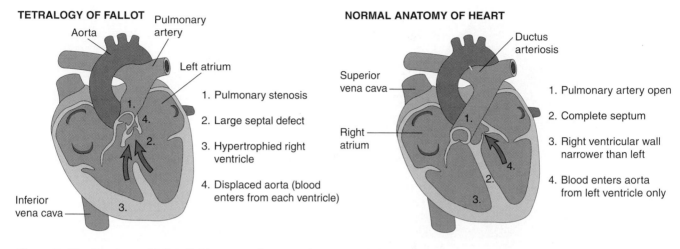

**TETRALOGY OF FALLOT**

1. Pulmonary stenosis
2. Large septal defect
3. Hypertrophied right ventricle
4. Displaced aorta (blood enters from each ventricle)

**NORMAL ANATOMY OF HEART**

1. Pulmonary artery open
2. Complete septum
3. Right ventricular wall narrower than left
4. Blood enters aorta from left ventricle only

**Figure 7–15** Tetrology of Fallot (left) compared to normal anatomy (right).

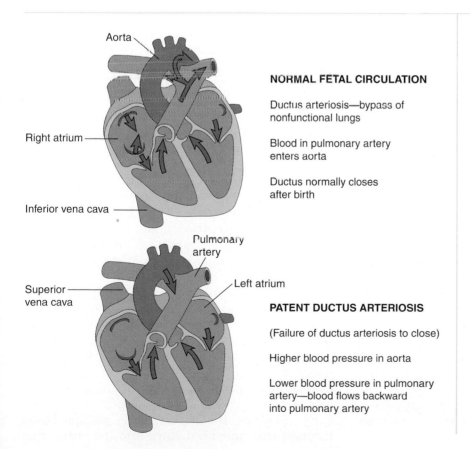

**NORMAL FETAL CIRCULATION**

Ductus arteriosis—bypass of nonfunctional lungs

Blood in pulmonary artery enters aorta

Ductus normally closes after birth

**PATENT DUCTUS ARTERIOSIS**

(Failure of ductus arteriosis to close)

Higher blood pressure in aorta

Lower blood pressure in pulmonary artery—blood flows backward into pulmonary artery

**Figure 7–16**
Patent ductus arteriosus.

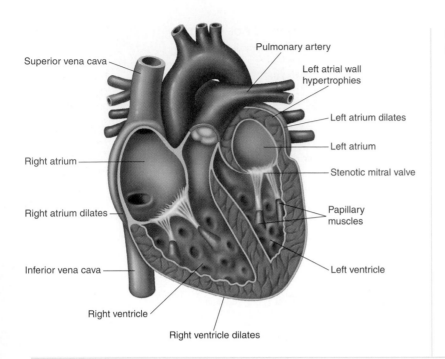

Superior vena cava

Right atrium

Right atrium dilates

Inferior vena cava

Right ventricle

Right ventricle dilates

Pulmonary artery

Left atrial wall hypertrophies

Left atrium dilates

Left atrium

Stenotic mitral valve

Papillary muscles

Left ventricle

**Figure 7–17**
Effect of mitral valve stenosis on the heart.

tion causes cyanosis because an inadequate amount of oxygen is reaching the tissues. The backup of blood and congestion cause the heart to become exhausted and may lead to congestive heart failure. Another complication of a valve defect is the increased risk for a thrombus (blood clot) to form on the valve. If the thrombus becomes detached, it travels as an embolism and may occlude a blood vessel supplying the brain, kidney, or other vital organ. Mitral stenosis often follows rheumatic fever and is more common in women than in men.

Stenotic valves may be widened to restore bloodflow with valvuloplasty, a surgical technique similar to angioplasty. A complication of the surgery may be a leaky valve, in which case the valve may be surgically replaced with metal alloy or pig valve.

In mitral insufficiency, also called mitral incompetence, the valve is unable to close completely, which allows blood to leak into the atrium each time the ventricle contracts. As the volume of blood and pressure in the left atrium increases, blood pressure increases in other vessels, including the vessels leading from the lungs to the heart, resulting in lung congestion. The insufficiency is exacerbated by sclerosis and retraction of the valve cusps.

Another cause of insufficiency is the failure of specialized valve muscles in the ventricle, called papillary muscles. These muscles attach to the underside of the cusps by means of small cords (chordae tendinae) that normally prevent the cusps from flipping up into the atria when the ventricles contract. If the papillary muscles fail to contract, the cusps open upward toward the atria under the force of expelled ventricular blood. This failure is commonly called mitral valve prolapse (MVP).

Most individuals with MVP are asymptomatic and lead normal lives. Those who have moderate or more severe cases of MVP take antibiotics like amoxicillin to prevent bacteria from colonizing in the defective valves. If the prolapse becomes severe, it may be corrected with surgical reconstruction or replacement.

**Aortic stenosis**, the narrowing of the valve leading into the aorta, occurs more often in men than in women and most frequently in men over 50 years old. It may result from rheumatic fever, a congenital defect, or with arteriosclerosis. Aortic stenosis is characterized by rigid cusps that adhere together and deposits of hard, calcified material, giving a warty appearance to the valve. Because the left ventricle pumps blood through this narrowed valve into the aorta, this chamber hypertrophies. Even with enlarged ventricles inadequate bloodflow to the brain persists and can cause syncope (fainting). This valve defect, like others, can be corrected surgically.

In aortic insufficiency, the valve does not close properly. With each relaxation of the left ventricle, blood flows back in from the aorta. Backflow of blood causes the ventricle to dilate, become exhausted, and eventually fail. This condition can result from inflammation within the heart, endocarditis, or a dilated aorta.

## Rheumatic Heart Disease

Rheumatic heart disease is a sequela of infection by group A hemolytic streptococci of skin, throat, or ear, although the organisms are no longer present when the disease presents itself. Approximately 2 weeks following the streptococcal infection, rheumatic fever develops, characterized by fever, inflamed and painful joints, and sometimes a rash.

Rheumatic fever is an autoimmune disease that results from a reaction between streptococcal antigens and the patient's own antibodies against them. All parts of the heart may be affected, frequently including the mitral valve. Blood clots deposit on the inflamed valves, forming nodular structures called vegetations along the edge of the cusps. The normally flexible cusps thicken and adhere to each other. Later, fibrous tissue develops, which has a tendency to contract.

If the adhesions of the cusps seriously narrow the valve opening, the mitral valve becomes stenotic. If sufficiently damaged, the cusps may not be able to meet properly, resulting in mitral valve insufficiency.

The incidence of rheumatic fever is highest among children and young adults. Prompt treatment of the streptococcal infection with antibiotics can prevent rheumatic fever and its complications.

## Infectious Endocarditis

Infectious endocarditis was once considered fatal but responds well to antibiotics if treated early. Endocarditis is an inflammation of the internal lining of the heart commonly caused by a streptococcus. These organisms can enter the bloodstream from infections at sites such as a tooth, the skin, or the urinary tract. Various routes of

bacterial invasion are illustrated in Figure 7–18. This inflammation occurs on previously damaged valves or congenital heart defects.

The nodules or vegetations that form in endocarditis are larger than those of rheumatic fever. They are also friable, tending to break apart easily and enter the bloodstream. These vegetations are filled with bacteria, unlike rheumatic fever vegetations. Typical lesions of endocarditis are shown in Figure 7–19. As fragments of the vegetations break apart, they enter

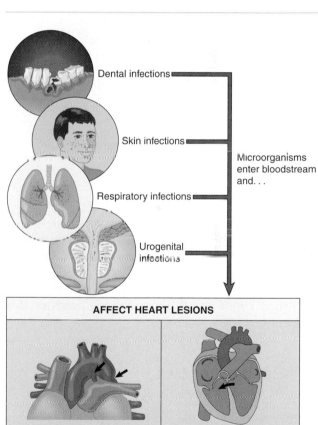

**Figure 7–18** Infections resulting in bacterial endocarditis.

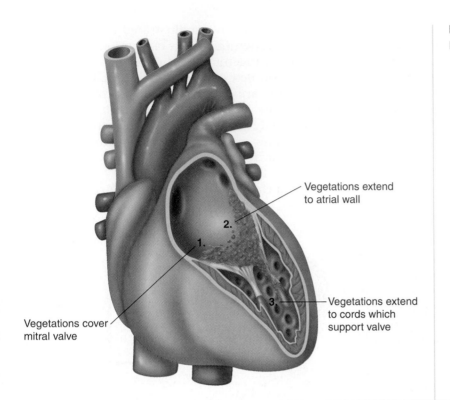

Vegetations extend
to atrial wall

Vegetations extend
to cords which
support valve

Vegetations cover
mitral valve

**Figure 7–19**
Bacterial endocarditis.

the bloodstream to form emboli, which can travel to the brain, kidney, lung, or other vital organs, causing a variety of symptoms. The emboli can lodge in small blood vessels of the skin or other organs and cause the blood vessels to rupture. These small hemorrhages produce tiny red spots called petechiae.

## ▶ Vascular Diseases

Both arteriosclerosis and atherosclerosis were discussed at the beginning of this chapter. This section focuses on other diseases of the blood vessels.

### Thrombosis and Embolism

Thrombosis, the formation of blood clots on blood vessel walls, is caused by slow bloodflow, and because blood flows more slowly in veins than in arteries, veins are common sites of thrombus formation. Thrombi are also likely to form where there is turbulence in the bloodflow, such as near heart valves, and a diseased valve is a likely site for a clot formation. Increased viscosity of the blood also leads to thrombosis. Dehydration, polycythemia (extra red blood cells), or high platelet levels increase viscosity and the tendency for thrombosis. Figure 7–20 illustrates thrombus formation.

If the thrombus breaks free, it becomes an embolus. These traveling clots typically lodge into the coronary arteries or lung or brain vessels. An embolism containing pyogenic bacteria is called a septic embolism. Should such an embolism lodge in a small vessel of the foot or leg, the tissue dies and becomes necrotic, leading to gangrene.

Anticoagulants prevent or reduce clot formation and promote bloodflow. Sepsis (blood infection) is a serious complication that occurs in 200,000 individuals annually in the United States.

### Aneurysms

A weakening in the wall of a blood vessel can cause local dilation known as an aneurysm. Aneurysms most commonly occur in the abdom-

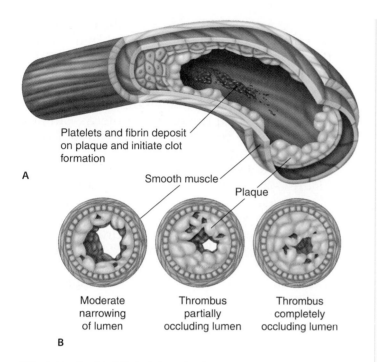

A

Platelets and fibrin deposit on plaque and initiate clot formation

Smooth muscle

Plaque

Moderate narrowing of lumen

Thrombus partially occluding lumen

Thrombus completely occluding lumen

B

**Figure 7–20**
Thrombus formation in an atherosclerotic vessel. Depicted are the initial clot formation (A) and the varying degrees of occlusion (B).

inal aorta or brain and result primarily from arteriosclerosis. The danger of an aneurysm is the tendency to increase in size and rupture, resulting in hemorrhage, possibly in a vital organ such as the heart, brain, or abdomen.

Aneurysms usually produce no symptoms and are detected by an x-ray or routine physical exam. Ultrasound techniques can diagnose and measure aneurysms. A computed tomography or CT scan is accurate in determining the shape and size of an aneurysm. Early detection prevents rupture.

Surgical procedures have been very successful in repairing blood vessels affected by aneurysm. The diseased area of the vessel is removed and replaced with an artificial graft or segment of another blood vessel. This procedure reduces the risk of hemorrhage and thrombus formation.

## Raynaud's Disease

Raynaud's disease is a condition in which small arteries or arterioles in the fingers and toes constrict. Symptoms are spasms including numbness, discoloration of the local skin of the fin-

gers and toes, and pain (see Figure 7–21). Spasms are intermittent and are commonly triggered by cold. As vessels constrict, bloodflow temporarily decreases, causing the fingers and toes to turn white. As the episode resolves, the affected areas may turn pink or blue.

Raynaud's disease can be controlled by protection from cold. Smoking should be avoided, as it constricts blood vessels regardless of environmental conditions. Relaxation techniques can help reduce stress, which may bring about an attack.

## Phlebitis

Phlebitis is inflammation of a vein. Any vein may be affected, but phlebitis usually occurs in deep veins of the leg. The greatest danger in the deep veins is thrombosis, a condition called thrombophlebitis (Figure 7–22). Edema develops once a vein becomes occluded because increased internal pressure causes fluid to leak out of the vessel. A major complication of thrombophlebitis is an embolism.

Causes of phlebitis include injury, infection, poor circulation, and obesity. Phlebitis is

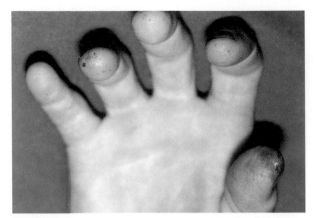

**Figure 7–21** Raynaud's disease. (Courtesy of Jason L. Smith, MD)

treated with anticoagulants, including aspirin, and antibiotics. Surgery may be required to remove the thrombus.

## Varicose Veins

Varicose veins are dilated, distorted veins that usually develop in the superficial veins of the leg, such as the greater saphenous vein. The veins become swollen and painful, and appear knotty under the skin. Varicose veins are caused by blood pooling within the veins because of decreased, stagnated bloodflow. Varicose veins can be an occupational hazard related to long periods of sitting or standing. Normally, the leg muscle movement moves blood up within the vein from one valve to the next. In the absence of this

"milking action" of the muscles, the blood exerts pressure on the closed valves and thin walls of the veins. The veins dilate to the extent that the valves are no longer competent. The blood collects and becomes stagnant, and the veins become more swollen and painful.

Pregnancy or a tumor in the uterus can also cause varicose veins because pressure on veins causes resistance to bloodflow. Heredity and obesity are also associated with varicose veins. Figure 7–23 illustrates the flow of blood through normal veins and varicose veins.

Complications of varicose veins include ulcers and infection, due to poor circulation, and hemorrhage, caused by weakened vein walls.

Treatment depends on the severity of the symptoms. An elastic bandage or support hose may increase circulation and provide relief from discomfort. Symptoms can be relieved by walking, elevating the legs when seated, and weight reduction. A surgical procedure called "stripping the veins" is very successful. The surgery involves removing the veins and tying off the remaining open ends. Collateral circulation tends to develop to compensate for the loss of the vein segment.

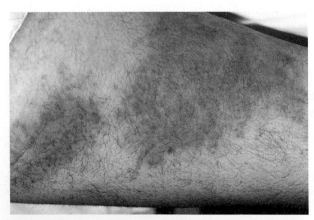

**Figure 7–22** Thrombophlebitis. (Courtesy of Jason L. Smith, MD)

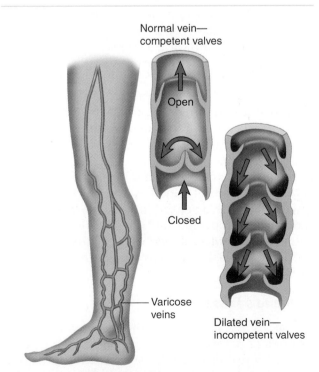

**Figure 7–23** Development of varicose veins.

Small, dense, red networks of veins, called spider veins, can be treated with laser. The light heats and scars the tiny superficial veins, which closes them off to blood flow (Figure 7–24). Another treatment is compression sclerotherapy in which a strong saline solution is injected into specific sites of the varicose veins. The irritation causes scarring of the inner lining and fuses the veins shut. The procedure is followed by uninterrupted compression for several weeks to prevent reentry of blood. A daily walking program during the recovery period is required to activate leg muscle venous pumps.

Hemorrhoids are varicose veins in the rectum or anus that cause pain, itching, and bleeding. Like varicose veins in the leg, hemorrhoids can develop from pressure on the veins. Straining due to constipation, pressure on the veins from a pregnant uterus, or a tumor may promote their development.

Esophageal varices, or varicose veins of the esophagus, frequently accompany cirrhosis of the liver. They result from pressure that develops within the veins as they try to empty. Because of blocked blood vessels within the damaged liver, there is a backup of blood and general congestion. The major complication from these varices is a fatal hemorrhage.

A relatively new procedure for treating esophageal varices is called endoscopic sclerotherapy. In this procedure, a retractable needle is guided into the esophagus by means of a fiberoptic endoscope. The gastroenterologist punctures the varicosities and injects a caustic

sclerosis (hardening) solution to occlude the swollen veins. This prevents engorgement, rupture, and hemorrhage, or stops a hemorrhage that has already begun.

## ▶ Hypertension

Hypertension is abnormally high blood pressure in the arteries. Called the "silent killer," hypertension is often asymptomatic and usually not diagnosed until complications arise. The causes of primary hypertension, also called essential hypertension, are not known, although the disease appears to be inherited. Primary hypertension is exacerbated by obesity, lack of exercise, and excessive alcohol and salt intake. Secondary hypertension results from other diseases, such as brain tumors, kidney disease, and endocrine disorders. Hypertension may have a gradual onset and continue for a long time, or it may be malignant, with sudden onset and rapid progression resulting in death if not treated immediately.

A blood pressure measurement consists of two values that correspond to the two phases of heart activity: the systolic and diastolic pressure. The systolic pressure is the highest pressure in the arteries caused by the force of contraction of the ventricles. Diastolic pressure corresponds to the pressure in the arteries when the ventricles are relaxing and refilling. The blood pressure of an average normal adult is 120 mm Hg (systolic) and 80 mm Hg (diastolic), often expressed as 120/80 mm Hg.

Blood pressure normally varies throughout the day, increasing with activity and decreasing with rest. Because of these fluctuations, high blood pressure is not considered abnormal unless there are three sequential elevated readings, each recorded at different times under similar conditions. Generally, pressures that are consistently greater than 140/90 mm Hg are considered high. Tables 7–3 and 7–4 show recent blood pressure guidelines.

The kidneys and the nervous system regulate blood pressure. Blood pressure increases are brought about by increased force of heart contraction and by constriction of arteries and arte-

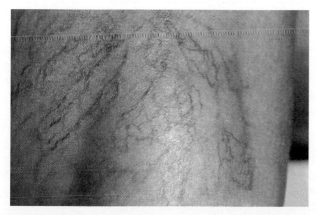

**Figure 7–24** Spider veins. (Courtesy of Jason L. Smith, MD)

| Table 7–3 | Blood Pressure Guidelines |
|---|---|
| Healthy (normal) | Below 120/80 mm Hg |
| Prehypertension | 120/80 to 139/89 mm Hg |
| Stage 1 hypertension | 140/90 to 159/99 mm Hg |
| Stage 2 hypertension | 160/100 mm Hg |

rioles. As more blood enters the vascular system, the blood pressure increases. The kidney also increases blood pressure by secreting a substance called renin, which activates angiotensin, a hormone that causes the walls of the arteries to constrict and increases blood pressure. Angiotensin also triggers the release of another hormone, aldosterone, which causes the kidneys to retain salt (sodium) and water, expanding blood volume and increasing blood pressure.

When blood volume is high, the pressure in the arteries forces fluid through the walls of capillaries into tissue spaces, reducing blood volume and blood pressure. Dilation of arteries and excretion of excess fluid by kidneys reduce blood pressure.

## Hypertensive Heart Disease

This condition is caused by chronic hypertension. Over time, the heart adapts to hypertension by enlarging. Enlargement fails to compen-

| Table 7–4 | Risk of Stroke and Heart Disease Increase with Increasing Blood Pressure |
|---|---|
| **Blood Pressure** | **Risk** |
| 115/75 | Normal |
| 135/85 | 2 times normal |
| 155/95 | 4 times normal |
| 175/105 | 8 times normal |

sate, however, and the left ventricle eventually becomes so weak that it fails to pump blood adequately.

## Hypertension and Kidney Disease

Hypertension contributes to kidney disease, and kidney disease contributes to hypertension. Decreased function of the kidneys leads to water and salt retention, causing increased blood volume and elevated blood pressure levels. Long-standing hypertension causes arteriosclerosis of the renal artery, which reduces blood flow to the kidneys and damages them.

Primary hypertension cannot be cured, but it can be treated to prevent complications. A combination of medication, diet changes, and exercise is the ideal method for controlling high blood pressure. Because there are usually no symptoms of high blood pressure, treatments that make people feel bad or interfere with lifestyle are avoided.

Overweight individuals are advised to reduce their weight. Changes in diet for those who have diabetes and high cholesterol levels are important for overall cardiovascular health. Cutting down on salt and alcohol intake may make drug therapy for high blood pressure unnecessary. Moderate exercise can help control weight and improve circulation.

Drug therapy can help reduce blood pressure. In general, drug therapy is used if lifestyle modification is not effective or produces an inadequate response. One or more drugs with different actions may be used to control blood pressure. For example, a diuretic like Lasix that controls blood volume in combination with a drug that blocks sympathetic stimulation may be prescribed. A drug that blocks the renin-angiotensin-aldosterone cascade is the ACE inhibitor (angiotensin-converting enzyme inhibitor). The best combination of drug therapy generally is one that fits the patient's lifestyle with minimal side effects.

Treatment of secondary hypertension depends on the underlying cause. For example, treatment of kidney disease, when recognized, can help normalize and lower blood pressure. If angiography reveals partially occluded vessels, then angioplasty may be used.

## Prevention ✚ PLUS!

### Take Action to Reduce Your Blood Pressure and Save Your Life

| | |
|---|---|
| Lose weight | Weight loss is the single most effective nondrug method to reduce blood pressure. |
| Exercise | Thirty to 35 minutes of exercise three times per week can decrease blood pressure, especially when combined with weight loss. |
| Limit alcohol | Alcohol raises blood pressure even without hypertensive disease. |
| Eat a low-fat, high-fruit and vegetable diet | A diet high in vitamins and low in fats is associated lower blood pressure. |
| Reduce dietary salt | Keep salt intake below 2400 mg per day, or less than 1 tsp. |

## ▶ Abnormalities of Heart Conduction

The conduction system of the heart can fail, a condition known as heart block. Heart block can result from scar tissue interfering with the conduction tissue, and it may be necessary to implant an electric pacemaker if the block is complete.

Heart block is graded as first, second, or third degree. First-degree heart block is characterized by slightly delayed conduction to the ventricles and usually produces no symptoms. In second-degree heart block, not every impulse from the atria reaches the ventricles. Some forms of second-degree heart block progress to third-degree heart block in which impulses from the atria are completely blocked. The ventricle beats slowly and less efficiently. Eventually, heart failure ensues.

At times, the impulse for contraction spreads over the atria and the ventricle in an uncoordinated fashion. Atrial fibrillation and atrial flutter are very fast, uncoordinated impulses. These fast impulses produce rapid and incompetent contraction of the ventricles. Medications can be administered to slow the conduction through the AV node to the ventricles. This allows the ventricles to fill properly before contraction.

Ventricular fibrillation is far more serious than atrial fibrillation, and it is potentially fatal. A series of uncoordinated impulses spread over the ventricles, causing them to twitch or quiver rather than contract. The ventricle does not carry out effective coordinated contractions. Because no blood is pumped from the heart, ventricular fibrillation is a form of cardiac arrest. Immediate attempts at resuscitation must be made, or death will result. Permanent damage to other organs, particularly the brain, results when blood supply to them is compromised. A machine called an automated external defibrillator (AED) delivers electrical shocks and is used to re-establish normal heart rhythm. Defibrillators implanted under the skin of the shoulder resynchronize the heart on a daily basis, similarly to a pacemaker device. There are also combination devices with built-in pacemakers. In addition, there are multilead pacemakers with biphasic current that give a more complete signal to the heart chambers to initiate heart timing and contraction.

Irregular heartbeat rhythm is known as cardiac arrhythmia or dysrhythmia. Abnormal rhythms include skipped beats, extra beats, and premature beats; the latter are called premature ventricular contractions (PVCs). Additional irregularities include significant increases in heart rate, tachycardia, or abnormally slow hearts rate, bradycardia. Medications typically control the irregularities.

## ▶ Shock

Shock is a life-threatening condition in which blood pressure drops too low to sustain life. Any condition that reduces the heart's ability to pump effectively or decreases venous return can cause shock. This low blood pressure causes an inadequate blood supply to the cells of the body.

The cells can be quickly and irreversibly damaged and die. Hypovolemic shock (hemorrhagic) results from fluid volume loss after severe hemorrhage or loss of plasma in burn patients. Treatment includes administration of plasma or whole blood. Neurogenic shock is due to generalized vasodilation, resulting from decreased vasomotor tone. The reduced blood pressure causes poor venous return to the heart and, hence, poor cardiac output. The decreased vasomotor tone may be due to spinal anesthesia, spinal cord injury, or certain drugs. Anaphylactic shock accompanies a severe antigen-antibody reaction. Cardiogenic shock is the result of extensive myocardial infarction. It is often fatal, but drugs to combat it are sometimes effective. The types of shock are summarized in Figure 7–25.

## ▶ Age-Related Diseases

Congenital diseases may be first detected in newborns, but may not be revealed until much later. Common congenital defects include holes in the heart septum, patent ductus arteriosus, and coarctation of the aorta. The incidence of rheumatic fever is highest among children. With aging, the lifetime effects of diet, family history, and behavior influence the risk for heart attacks and strokes.

With age, the heart, coronary arteries, and peripheral vessels lose strength and elasticity. The incidence of atherosclerosis, arteriosclerosis, and aneurysms increases with age, and about half of the elderly population have signs of heart disease.

The incidence of hypertension also increases with age. As a result, the average elderly person's heart exhibits approximately 30% thickening in the left ventricle walls.

Except for blood pressure, other cardiac functions show few age-related changes. An age-related decrease in maximum attainable heart rate during exercise or stress is a sign of decreased heart function. The cumulative effects of hypertension, atherosclerosis, and arteriosclerosis lead to an increased incidence of congestive heart disease in elderly persons.

## Diagnostic Procedures

Many techniques for diagnosing and treating heart problems exist. Auscultation, listening through a stethoscope for abnormal sounds, and the electrocardiogram (ECG) provide valuable information regarding heart condition. The electrocardiogram is an electrical recording of heart action and aids in the diagnosis of coronary artery disease, myocardial infarction, valve disorders, and some congenital heart diseases. It is also useful in diagnosing arrhythmias and heart block. Echocardiography (ultrasound cardiography) is also a noninvasive procedure that utilizes high-frequency sound waves to examine the size, shape, and motion of heart structures. It gives a time-motion study of the heart, which permits direct recordings of heart valve movement, measurements of the heart chambers, and changes that occur in the heart chambers during the cardiac cycle. Color Doppler echocardiography explores bloodflow patterns and changes in velocity of bloodflow within the heart and great vessels. It enables

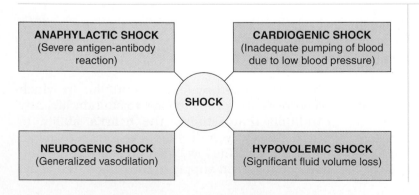

**Figure 7–25**
Various types of shock.

ANAPHYLACTIC SHOCK
(Severe antigen-antibody reaction)

CARDIOGENIC SHOCK
(Inadequate pumping of blood due to low blood pressure)

SHOCK

NEUROGENIC SHOCK
(Generalized vasodilation)

HYPOVOLEMIC SHOCK
(Significant fluid volume loss)

the cardiologist to evaluate valve stenosis or insufficiency.

An exercise tolerance test is used to diagnose coronary artery disease and other heart disorders. This test monitors the ECG and blood pressure during exercise. Problems that normally do not occur at rest are revealed.

Cardiac catheterization is a procedure in which a catheter is passed into the heart through blood vessels to sample the blood in each chamber for oxygen content and pressure. The findings can indicate valve disorders or abnormal shunting of blood, and aids in determining cardiac output.

X-rays of the heart and great vessels, the aorta, and the pulmonary artery, in conjunction with angiocardiography, in which a contrast indicator (dye) is injected into the cardiovascular system, can detect blockage in vessels. Coronary arteriography employs a selective injection of contrast material into coronary arteries for a film recording of blood vessel action.

plained. It was noted that a congenital defect is frequently the site of a bacterial infection.

Valve disorders such as stenosis and insufficiency cause heart murmurs. Rheumatic heart disease is a common cause of valve disease. Surgical techniques may be required to correct diseased valves.

Antibiotics have reduced the danger of endocarditis and the frequency of rheumatic heart disease.

Abnormalities of heart action, heart block, fibrillation, and arrhythmia were described. Diagnostic procedures include auscultation, electrocardiography, ultrasound cardiography (echocardiography), cardiac catheterization, and exercise tolerance testing. The condition of coronary arteries and the great vessels can be evaluated through angiocardiography and coronary arteriography. Surgical procedures are available to correct congenital heart defects, replace valves, and implant electric pacemakers or defibrillators. Coronary bypass surgery and angioplasty with stent implants reduce heart damage by increasing coronary circulation. Diet and exercise in moderation continue as major benefits to a healthy cardiovascular system.

## CHAPTER SUMMARY

After reviewing the normal structure and function of the heart, heart diseases such as coronary artery disease, myocardial infarction, and angina pectoris were discussed. Myocardial infarction and angina pectoris cause severe chest pain or referred pain in the arm or neck. Dyspnea is a common symptom of many heart diseases; the lack of oxygen in the tissues stimulates the respiratory center, causing the person to experience difficulty in breathing or shortness of breath. Fainting or loss of consciousness occurs when the brain is deprived of an adequate blood supply. All of the tissues and organs are affected by poor circulation. Cyanosis occurs when blood is not properly oxygenated and fluid accumulates in the tissues, causing edema when veins become congested.

Hypertensive heart disease develops from long-standing hypertension, and cor pulmonale results from chronic lung disease. Congestive heart failure is characterized inadequate pumping of blood to meet the needs of the body.

Congenital heart diseases, tetralogy of Fallot, patent ductus arteriosis, and coarctation of the aorta were ex-

## RESOURCES

Beers, M. H., et al. *The Merck Manual of Medical Information,* 2nd ed. Merck Research Laboratories, 1999.

Braunwald, E., P. Libby, D. P. Zipes. *Heart Disease: A Textbook of Cardiovascualr Medicine,* 6th ed. Saunders, 2001.

Damjanov, Ivan. *Pathology for the Health-Related Professions.* Saunders, 1996.

*Diseases,* 3rd ed. Springhouse, 2001.

Martini, F. H., M. J. Timmons, R. B. Tallitsch, *Human Anatomy,* 5th ed. Prentice Hall, 2003.

*New England Journal of Medicine,* Vol. 349:1315–1323, No. 14, October 2, 2003.

*Northwest Herald,* "American Profile," 14 February 2004.

*Northwest Herald,* "Dr. Gott," 31 December 2003.

Tamparo, C. D., M. A. Lewis, *Diseases of the Human Body,* 3rd ed. F. A. Davis, 2001.

World Health Organization: www.who.org.

# DISEASES AT A GLANCE

## Cardiovascular System

| DISEASE | ETIOLOGY | SIGNS AND SYMPTOMS |
| --- | --- | --- |
| Endocarditis | Streptococcus infection, drugs | Fever, anorexia, weight loss, back pain, night sweats, petechiae, heart murmur |
| Rheumatic disease | Streptococcus pyogenes, autoimmune to heart | Follows infection by Group A hemolytic streptococci; latent period followed by fever, inflamed and painful joints, rash, heart murmur |
| Coronary artery disease | Plaque, arteriosclerosis | Angina pectoris following exercise, stress, heavy meal |
| Myocardial infarct (MI) | Plaque, arteriosclerosis | Chest pain radiating to jaw, neck, left arm, back; feeling of tightness; suffocation; nausea and vomiting may occur; may be "silent" (no symptoms) |
| Hypertensive heart disease | Essential hypertension, kidney disease | Long-standing High blood pressure, enlargement of heart, later pulmonary edema with dyspnea, dilation and weakness of ventricles |
| Congestive heart failure | Rheumatic disease, hypertension, myocardial infarction | Fatigue, difficulty breathing; left-side failure leads to pulmonary edema, right-side failure leads to systemic edema; both may occur |
| Cor pulmonale | Chronic hypertensive lung | Chronic lung disease, right-side heart failure with systemic edema, fatigue, rapid heart rate |
| Mitral stenosis | Infection, congenital | Heart murmur, dyspnea, fatigue, lower oxygen in arteries; pulmonary edema may develop |
| Mitral insufficiency (mitral prolapse) | Idiopathic, infection, weak papillary muscles | Heart murmur, may be asymptomatic; palpitations, fatigue, dyspnea may develop |
| Aortic stenosis | Congenital, infection | Lower output of blood with syncope, heart murmur |
| Aortic insufficiency | Congenital, idiopathic | Heart murmur, backflow into ventricle, enlarged ventricle |

| DIAGNOSIS | TREATMENT |
| --- | --- |
| Echocardiography | Antibiotics |
| Patient history of strep infection; physical exam, strep antibody test | Anti-inflammatory drugs, steroids, diuretics, bed rest |
| Angiocardiography, coronary arteriography | Drug therapy, nitroglycerin, angioplasty, bypass surgery |
| ECG, blood test (serum enzymes), physical exam | Drug therapy, oxygen, reduced activities, rest |
| enlarged heart, x-ray, physical exam | Drug therapy, oxygen |
| Physical exam, x-ray, scans show enlarged heart | Drug therapy, diuretics, oxygen |
| Patient history, physical exam | Bronchodilators, ventilator |
| Echocardiography, auscultation | Valve replacement surgery |
| Echocardiography, auscultation | Valve replacement surgery only if severe |
| Echocardiography, auscultation | Valve replacement surgery |
| Echocardiography, auscultation | Valve replacement surgery |

# DISEASES AT A GLANCE (*continued*)

## Cardiovascular System

| DISEASE | ETIOLOGY | SIGNS AND SYMPTOMS |
| --- | --- | --- |
| Heart block | Atherosclerois, scar tissue in conducting pathway | Reduced pulse, palpitations or irregular beat |
| Atrial fibrillation | Drugs, electrolytes imbalance, hypertrophy | Palpitations, as ventricle contraction is affected |
| Ventricular fibrillation | Electrical shock, myocardial infarction | Collapse, since bloodflow stops; cardiac arrest |
| Cardiac arrthymia | Myocardial infarction, drugs, electrolyte imbalance | Palpitations, as beat is uncoordinated |
| Tachycardia | Congenital, idiopathic | Rapid heart rate, not due to exercise |
| Bradycardia | Congenital, idiopathic | Slow heart rate, not increasing with exercise |
| Atrial septal defect (ASD) | Congenital | Small ASDs without symptoms; large ASDs may lead to pulmonary hypertension |
| Ventricular septic defect (VSD) | Congenital | Loud murmur during contraction of ventricles; right-side heart failure may occur with large defect; cyanosis if blood shunts right to left |
| Tetralogy of Fallot | Congenital | Cyanotic "blue baby," murmurs, excess number of red cells, dyspnea, fingers and nails clubbed |
| Patent ductus arteriosus (PDA) | Congenital | Murmur develops |
| Coarctation of aorta | Congenital | Blood Pressure low in legs, high in arms; congestive heart failure can result |
| Hypertension | Idiopathic, atherosclerosis | None obvious: "silent killer" |

| DIAGNOSIS | TREATMENT |
| --- | --- |
| ECG | Artificial pacemaker |
| ECG | Medication such as lanoxin |
| ECG | Cardiopulmonary resuscitation, defibrillation |
| ECG | Medication |
| ECG | Medication |
| ECG | Pacemaker may be needed |
| Chest x-ray, ECG | Large defects surgically repaired |
| Chest x-ray, ECG, cardiac catheterization, angiography, or echocardiography | Large defects surgically repaired; small ones may spontaneously close |
| Chest x-ray, ECG, cardiac catheterization, angiography | Surgical repair |
| Chest x-ray, cardiac catheterization, angiography | Medication, ligation (tying shut) of defect |
| Chest x-ray, cardiac catheterization | Surgery |
| Blood pressure measures consistently high | Weight loss, reduced salt and fat in diet, exercise, smoking cessation, medication |

# DISEASES AT A GLANCE (*continued*)

## Cardiovascular System

| DISEASE | ETIOLOGY | SIGNS AND SYMPTOMS |
| --- | --- | --- |
| Hypovolemic | Blood loss due to hemorrhage | Severe hemorrhage, severe and extensive burns |
| Neurogenic shock | CVA, loss of vascular tension | Falling blood pressure, slow heart rate |
| Anaphylactic shock | Allergic reaction | Hives, itching, wheezing, increased heart rate, increased respiratory rate |
| Cardiogenic shock | Myocardial infarction, electrical shock | Myocardial infarction; fast heart rate; cool, clammy skin |
| Raynaud's disease | Idiopathic, smoking | Numbness, discoloration, pain, cold digits |
| Arteriosclerosis, Atherosclerosis | Genetic, diet, idiopathic | Varies with arteries affected and severity; thrombus (clot) may block artery; embolus (traveling clot) may be released and blo artery elsewhere |
| Aneurysm | Congenital, hypertension | No symptoms until rupture |
| Thrombophlebitis | Stagnant blood, CHF | Pain, edema, inflammation, thrombus (clot) formation |
| Varicose veins | Excess weight, continuous standing | Swelling of veins, stasis, rupture may occur; spider veins, hemorrhoids, esophageal varices |

| DIAGNOSIS | TREATMENT |
| --- | --- |
| Physical exam | Fluid replacement, transfusion |
| Physical exam, cardiovascular monitoring | Elevation of legs, compressive stockings, drugs, fluids |
| Physical exam | Epinephrine, steroids, fluids |
| Physical exam, cardiovascular monitoring | Treatment of heart failure, drugs |
| Physical exam | Protection from cold, smoking cessation |
| Ultrasound arteriography, Doppler imaging | Low cholesterol diet, exercise, weight loss, smoking cessation; balloon angiography, bypass surgery |
| X-ray, MRI, ultrasound | Surgical repair |
| Physical exam | Anticoagulants, antibiotics, surgery |
| Physical exam | Compression sclerotherapy, support hose, surgery |

# Interactive Activities

## Cases for Critical Thinking

1. A 59-year-old male calls paramedics after experiencing an episode of chest pain while shoveling snow. He describes his pain as a crushing, tight feeling that radiates to his left arm and jaw. What type(s) of heart disease is this patient experiencing?

2. A 60-year-old male has been experiencing an increase in shortness of breath, a productive cough, and tiredness over the past few months. On examination, the doctor hears congestion in the lungs. What type of heart failure is this patient currently experiencing?

3. A 12-year-old child experiences high fever and chills. He also says that his heart feels like it's pounding. Two weeks before these symptoms, the child fell off his bike and skinned his knee. This child also has a history of a heart murmur. What disease should we consider?

## Multiple Choice

1. Congestive heart failure and shortness of breath due to pulmonary edema result from failure of which heart structure?

   a. right ventricle     c. septum
   b. left ventricle      d. right auricle

2. Which four defects in the list below are associated with the tetralogy of Fallot?

   (1) mitral insufficiency
   (2) hypertrophy of right ventricle
   (3) atrial septal defect
   (4) pulmonary stenosis
   (5) aortic stenosis
   (6) ventricular septal defect
   (7) misplaced aorta
   (8) hypertrophy of left ventricle
   a. (1), (2), (4), (8)     c. (2), (3), (5), (7)
   b. (3), (5), (7), (8)     d. (2), (4), (6), (7)

3. What causes cyanosis?

   a. failure of the foramen ovale to close
   b. failure of the ductus arteriosus to close
   c. pulmonary stenosis
   d. large septal hole

4. Which of the following requires immediate attempts at resuscitation to prevent cardiac arrest?

   a. atrial fibrillation     c. bradycardia
   b. ventricular            d. tachycardia
      fibrillation

5. Hypertension in a patient's arms but no femoral pulse indicates_____.

   a. tetralogy of Fallot
   b. coarctatin of the aorta
   c. patent ductus arteriosus
   d. failure of the foramen ovale to close

6. The depositing of fatty plaques within the arteries is called _____.

   a. arteriosclerosis     c. petechiae
   b. atherosclerosis      d. stasis

7. Phlebitis is an inflammation of the _____.

   a. veins          c. aorta
   b. arteries       d. pulmonary valve

8. A bubble-like protrusion of an arterial wall is called _____.

   a. hematoma       c. aneurysm
   b. petechia       d. angioplasty

9. An embolus traveling from the leg to the heart would be more likely to block the _____.

   a. aorta             c. mitral valve
   b. pulmonary artery  d. kidney artery

10. What is the action of renin on arterioles?

    a. constriction     c. no change
    b. dilation         d. blockage

## True or False

_____ 1. The left atrium hypertrophies and dilates when the mitral valve becomes stenotic.

_____ 2. Pain of a myocardial infarction is relieved by nitroglycerin.

_____ 3. Tachycardia refers to a decreased heart rate.

_____ 4. Aortic insufficiency causes backflow of blood from aorta to the left ventricle.

_____ 5. Long-standing hypertension causes the left ventricle to hypertrophy.

_____ 6. Embolisms to the brain can result from a thrombus on the mitral valve.

_____ 7. Neurogenic shock results from severe fluid-volume loss.

_____ 8. After a severe hemorrhage, blood pressure increases.

_____ 9. Women have less chance of myocardial infarction after age 60.

_____ 10. Angioplasty is less invasive than a bypass surgery.

## Fill-Ins

1. _____ uses high-frequency sound waves to examine the heart.

2. Enlargement of the walls of the heart is _____.

3. Oxygen-poor blood flows from the body through the _____ artery and to the _____ .

4. The left ventricle pumps blood to the body via the _____.

5. Raynaud's disease results in _____ of the arterioles.

6. The highest pressure in a blood pressure reading reflects _____.

7. Anticoagulant medication is administered to prevent a thrombus from becoming an _____ .

8. In primary or essential hypertension, the causes are _____.

9. A common drug for anticoagulant use is _____.

10. An implanted device or external instrument that corrects heart rhythm is the _____ .

## MedMedia Wrap-Up

**www.prenhall.com/mulvihill**
Remember to visit this website for extra study practice, including exercises, Internet links, news updates, and an audio glossary.

**Activity CD-ROM**
Check out the CD-ROM in the back of this book. You will find games, exercises, puzzles, and videos to help enhance your understanding of this chapter.

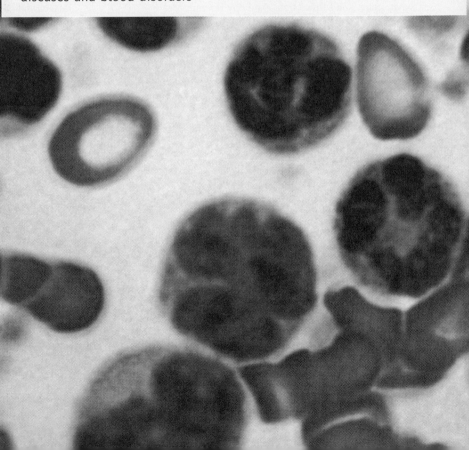

Peripheral blood smear showing blast crisis of chronic myelogenous leukemia. (Courtesy of the CDC/Stacy Howard, 1994.)

# Diseases of the Blood

## Learning Objectives

After studying this chapter, you should be able to

■ Distinguish between formed elements and fluid portions of the blood

■ Delineate the function of red blood cells, white blood cells, and platelets

■ Identify the causes, signs, and symptoms of anemia, bleeding disorders, platelet disorders, and white blood cell disorders

■ Describe various treatment modalities for anemia, bleeding disorders, platelet disorders, and white blood cell disorders

■ Explain the role of various diagnostic tests in identifying systemic diseases and blood disorders

## Fact or Fiction?

Sickling of red blood cells results from inadequate oxygen saturation of red blood cells.

*Fact:* In 1948, using the new technique of protein electrophoresis, Linus Pauling and Harvey Itano showed that abnormal hemoglobin, the oxygen-binding protein in red blood cells, was responsible for sickle cell disease. Under low oxygen conditions, the abnormal hemoglobin causes red blood cells to sickle. Sickle cell disease was the first disorder linked to the presence of a specific abnormal protein.

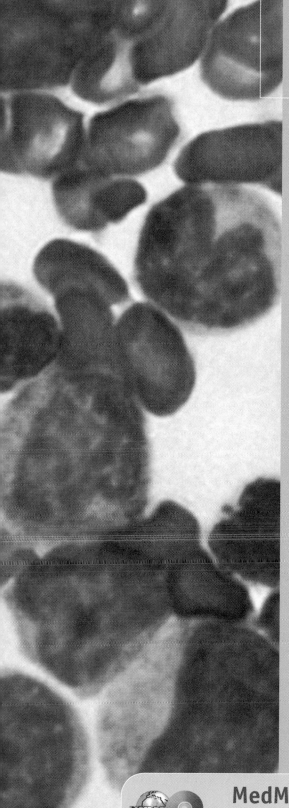

# Disease Chronicle

## Four Body Humors

Prior to the time of Hippocrates (460–377 BCE), all illnesses were attributed to one disease with variable symptoms. Careful clinical observations by Hippocrates led to the recognition of specific disease states with identifying symptoms. It was during this time that the concept of body humors developed. The four fluid substances (humors) of the body were blood, phlegm, yellow bile, and black bile. Health depended on the proper balance of these humors. Bloodletting was a method used for adjusting one of the humors to proper balance. It was thought that blood carried the vital force of the body and was the seat of the soul; body weakness and insanity were ascribed to a defect in this vital fluid. Blood spurting from fallen gladiators was drunk with the hope that it would transfer strength to the recipient. Caspar Bartholin, MD, (1655–1738) described an epileptic girl in Breslau who drank the blood of a cat. The girl, so the report goes, became endowed with the characteristics of a cat. She climbed on the roofs of houses and imitated the manner of a cat by jumping, scratching, and howling. Not content with that, she would sit for hours gazing into a hole in the floor.

## MedMedia
www.prenhall.com/mulvihill

Use the web address to the left to access the free, interactive Companion Website created for this textbook. It features chapter-specific exercises, Internet links, news links, and an audio glossary. Additionally, explore the CD-ROM that accompanies this book to discover Disease Focus videos and a rich array of activities that accompany this chapter.

## ▶ Introduction

The blood serves as the body's major transport system. It is the medium for transporting oxygen from the lungs to the cells, and carbon dioxide waste from the cells to the lungs. Components of the blood protect the body from disease by recognizing and engulfing microorganisms and foreign molecules in the blood. Other components of the blood transport metabolic waste from the cells to the kidneys, nutrients from the digestive system to the cells, and hormones throughout the body.

The cellular components or formed elements of blood are red blood cells or erythrocytes, white blood cells or leukocytes, and clotting cells or platelets. Blood cells are suspended in the plasma or the fluid portion of circulating blood. Formed elements comprise about 45% of the blood, and plasma comprises the remaining 55%. The ratio of red blood cell–volume to whole blood is called hematocrit.

The plasma is the fluid portion of the blood. It contains water, proteins, potassium, sodium, chloride, potassium, and bicarbonate. It also contains metabolic waste products, hormones, nutrients, proteins, and gases. When platelets are removed from the plasma, the remainder is known as serum.

## ▶ Red Blood Cells

The red blood cells make up about half of the blood's volume. Unlike other cells in the body, red blood cells are biconcave sacs filled with hemoglobin that enables them to carry oxygen from the lungs to all the body tissues. Erythrocytes normally number about 5 million/mm$^3$ of blood in males and 4.5 million/mm$^3$ in females.

Red blood cells are produced in the red marrow of bones such as the vertebrae, ribs, and body of the sternum. The process of red blood cell formation, called erythropoiesis, is regulated by the hormone erythropoietin. Red blood cell synthesis begins with large, nucleated stem cells that progress through many stages before emerging as mature red blood cells. In the process, hemoglobin accumulates within the cytoplasm and the nucleus disappears. Mature red blood cells emerge from the bone marrow as reticulocytes.

Iron, vitamin B$_{12}$, and folic acid are critical nutrients for red blood cell synthesis and red blood cell integrity. Nutrient deficiencies, the presence of immature red blood cells, as well as the characteristic color and volume of red blood cells, are laboratory variables used to distinguish different types of anemia.

## ▶ Anemia

Anemia is the condition of reduced numbers of red blood cells. Hemorrhages, excessive destruction, or impaired synthesis of red blood cells, and chronic diseases reduce the number of red blood cells and oxygen delivery to cells and tissues. Thus symptoms of anemia are due to tissue hypoxia or lack of oxygen. General symptoms of anemia include pallor or deficiency of color, fatigue, dizziness, headaches, decreased exercise tolerance, rapid heartbeat, and shortness of breath. Untreated anemia may progress to death from heart failure or cardiovascular collapse or shock.

### Iron Deficiency Anemia

Iron deficiency is one of the most common causes of anemia. Increased iron requirements, impaired iron absorption, or hemorrhage may cause iron deficiency anemia. Without enough iron, the body fails to synthesize hemoglobin, and the ability to transport oxygen is reduced.

Iron requirements are greatest during the first two years of life. Adolescent girls may become iron deficient due to inadequate dietary iron, increased growth requirements, and the onset of menstruation. Likewise, a sudden growth spurt in adolescent boys may significantly increase physiological demands for iron, resulting in iron deficiency anemia. Supplemental iron is needed during pregnancy as iron is provided to the developing fetus.

Decreases in iron absorption occur with malabsorption syndromes and chronic disease. Iron absorption requires an intact gastrointestinal tract with healthy intestinal mucosal cells. Chronic disease, removal of the stomach, and bowel disorders limit availability of iron required for the synthesis of hemoglobin.

Symptoms specific to iron deficiency include a craving for ice, swelling of the tongue, and dry lips. The diagnosis of iron deficient anemia is confirmed by microscopic examination of the blood. Red blood cells are reduced in number and appear hypochromic, or lighter than normal, due to a lack of hemoglobin.

The first step in treating iron deficiency anemia is to identify and correct any causes of bleeding. Oral supplements are effective in those with an intact gastrointestinal tract. The addition of vitamin C enhances iron absorption. Injectable iron supplements are available for individuals with malabsorption or those who cannot tolerate oral supplementation.

## Anemia of Chronic Disease

Anemia of chronic disease is the second leading cause of anemia worldwide. Chronic disease such as heart disease, cancer, arthritis, and infectious disease induce inflammatory changes that suppress red blood cell synthesis in the bone marrow and shorten survival of red blood cells already within the systemic circulation. The chronic nature of the disease usually parallels the severity of the anemia.

## Vitamin $B_{12}$ Deficiency Anemia

Vitamin $B_{12}$ deficiency anemia, or pernicious anemia, is caused by inadequate absorption or intake of Vitamin $B_{12}$ or a deficiency in a protein called intrinsic factor. Intrinsic factor is produced in the stomach and is essential for the absorption of vitamin $B_{12}$ from the small intestine. Without vitamin $B_{12}$ and intrinsic factor, the membranes of immature red blood cells rupture easily within the chemical environment of the blood stream. The result is fewer than normal red blood cells and consequently a reduced oxygen-carrying capacity.

Causes of pernicious anemia include inadequate diet, inadequate absorption, inadequate utilization, increased requirements, and increased excretion of vitamin $B_{12}$. Principal dietary sources of vitamin $B_{12}$ come from animal products. Strict vegetarians who restrict all animal products develop pernicious anemia unless they consume vitamin $B_{12}$ supplements. Abnormal bacterial growth in the small intestine and bowel disorders induce pathological changes that either impair absorption or enhance elimination of vitamin $B_{12}$. Removal of the stomach or the bowel impairs availability of intrinsic factor and limits absorption of vitamin $B_{12}$.

Symptoms of pernicious anemia include abdominal distress such as nausea and vomiting, and burning of the tongue. Neurological disturbances include numbness, weakness, and peculiar yellow and blue color blindness.

Vitamin $B_{12}$ supplementation effectively reverses the effects of pernicious anemia. Because vitamin $B_{12}$ cannot be absorbed into the bloodstream, it must be replaced by injection. Vitamin $B_{12}$ supplementation is required for life for strict vegetarians and for those with chronic bowel disorders or individuals who have had their stomach or bowel partially or fully removed.

## Folic Acid Deficiency Anemia

Folic acid deficiency anemia is common in the Western world where consumption of raw fruits and vegetables is low. Inflammation of the bowel as in Crohn's disease and adverse effects certain medications impair absorption of folic acid. Body stores of folic acid are small and as such folic acid deficiency anemia occurs within a few months. Pregnant and lactating females, alcoholics, and individuals with kidney disease are especially susceptible to folic acid deficiency anemia owing to increased metabolic demands.

Measurement of serum folic acid levels is conclusive for folic acid deficiency anemia. Oral folic acid supplementation is effective in replacing folic acid and meeting increased requirements for those with increased metabolic demands.

## Hemolytic Anemia

Hemolytic anemia is a reduction in circulating red blood cells that is caused by pathological conditions that accelerate destruction of red blood cells. Inherited abnormalities such as hemoglobin defects, enzyme defects, and membrane defects impair intrinsic physical properties that are needed for optimal red blood cell survival. Infectious agents, certain medications, and immune disorders may also reduce red blood cell survival.

Significant red blood cell destruction produces symptoms similar to those of other anemias. Unlike other anemias, hemolytic anemia produces increased serum levels of bilirubin that result from the degradation of heme in destroyed red blood cells. Accumulation of bilirubin causes a jaundiced or yellow-orange appearance in the tissues, urine, and feces.

## ▶ Anemia Caused by Defective Hemoglobin Synthesis

### Hemoglobin

Hemoglobin is composed of four protein chains: two alpha chains and two beta chains. Each chain is attached to a heme group that contains iron. Oxygen molecules bind to the heme portion of the hemoglobin to form oxyhemoglobin. Since single hemoglobin has four heme groups, it can transport four oxygen molecules. Hemoglobin also transports a small amount of carbon dioxide.

### Sickle Cell Anemia

Sickle cell anemia is a genetically transmitted disorder marked by severe hemolytic anemia, episodes of painful crisis, and increased susceptibility to infections. Approximately 10% of African Americans have the sickle cell trait or are heterozygous for the disorder. Those with the disease are homozygous or have inherited two genes (one from each parent).

In sickle cell disease, red blood cells contain an abnormal form of hemoglobin, or hemoglobin S. As the red blood cell deoxygenates, hemoglobin S forms cross-links with other hemoglobin S molecules, and long crystals develop. Crystals continue to form as oxygen is released, and the red cells assume a sickled shape.

Sickled red blood cells are inflexible and rigid, and cause mechanical obstruction of small arterioles and capillaries, leading to pain and ischemia. Sickled cells are also more fragile than normal, leading to hemolysis. Tissue death secondary to ischemia causes painful crises that progress to organ failure with repeated occlusive episodes.

Sickle cell anemia cannot be cured. Treatment is aimed at preventing sickle cell crisis, controlling the anemia, and relieving painful symptoms. Painful crises are adequately managed with narcotic analgesics. Blood transfusions and fluid replacement expand blood volume and oxygen exchange needed for reperfusion of occluded vessels.

### Thalassemia

Thalassemia is a group of inherited blood disorders in which there is deficient synthesis of one or more alpha or beta chains required for proper formation and optimal performance of the hemoglobin molecule. Several different categories of thalassemia produce mild to severe symptoms (Table 8–1).

The most severe forms of thalassemia produce severe, life-threatening anemia, bone marrow hyperactivity, and enlargement of the spleen, growth retardation, and bone deformities. Blood transfusions are required to sustain life, and life expectancy is reduced.

## ▶ Bleeding Disorders

### Platelets and Clotting Factors

Bleeding disorders result from platelet dysfunction or deficiency, vitamin K deficiency, and clotting factor deficiencies. Platelets are blood elements produced in the bone marrow that are essential for blood clotting in response to immediate injury, and for the mobilization of clotting factors. Clotting factors are formed in the liver and released in response to tissue injury and platelet fragments to form insoluble fibrin clots. Vitamin K is required for the synthesis of the prothrombin and fibrinogen, clotting factors. Platelets, clotting factors, vitamin K, and cal-

## Table 8–1  Categories of Thalassemia

### Alpha Thalassemia

| Thalassemia | Affected Protein Chain | Severity | Cultural Prevalence |
|---|---|---|---|
| Silent carrier state | Alpha chain | Mild anemia | Africa, Middle East, India, Southeast Asia, Southern Asia, occasionally in the Mediterranean region |
| Hemoglobin Constant spring | Mutation of the alpha chain | Mild anemia | |
| Mild alpha Thalassemia | Slight deficiency of alpha protein | Mild anemia | |
| Hemoglobin H disease | Severe deficiency of alpha protein forms H hemoglobin | Severe disease, hemoglobin destroys red blood cells | |
| Hemoglobin H constant spring disease | Deficiency in alpha protein is greater than in hemoglobin H disease | Severe anemia, greater destruction of red blood cells than in hemoglobin H disease | Mediterranean region |
| Homozygous constant spring | Similar to hemoglobin H disease | Generally less severe than hemoglobin H | |
| Alpha thalassemia major, or hydrops fetalis | Complete lack of alpha chains | Death at birth or lifelong transfusions with constant medical care | |

### Beta Thalassemia

| Thalassemia | Affected Protein Chain | Severity | Cultural Prevalence |
|---|---|---|---|
| Thalassemia minor or thalassemia trait | Lack beta protein | Mild symptoms | Mediterranean descent: Greeks, Italians; Arabian Peninsula, Iran, Africa, southeast Asia, Southern China |
| Thalassemia intermedia | Lack beta protein | Moderately severe anemia | |
| Thalassemia major or Cooley's anemia | Complete lack of beta protein | Severe life threatening anemia | |

cium are essential for hemostasis, or the arrest of bleeding.

## Vascular Bleeding Disorders

**Purpura Simplex**  Purpura simplex, or easy bruising, usually affects women and appears to have a hereditary predisposition. Bruises develop without an apparent cause, and the vascular appears fragile. The number of platelets as well as the platelet activity is normal, and the condition is generally not serious. Bedrest and avoidance of products containing aspirin, which can suppress platelet function, is recommended.

**Hereditary Hemorrhagic Telangiectasia**  Hereditary hemorrhagic telangiectasia is a disorder characterized by malformations of the vasculature. This hereditary disorder affects both men and women. Red to violet telengiectatic lesions appear on the face, lips, oral and nasal mucosa, as well as on the tips of the fingers and toes. Telengiectatic lesions are due to abnormal dilation of existing or small vessels. These vessels rupture easily and form artificial shunts, or fistulas, to critical organs of the body. Mild disease is characterized by recurrent nosebleeds. With severe disease, extensive fistulas develop to the lungs, resulting in shortness of breath and fatigue due to deficient oxygenation. Infected emboli also develop in telengiectatic vessels, resulting in strokes or ischemia to brain.

Telengiectases in the nose and gastrointestinal tract may be treated with laser ablation. Large fistulas usually require surgical resection. Multiple blood transfusions and continuous iron therapy may be needed if blood loss is excessive.

## Platelet Disorders

**Thrombocytopenia** An abnormally small number of platelets, or thrombocytopenia, result from conditions that either impair production, increase destruction, or cause sequestration of platelets. Regardless of cause, prolonged bleeding results from minor and major trauma. Spontaneous hemorrhages are often-visible on the skin as small, flat, red spots called petechiae, or as larger purplish patches called ecchymosis. Spontaneous hemorrhages may also occur in the mucous membranes of the mouth and internal organs.

Suppression of the bone marrow by certain medications or cancer may diminish platelet production. Autoimmune disorders may increase platelet destruction or impair platelet function. Massive blood transfusions dilute circulating platelets and decrease platelet viability.

Thrombocytopenia can usually be corrected by treating the underlying cause. Preventative measures such as bedrest to avoid accidental trauma are highly recommended until platelet counts increase to acceptable levels. Platelet transfusions are reserved for severe thrombocytopenia or in cases of severe bleeding.

**Primary Thrombycythemia** Primary thrombocythemia is a marked increase in circulating platelets due to unknown causes. Primary thrombocythemia occurs most frequently in adult men and women during the sixth or seventh decade of life. Symptoms are related to abnormal platelet function and thrombosis. Thrombosis causes ischemia to the central nervous system, the peripheral extremities, and vital organs of the body. Symptoms include dizziness, visual problems, headaches, difficulty breathing, and extreme pain in the extremities. Bleeding may result in some cases due to abnormal platelet function.

## Disorders of Platelet Ahesion

**von Willebrand's Disease** A mutation in the von Willebrand factor gene causes a severe disorder characterized by a tendency to bleed from mucous membranes despite adequate levels of circulating platelets. A deficiency in the von Willebrand clotting factor as well as defective platelet aggregation and adherence lead to excessive and prolonged bleeding and anemia.

Chronic medical treatment is generally not required for most individuals with platelet-function disorders. The avoidance of aspirin that inhibits platelet function is recommended, as are preventive measures prior to invasive medical, surgical, or dental procedures. The most definitive treatment for severe bleeding is platelet transfusion.

## Blood Coagulation Disorders

**Hemophilia** Hemophilia is a sex-linked, inherited coagulation disorder caused by a deficiency of clotting factors. Because hemophilia is an X-linked disorder, almost all symptomatic individuals are males. Daughters of affected males have a 50:50 chance of being carriers, whereas sons of carriers have a 50:50 chance of having hemophilia.

The severity of hemophilia depends on how the gene affects the activity of the clotting factors, the number of bleeds and whether the bleeds occur spontaneously or with trauma. Severely affected individuals may have two or three bleeding episodes per month, may spontaneously bleed without noticeable trauma, or may bleed profusely without immediate treatment. Moderately affected individuals bleed approximately five or six times per year but may have prolonged periods free of bleeding, and usually bleed only with trauma. Mildly affected individuals bleed rarely, unless provoked by significant trauma or surgery.

Severely affected individuals require regular transfusion to replace deficient clotting factors. Mildly affected individuals may occasionally need transfusions. In all cases, situations that might provoke bleeding should be avoided, and preventative medications can be administered prior to dental procedures and surgery.

## ▶ White Blood Cells

Leukocytes, or white blood cells, include neutrophils, eosinophils, basophils, monocytes, and lymphocytes. White blood cells are synthesized in the bone marrow from their respective stem cells. The primary function of leukocytes is to defend tissues against infections and foreign substances. Quantitative abnormalities, inherited acquired defects, and neoplastic alterations result in disease and disability.

### Disorders of White Blood Cells

**Neutropenia** A reduction of circulating neutrophils increases the risk for bacterial and fungal infections. Because neutrophils are responsible for most clinical findings during an acute infection, the classic signs of infection may be diminished or absent in a severely neutropenic individual.

Neutropenia is a frequent complication of medication used for cancer chemotherapy or medications used for immune suppression. These medications suppress cellular proliferation within in the bone marrow. Infectious complications depend on the severity of neutropenia and are usually profound and severe in cancer patients.

Immune destruction of neutrophils occurs with rheumatoid arthritis or as a primary condition with unknown causes. Neutropenia may be either mild or severe, and infectious complications are variable. Chronic and severe cases require medical treatment with medications that increase neutrophil proliferation or medications that suppress immune function.

### Neoplastic Abnormalities of Leukocytes

**Leukemia** Leukemia, or cancer of the white blood cells, results in production of a large number of abnormal leukocytes. Overproduction of malignant white cells suppresses the production of red blood cells and platelets. Organs where blood is stored, such as the liver and the spleen, become greatly enlarged with infiltration of malignant white blood cells.

The cause of leukemia is unknown, but it may be due to a virus or exposure to radiation. A high incidence of leukemia has been reported in areas around the world exposed to fallout from nuclear energy. Heredity may also play a part in its etiology. Table 8–2 compares the types of leukemias.

Signs and symptoms of leukemia include fever, swollen lymph nodes or lymphadenopathy, joint pain, abnormal bleeding, and weight loss. Anemia with its manifestations of weakness, shortness of breath, and heart palpitations accompanies leukemia. Blood clotting is reduced with a reduction of platelets, causing a tendency to bruise and hemorrhage. White blood cells are produced faster than they mature and are ineffective in fighting infections.

The two main types of leukemia are named for the site of the malignancy. If the cancer originates in the bone marrow, it is called myelogenous leukemia because the primitive white cells in this tissue are called myelocytes. In myelogenous leukemia, neutrophil production is greatly increased, and both red blood cells and platelets production is suppressed.

The other type of leukemia is a lymphocytic leukemia and results from malignancy of the lymphatic cells, found both in the bone marrow and lymph nodes. The lymphocytes in this case are the only blood cells that are increased; however, they become disproportionately high in number and are immature and ineffective.

Both types of leukemia can be chronic or acute. Acute lymphocytic leukemia is the more common form in children. It has an abrupt onset and progresses rapidly. Immature lymphocytes with diminished activity accumulate

## Table 8–2 Comparison of Leukemia Types

| Type | Incidence | Signs and Symptoms | Prognosis | Malignant Cells |
|------|-----------|--------------------|-----------|-----------------|
| Acute myelogenous leukemia (AML) | Most common nonlymphocytic leukemia Usually develops in persons between ages 30 and 60 Slightly more common in men | Usual: anemia, pallor, fatigue, weakness, fever Possible: bleeding, bruising, bond and joint pain, headache, enlarged lymph nodes, liver and spleen, recurrent infections | Generally poor; death usually results from infection or hemorrhage | Granulocytes (neutrophils, eosinophils, and basophils) |
| Acute lymphocytic leukemia (ALL) | Most common cancer in children Usually diagnosed before age 14 (peak incidence between ages 2 and 9) Males slightly more affected than females | Usual: anemia, pallor, fatigue, weakness, swollen lymph nodes recurrent infections Possible: bleeding, bruising, and headache | Generally good (initial treatment usually induces remission in 95% of patients) Overall cure is 50% | Lymphocytes |
| Chronic myelogenous leukemia (CML) | About 20% of blood cancers Usually affects adults between ages 40 and 60 | Usual: loss of appetite, weight loss, fatigue, weakness, enlarged spleen and liver Possible: bleeding, bruising, bone and joint pain, fever, enlarged lymph nodes | Generally poor Average survival time of 3 years No treatment produces satisfactory results | Granulocytes |
| Chronic lymphocytic leukemia (CLL) | Most common form of blood cancer in industrial countries Affects primarily older adults, males more frequently than females | Usual: weight loss, enlarged lymph nodes and spleen Possible: fever | Depends on patient's age, signs, and symptoms Median survival time is 4 to 6 years | B lymphocytes |

in the systemic circulation, and symptoms appear rapidly.

Acute myelogenous leukemia is more common in adults. Chronic forms of leukemia produce cells that undergo some maturation and are at least partially functional. Because the cells do function, the disease is slow to develop

and is often discovered by accident, during routine blood tests.

Progress is being made in controlling and finding a cure for leukemia. Treatment goals include eliminating leukemic cells by inhibiting their growth, maintaining remission, and preventing complications from the disease and its treatments. Chemotherapy medications inhibit the growth of malignant cells and healthy cells. The side effects of chemotherapy are due in part to growth suppression of healthy cells. The ability of the patient to tolerate adverse medication effects determines the intensity of the chemotherapy. Remission is possible in 50% to 90% of patients.

## Abnormalities of Monocytes

**Myelomonocytic Leukemia** Myelomonocytic leukemia is a variation of acute myelogenous leukemia most commonly seen in adults. Common symptoms are fever, weight loss, lymphadenopathy, enlarged spleen, anemia, and thrombocytopenia. This disorder is rapidly fatal if left untreated. With treatment, current survival is approximately 40%.

## Abnormalities of Eosinophils and Basophils

**Idiopathic Hypereosinophilic Syndrome** The onset of idiopathic hypereosinophilic syndrome occurs between the ages of 20 and 50 years, and there is a strong male predominance. Persistent increases in blood eosinophils and associated involvement of the heart and nervous system are responsible for the most important clinical symptoms. Cardiac involvement produces congestive heart failure, valvular dysfunction, conduction defects, and myocarditis. Congestive heart failure is a frequent cause of death. Neurologic findings may include altered behavior and cognitive function, spasticity, and ataxia.

Prognosis in the idiopathic hypereosinophilic syndrome historically has been poor, with median survival of approximately 1 year. However, chemotherapy has recently been reported to produce 70% survival at 10 years.

**Eosinophilia-Myalgia Syndrome** A recently described disorder, eosinophilia-myalgia syndrome is a chronic, multisystem disease with a spectrum of clinical symptoms ranging from self-limited myalgias, or muscle pain, and fatigue to a progressive and potentially fatal illness characterized by skin changes, nervous system abnormalities, and pulmonary hypertension. Elevation of circulating levels of eosinophis is a universal feature of this disorder, and the illness has been related to ingestion of the dietary supplement L-tryptophan.

## ▶ Diagnostic Tests

Blood tests are diagnostic for systemic diseases as well as specific blood disorders. Blood analysis measures total blood counts (red blood cells, white blood cells, and platelets), hemoglobin, hematocrit, serum chemistry, and enzyme and hormone levels within the body. Differential blood analysis provides qualitative information such as size, shape, and ratio of one cell type to another.

A bone marrow smear is used to diagnose malignant blood disorders and increases or decreases in blood counts without any apparent cause. Bone marrow samples are obtained by needle aspiration of the bone marrow from the bone marrow cavity. Bone marrow analysis provides information on the function of the bone marrow and the qualitative characteristics of stem cells that give rise to all blood cells.

## CHAPTER SUMMARY

The blood is the connective tissue that transports red blood cells, platelets, white blood cells, proteins, and nutrients. Normal amounts of all blood cells are essential for life. Elevations or deficiencies in blood cells are due to conditions that suppress or enhance growth and differentiation, including malignancies, certain medications, environmental exposures, nutrient deficiencies, and inherited genes.

## RESOURCES

Beers, M. H., & R. Berkow. *The Merck Manual of Diagnosis and Therapy,* 17th ed. John Willey & Sons, 1999.

*Professional Guide to Diseases,* 6th ed. Springhouse, 1998.

# DISEASES AT A GLANCE

## Diseases of the Blood

| DISEASE/DISORDER | ETIOLOGY | SIGNS AND SYMPTOMS |
| --- | --- | --- |
| Iron deficiency anemia | Increased iron requirements<br>Impaired iron absorption<br>Hemorrhage<br>Chronic disease | Pallor<br>Fatigue<br>Shortness of breath |
| Vitamin $B_{12}$ deficiency anemia | Malnutrition<br>Strict vegetarianism<br>Deficiency of intrinsic factor | Pallor<br>Fatigue<br>Shortness of breath<br>Burning of the tongue<br>Abdominal distress, nausea and vomiting |
| Folic acid deficiency anemia | Inflammation of the bowel<br>Certain medications that impair absorption of folic acid<br>Pregnancy and lactation<br>Alcoholism<br>Kidney disease | Pallor<br>Fatigue<br>Shortness of breath |
| Sickle cell anemia | Genetics: results in formation of abnormal hemoglobin | Pallor<br>Fatigue<br>Shortness of breath<br>Painful sickle cell crisis |
| Thalassemia | Genetics: results in formation of defective hemoglobin | Pallor<br>Fatigue<br>Shortness of breath |
| Purpura simplex | Genetics<br>Hereditary disorder<br>Unknown causes | Easy bruising |
| Hereditary hemorrhagic telangiectasia | Genetics<br>Hereditary disorder | Red to violet lesions on the face, lips, oral, and nasal mucosa and on the tips of the fingers and toes |

| DIAGNOSIS | TREATMENT |
| --- | --- |
| Blood test | Iron supplementation<br>Treatment of hemorrhage |
| Blood test | Vitamin $B_{12}$ supplementation |
| Blood test | Folic acid supplementation |
| Genetic testing<br>Blood test | Prevention of sickle cell crisis<br>Supportive care during crises<br>Blood transfusion |
| Genetic testing<br>Blood test | Supportive care<br>Blood transfusions if anemia is severe<br>Treatment of iron overload for frequent transfusions |
| Blood test<br>Rule out other disorders<br>Family history | Bedrest<br>Avoidance of aspirin or products that suppress platelet function |
| Rule out other disorders<br>Family history | Laser ablation<br>Surgical resection<br>Blood transfusions<br>Iron therapy if blood loss is excessive |

# DISEASES AT A GLANCE (*continued*)

## Diseases of the Blood

| DISEASE/DISORDER | ETIOLOGY | SIGNS AND SYMPTOMS |
|---|---|---|
| Thrombocytopenia | Conditions that impair production or cause sequestration of platelets | Bleeding<br>Spontaneous hemorrhage |
| Thrombocythemia | Unknown | Clotting<br>Central nervous system damage |
| von Willibrand's disease | Genetic hereditary disease | Bleeding tendency despite adequate levels of circulating platelets |
| Hemophilia | Genetic hereditary disease | Bleeding tendency |
| Neutropenia | Immune suppression<br>Chemotherapy<br>Radiation therapy | Infections<br>Fever |
| Leukemia | Unknown<br>Virus<br>Radiation | Fever<br>Swollen lymph nodes<br>Anemia |
| Myelomonocytic leukemia | Unknown<br>Virus<br>Radiation | Fever<br>Swollen lymph nodes<br>Anemia |
| Idiopathic hypereosinphilic syndrome | Unknown<br>Virus<br>Radiation | Congestive heart failure<br>Valvular defects<br>Myocarditis |
| Eosinophilia myalgia syndrome | Unknown<br>Ingestion of L-tryptophan | Muscle pain<br>Weakness |

| DIAGNOSIS | TREATMENT |
| --- | --- |
| Blood test | Platelet transfusions |
| Blood test | Medical treatment to prevent complications |
| Blood test Genetic testing | Platelet transfusion |
| Blood test Genetic testing | Transfusion of deficient clotting factor(s) |
| Blood test | Medications that increase production of neutrophils |
| Blood test | Chemotherapy Radiation |
| Blood test | Chemotherapy Radiation |
| Blood test | Chemotherapy Radiation |
| Blood test | Avoidance of potentially offending agents Pharmacotherapy for pain |

# Interactive Activities

## Cases for Critical Thinking

1. A 17-year-old male presents to the emergency room with severe abdominal pain and shortness of breath. The whites of his eyes appear yellow. A blood count reveals a low red blood cell count and impaired hemostasis. What disorders do you suspect this patient to have? What other information do you need to obtain from the patient to make a correct diagnosis?

2. A 37-year-old female seeks medical attention for increasing fatigue and several bruises that appeared on her legs for no apparent reason. Her blood differential reports the following results: elevated neutrophils with many immature cells, anemia, iron deficiency, and slightly decreased platelet counts. The nurse practitioner suspects that the patient has anemia and a bacterial infection from poor nutritional habits. Rest with iron therapy is prescribed. Do you agree or disagree with this assessment? What are some other possible causes for these symptoms? What additional information do you need to narrow down your diagnosis?

## Multiple Choice

1. The ratio of red blood cell–volume to whole blood is called _____.

   a. hematrocrit      c. monocytes
   b. thrombocytes     d. lymphocytes

2. Decreases in red blood cells are cause by _____.

   a. hemorrhages       c. chronic diseases
   b. excess destruction  d. all the above

3. Hemophilia is a deficiency of _____.

   a. platelets        c. clotting factors
   b. hematocrit       d. monocytes

4. The most severe forms of thalassemia are _____.

   a. beta thalassemia major
   b. hemoglobin H disease
   b. alpha thalassemia major
   c. all of the above

5. Compared to chronic leukemia, acute leukemia _____.

   a. is less severe     c. occurs abruptly
   b. is shorter in      d. progresses slowly
      duration

6. The most common cause of anemia is _____.

   a. iron deficiency       c. vitamin $B_{12}$ deficiency
   b. folic acid deficiency  d. intrinsic factor deficiency

7. Fever, swollen lymph nodes, and weight loss are common symptoms of _____.

   a. leukemia        c. thrombocythemia
   b. eosinophilia    d. neutropenia

8. Unlike other anemias, hemolytic anemia results in accumulation of _____.

   a. iron           c. heme
   b. bilirubin      d. folic acid

9. Absorption of vitamin $B_{12}$ in the absence of intrinsic factor results in _____.

   a. hypoxia         b. shortness of breath
   b. anemia          c. all of the above

10. Sickled red blood cells result in _____ and _____.

    a. iron deficiency and folic acid deficiency
    b. ischemia and hemolysis
    c. pain and inflammation
    d. immune suppression and hemorrhage

## True or False

_____ 1. von Willebrand's disease results in decreased platelet adherance.

_____ 2. Red blood cells in iron deficiency anemia are reduced in number and are hypochromic.

_____ 3. Measurement of serum folic acid levels is diagnostic for pernicious anemia.

_____ 4. Accelerated destruction of red blood cells with breakdown of heme is characteristic of platelet dysfunction.

_____ 5. In general, the severity of thalassemia is related to the number of affected beta chains.

_____ 6. Platelet production may be diminished by immune-suppressing agents.

_____ 7. The primary blood cells that are affected in lymphocytic leukemia are the lymphocytes.

_____ 8. Eosinophilia is related to ingestion of L-tryptophan.

_____ 9. Petechiae or ecchymosis is a frequent complication of anemia.

_____ 10. Primary thrombocythemia, or increases in circulating platelets, may be associated with bleeding.

## Fill-Ins

1. White blood cells are called _____.

2. Mature red blood cells are called _____.

3. Oxygen combines with hemoglobin to form _____.

4. Sickle cell disease causes formation of _____ that forms cross-links and sickling of red blood cells.

5. Hemoglobin consists of _____ and _____.

6. Cancer of the white blood cells that originates in the bone marrow is called _____.

7. Cancer chemotherapy frequently suppresses proliferation of white blood cells required to fight _____ and _____ infections.

8. Thrombocytopenia is a decrease in the circulating levels of _____.

9. Myalgias, fatigue, skin changes, nervous system abnormalities, pulmonary hypertension, and elevations of eosinophils are characteristic of _____.

10. Blood analysis measures _____ and _____ characteristics of blood cells.

# MedMedia Wrap-Up

**www.prenhall.com/mulvihill**

Remember to visit this website for extra study practice, including exercises, Internet links, news updates, and an audio glossary.

**Activity CD-ROM**

Check out the CD-ROM in the back of this book. You will find games, exercises, puzzles, and videos to help enhance your understanding of this chapter.

*Mycobacterium tuberculosis* bacteria from a sputum specimen, viewed with Ziehl-Neelsen stain. (Courtesy of the CDC, 1979.)

# Diseases of the Respiratory System

## Learning Objectives

After studying this chapter, you should be able to

- Describe the normal structure and function of the respiratory organs
- Compare upper respiratory tract infections with lower respiratory tract infections
- Define COPD/COLD and name examples, causes, and treatments
- Compare acute bronchitis with chronic bronchitis
- Describe the cause and prognosis of throat cancer
- Discuss the causes and treatments of emphysema
- Differentiate between influenza, the common cold, and allergies
- Describe the various forms of pneumonia and their causes and treatments
- Describe the causes and treatments of pleurisy
- Describe the signs, symptoms, diagnosis, treatment, and prevention of tuberculosis
- Understand the factors causing the recent re-emergence of tuberculosis

## Fact or Fiction?

Don't go out into the cold with wet hair, or you might catch cold!

*Fiction: Viruses cause colds. However, sleeping in a draft, getting soaked in rain, or getting chilled can lower one's resistance to infection.*

# Disease Chronicle

## Breathing Clean Air

At rest, adults breathe 12 to 20 times per minute, and clean, fresh air is preferred, but throughout history this has not always been possible in densely populated urban areas. In 61 AD, the Roman philosopher Seneca remarked that the heavy, smoke-filled air of Rome had a foul smell and tended to alter his disposition. During the 1800s, smothering fogs enveloped London numerous times. In December 1952, London suffered its worst single air pollution disaster. Between December 4 and 10, approximately 4,000 died (some estimates are as high as 12,000) while dense yellow smog cloaked the city, a deadly combination of fog from cold heavy air and coal smoke from trains, factories, and homes. Hospitals treated thousands of patients with chest ailments. The major symptom was choking caused by excessive mucus within the irritated respiratory tract. Toxic sulfur dioxide in the coal smoke mixed with water vapor, producing sulfuric acid (battery acid), which probably triggered the respiratory distress that caused so many deaths.

## ▶ Structure and Function of the Respiratory System

The respiratory system obtains oxygen from the air, delivers it to the blood for distribution, and removes carbon dioxide from the blood. Respiratory structures also warm and moisten inhaled air and make vocalization possible.

Air enters the nasal cavity or oral cavity, and passes back through the pharynx, and then down to the trachea. At the entrance to the trachea is the larynx. The trachea branches into two bronchi, one going to each lung. The bronchi branch further into smaller and smaller tubules called bronchioles, which lack cartilaginous rings. The branching structure resembles an inverted tree and is often called the bronchial tree.

The bronchioles terminate in the lungs as small air sacs called the alveoli. Figure 9–1 illustrates the respiratory system.

The alveoli are thin-walled sacs surrounded by blood capillaries and are the site of gas exchange. Oxygen that is inspired, or inhaled, diffuses from the alveoli into the blood capillaries. The hemoglobin molecules of the red blood cells become saturated with oxygen. Carbon dioxide, a waste product of cellular metabolism, diffuses from the blood capillaries into the alveoli to be expired, or exhaled. This exchange of gases is illustrated in Figure 9–2.

To deliver oxygen to the alveoli, air must be inspired into the lungs. The diaphragm and the muscles between the ribs called external intercostals are the main muscles of inspiration. Contraction of these muscles increases the vol-

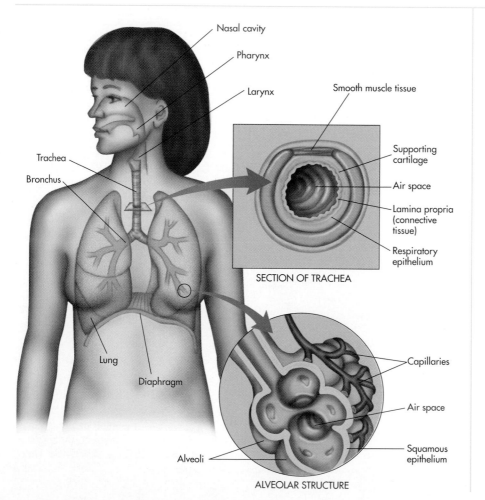

**Figure 9–1**
The respiratory system.

Nasal cavity
Pharynx
Larynx
Trachea
Bronchus
Lung
Diaphragm
Alveoli

Smooth muscle tissue
Supporting cartilage
Air space
Lamina propria (connective tissue)
Respiratory epithelium

SECTION OF TRACHEA

Capillaries
Air space
Squamous epithelium

ALVEOLAR STRUCTURE

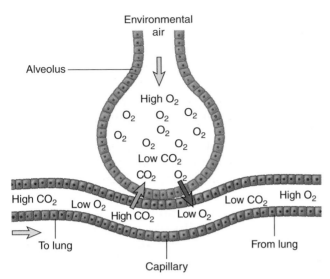

**Figure 9–2** Exchange of gases between lungs and blood. High concentration of $CO_2$ in blood capillary entering the lung diffuses into alveolus. High concentration of $O_2$ in alveolus diffuses into blood capillary leaving lung.

ume of the chest cavity, decreasing the pressure within the lungs, which allows air to rush in. When the same muscles relax, the volume of the chest cavity decreases, pressure within the lungs increases, and air is pushed out. Other muscles that assist exhalation include abdominal and internal intercostal muscles, which are utilized during labored breathing.

The lungs are encased by a double-membrane consisting of two layers called pleura. One layer of this membrane covers the lungs, and the other lines the inner chest wall or thoracic cavity. There is only a potential space, the pleural cavity, between them, containing a small amount of fluid. This fluid lubricates the surfaces, preventing friction as the lungs expand and contract. The fluid also reduces surface tension, which helps keep the lungs expanded. The airtight space between the lungs and the chest wall has a pressure slightly less than the pressure within the lungs. This difference in pressure acts as a vacuum and prevents the lungs from collapsing.

The entire respiratory tract is lined with a mucous membrane, the respiratory epithelium. Numerous hair like projections called cilia line the surface of this mucosa. The cilia exert a sweeping action, preventing dust and foreign particles from reaching the lungs. The breakdown of this mucous membrane paves the way for infection. The mucous membrane also protects the lungs by moistening and warming inhaled air.

## ▶ Common Symptoms of Respiratory Disease

Respiratory diseases are common, and some of their signs and symptoms are familiar.

- Breathing irregularities, including dyspnea (labored breathing) tachypnea (rapid breathing), and wheezing
- Coughs—dry, productive (produces mucus), hemoptysis (coughing blood)
- Cyanosis (blue color in skin and nails)
- Fever
- Pain
- Weakness

## ▶ Upper Respiratory Diseases

Upper respiratory diseases are infections occurring in sinuses, nose, and throat, and include common infections and allergies.

### The Common Cold

The common cold is familiar to everyone. Why is it so common? More than 200 strains of viruses, including adenoviruses, rhinoviruses, and a type of paramyxovirus, are capable of causing colds. Unlike many other diseases, infection provides no immunity because so many strains of virus exist.

A relatively contagious disease, a cold is an acute inflammation of the mucous membrane lining the upper respiratory tract. The virus infection triggers swelling of the nasal mucous membrane and mucous secretion, causing nasal congestion. There is no cure for the common cold, but symptoms can be treated. Aspirin lowers fever, and antihistamines relieve nasal congestion. Occasionally, secondary infections of sinuses occur, and if bacterial, these infections may be treated with antibiotics.

## Sinusitis

In the United States, approximately one person in seven has sinus problems at a cost of more than a billion dollars per year. The sinuses are air-filled spaces that reduce the weight of the skull and contribute resonance to the voice. The sinuses are referred to as paranasal sinuses because they all are connected to and drain their mucus secretions into the nasal cavity. The sinuses are named for the skull bone in which they are found: frontal, ethmoid, maxillary, and sphenoid.

In sinusitis, inflammation of the mucous membrane linings cause pressure, pain, and often a headache. Children tend to have ethmoid sinus inflammation more commonly than do adults (Figure 9–3).

Sinusitis is caused by viruses, bacteria, and allergens. Environmental conditions such as changes in barometric pressure, airplane flight, swimming, or diving activities may precipitate sinusitis. Inflammation also may follow a tooth extraction or dental work. Nasal congestion accompanying a cold may block sinus drainage and cause sinusitis.

Sinusitis may be diagnosed using physical exam, patient history, x-ray, and endoscopic sinuscopy. Nasal discharge may be sent to the laboratory to confirm or rule out bacterial infections.

Over-the-counter drugs like decongestants and antihistamines are common, inexpensive measures to treat sinusitis. These agents cause swollen mucous membranes to shrink. If pressure becomes chronic and painful, the sinuses may be drained with a sinus tap under local anesthesia.

## Nasal Polyps

Nasal polyps are noncancerous growths within the nose or sinus passageway. The exact cause of these growths is unknown. Certain chemicals found within these polyps may be the cause. Typically, nasal polyps form along with a sensitivity or allergic response to aspirin and some aspirin-like substitutes. Individuals with asthma and chronic rhinitis (nasal inflamma-

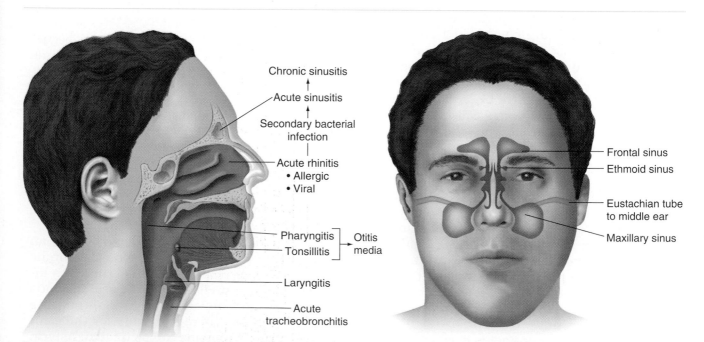

**Figure 9–3** Paranasal sinuses are part of the upper respiratory system. From here, infections may spread via nasopharynx to the middle ear or bronchi.

tion) are susceptible, as are children with cystic fibrosis. Large polyps cause nasal drainage, interfere with smell capability, and on rare occasion may be linked to obstructive sleep apnea.

Treatment may include nasal sprays with cortisone-like drugs to control allergies and surgery if the polyps are troublesome. However, even if surgery clears the passageway, it may not prevent the recurrence of the polyps.

## Snoring and Obstructive Sleep Apnea

Obstructive sleep apnea is the most common sleep disorder. Apnea is the cessation of breathing during the night due to an obstruction, usually nasal polyps, uvula, deviated septum, or fatty tissues. The incidence of sleep apnea is highest among middle-age, overweight males, but anyone may have this condition. Obstructive apnea causes heavy, long, and loud snoring and snorting. Four or five episodes of sleep apnea per hour significantly affects quality of life, while 20 episodes per hour is severe. Extreme cases reach 100 to 500 apneas in a single night. Without proper sleep, individuals awake tired and feel drowsy most of the day while functioning at low capacity. In 75% of cases, decreased bloodflow to the brain occurs. Therefore, the potential for cerebral stroke is increased, especially in moderate and severe apnea cases.

Treatment depends on the cause. If sinuses or nasal cavities are misshaped or blocked, they need repair. Some patients find relief with pharyngoplasty, the trimming of the uvula to prevent blockage of the breathing passageway.

## Hay Fever (Seasonal Allergic Rhinitis)

Hay fever, also called seasonal allergic rhinitis, is characterized by sensitivity to airborne allergens, especially pollens of ragweed and grasses. Allergens trigger respiratory mucosa to secrete excessive mucus, causing a runny nose and congestion. Mucosal surfaces of the eyes react to the allergens, causing redness, tearing, and itching.

Because the release of histamine causes these signs and symptoms, treatment includes antihistamine medications. Antihistamines do have side effects, such as drowsiness, dizziness, or muscular weakness. Many hay fever suffer-

ers take allergy injections to **desensitize** them to pollen or other allergens. Desensitizing works by administering small doses of antigen and gradually increasing the dosage, allowing the person to produce antibodies against it. These antibodies can inactivate the pollen before it interacts with the nasal mucosa.

## Tonsillitis, Pharyngitis, Laryngitis

The tonsils, pharynx, and larynx can be infected with bacteria, viruses, or other pathogens. Infections of these tissues lead to difficulty swallowing and redness and pain in the throat.

In the midsection of the throat (oropharynx) lie the palatine tonsils (Figure 9–4), masses of lymphatic tissue embedded into the lateral mucous membranes of the oropharynx. When infected the tonsils may swell and become painful, making swallowing very difficult. If infections are severe and recurrent, the tonsils may be surgically removed (tonsillectomy).

Pharyngitis, an inflammation of the pharynx, is characterized by pain in the throat. Foreign objects, hot liquids, or spicy foods may contribute to short-term pharyngitis. Breathing through the mouth due to nasal congestion or falling asleep with an open mouth dries the throat and can cause temporary discomfort. Strep throat is caused by streptococci and is characterized by a red, purulent throat. A throat

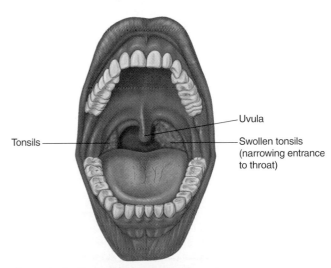

**Figure 9–4** Tonsils: normal and enlarged.

culture or a rapid immunological test that can be performed in the physician's office can confirm the presence of bacteria in the throat. Treatment includes antibiotics.

Laryngitis, an inflammation of the larynx or voice box, is characterized by hoarseness and aphonia. Bacteria, viruses, allergies, overuse of the voice, or exposure to caustic chemicals and smoke may cause a "lost voice." Antibiotics are used for bacterial infections. A viral infection called croup causes laryngitis in young children. Symptoms of croup or other laryngitis can be alleviated by resting the voice, drinking fluids, and using steam inhalations.

## Influenza

Influenza is a viral infection of the upper respiratory system. Many different strains of viruses cause influenza. Unfortunately, immunity for one strain does not protect against another strain.

The symptoms of flu are common and familiar. The onset is sudden, and within 2 days of exposure to the virus, symptoms develop, including chills, fever, cough, sore throat, runny nose, chest pain, muscle aches, and gastrointestinal disorders. The severity of flu cases varies from mild to severe, with pneumonia chief among the complications. The virus destroys the respiratory epithelium, and with the loss of this protection, the lungs become susceptible to pneumococci, streptococci, and staphylococci, all of which can cause pneumonia. Influenza is particularly serious in the elderly and chronically ill.

No medication cures influenza. Treatments are symptomatic and include rest, fluids, and aspirin to reduce fever. Antibiotics are prescribed to treat secondary bacterial infections.

Flu vaccines are available before the onset of the season, typically October and November, and are recommended for those considered at high risk: elderly and respiratory compromised. Unfortunately, these do not give immunity for all strains of the influenza virus.

Allergy, influenza, and cold share some characteristics, but actually are quite distinct (Table 9–1).

## ▶ Lower Respiratory Diseases

### Chronic Obstructive Pulmonary Disease

Chronic obstructive pulmonary disease (COPD), also known as chronic obstructive lung disease (COLD), includes a number of diseases in which the exchange of respiratory gases is ineffective. It includes chronic bronchitis, emphysema, and chronic asthma.

### Bronchitis

Bronchitis, inflammation of the bronchi, may be acute or chronic. The mucous membrane lining the bronchi becomes swollen and red, the typical inflammatory response. Irritants such as industrial fumes, automobile exhaust, viruses, and bacteria can cause acute bronchitis.

Acute bronchitis is most serious in small children, the chronically ill, and the elderly. The small bronchioles of children can become easily obstructed. The elderly or chronically ill are likely to have a secondary infection develop, such as pneumonia. Acute bronchitis is characterized by chest pains, dyspnea, cough, fever,

## Prevention ✚ PLUS!

### Influenza Vaccination

Who should get the flu vaccine? Why do we hear about the vaccine every year? Because the complications of influenza can be serious or fatal, those persons considered at risk should receive the vaccine. Those at risk include children, the elderly, persons with chronic debilitating diseases, persons with immune deficiencies, and health-care workers. The vaccine formula is different every year because the virus strains are different. The viruses are capable of mutation, and the immunity level an individual has one year may not protect against different strains that emerge the following year.

| Symptom/Sign | Allergy | Cold | Flu |
|---|---|---|---|
| Onset | Response to allergen | Slow | Fast |
| Duration | > Week | 1 week | 1–3 weeks |
| Season | Spring/Summer | Fall/Winter | Fall/Winter |
| Fever | None | Rare, < 100 | 102–104; lasts 3–4 days |
| Fatigue, weakness | Mild; varies | Quite mild | May last 2–3 weeks |
| Extreme exhaustion | Rare | Never | Early and prominent |
| General aches, pains | Varies | Slight | Usual; often severe |
| Headache | Usual | Rare | Prominent |
| Sneezing | Usual | Usual | Sometimes |
| Sore throat | Sometimes | Common | Sometimes |
| Stuffy nose | Common | Common | Sometimes |
| Nasal discharge | Clear | Yellow/greenish | Varies |
| Chest discomfort | Sometimes | Mild to moderate | Common; can be severe |
| Cough | None; dry | Yes | Yes; dry hacking |
| Vomit and/or diarrhea | Rare; varies | Rare | Common |

**Table 9–1 Comparison of Allergy, Cold, and Influenza**

and sometimes, chills. The sputum may contain pus. Depending on the cause, antibiotics may be administered. Viruses do not respond to antibiotics, but vapors, sprays, and cough medicines may give relief.

Chronic bronchitis is indicated by repeated attacks of acute bronchitis, and coughing with sputum production, lasting for at least 3 months for 2 consecutive years. It is more common in middle-aged men than in women.

The symptoms are the same as in acute bronchitis, but they persist. In chronic bronchitis, there is an excessive secretion of mucus from the mucous glands of the bronchial mucosa (lining). The mucous glands hypertrophy, and the mucosa itself is thickened and inflamed. The interference in the air passageway caused by the swelling and mucus reduces the person's oxygen level. Hypoxia, an insufficient oxygenation of the tissues, results. Poor drainage of the mucus sets the stage for bacterial infection. Parts of the respiratory tract can become necrotic, and fibrous scarring follows.

Chronic bronchitis may be a complication of another respiratory infection. It can result from long-term exposure to air pollutants or cigarette smoking. Respiratory diseases such as the flu or a common cold exacerbate chronic bronchitis. There is no cure for chronic bronchitis. The symptoms can be treated with antibiotics and moist vapors. A cigarette smoker should quit smoking, and clean air environments should be sought at all times.

## Bronchial Asthma

Bronchial asthma is characterized by hypersensitivity to various allergens like dust, mold, pollen, animal dander, and various foods. Eighty percent of asthmatic children and 50% of adult asthmatics have allergies. Asthma kills 15 people daily in the United States, according to the American Lung Association. The disease is increasing across the country; approximately 4 million Americans of all ages have the disease.

Constriction of smooth muscle in the walls of the bronchi and bronchioles narrows the lumen of the tubes. Recall the lack of cartilaginous rings in the bronchioles; this structural change allows spasms to occur. The spasm is caused by a sustained or intermittent contraction of the musculature, making breathing, particularly expiration, very difficult. Figure 9–5 shows the narrowed bronchi resulting from muscular contraction. The mucous membrane becomes swollen with fluid, also narrowing the lumen. Excessive secretion of mucus adds to the obstruction. Stale air becomes trapped, which decreases the

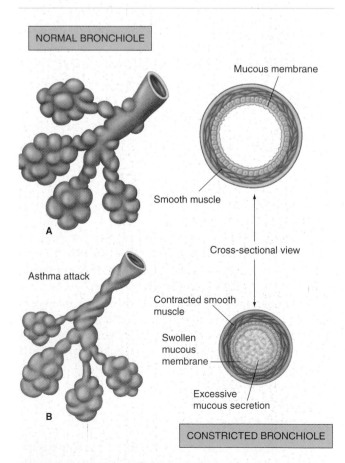

**NORMAL BRONCHIOLE**

Mucous membrane

Smooth muscle

A

Cross-sectional view

Asthma attack

Contracted smooth muscle

Swollen mucous membrane

Excessive mucous secretion

B

**CONSTRICTED BRONCHIOLE**

**Figure 9–5** Normal bronchiole (A) and one constricted (B) in asthma attack.

amount of fresh air that can enter the lungs. A characteristic wheezing sound results from air passing through the narrowed tubes.

Allergens typically trigger asthma. Nonallergic causes include anxiety, overexertion, infection, bronchitis, and exposure to cigarette smoke, aerosol sprays, or perfume. There is no cure for asthma, but attacks may become less severe with age. It is important to avoid the responsible allergens and other known triggers. Athletes should warm up before an event to prevent asthma caused by sudden overexertion.

Skin tests can show which allergens are responsible. Medication and allergy shots can reduce the incidence or severity of asthma attacks. Bronchodilators, ephedrine sprays, and epinephrine (adrenalin) injections are used to treat an acute attack. Cortisone drugs are sometimes used for prevention, but long-term use is associated with side effects. All medications used in the treatment of asthma must be carefully controlled and administered under close supervision of the physician. Antihistamines, although somewhat effective for hay fever, should not be used for asthma.

In the most severe form of asthma attack, called status asthmaticus, a tracheotomy, which is a surgical opening of the trachea, may be required. If not treated, status asthmaticus may end in respiratory failure and death.

## Emphysema

Emphysema is a crippling and debilitating obstruction and destruction of lung tissue. In emphysema, the alveolar walls break down, adjacent alveoli fuse, and the lungs lose their elasticity. Air cannot be adequately exhaled to allow oxygen to enter, and the lungs become filled with air that is high in carbon dioxide. Symptoms include a suffocating feeling and great distress from the inability to breathe. Severe pain accompanies the difficult breathing. To compensate for the reduced gas exchange, breathing becomes faster and deeper than normal. With the breakdown of alveolar walls, surrounding blood capillaries are damaged, and this causes obstruction of the pulmonary artery. The large air sacs, formed by the fusion of the alveoli, tend to rupture, allowing air into

## SIDE by SIDE ■ Emphysema

▲ Normal lung magnified 25x. (© J. Seibert/Custom Medical Stock Photo.)

▲ Emphysema. Note enlarged and fused alveoli in emphysema. (© C. Abrahams, M.D./Custom Medical Stock Photo.)

the pleural cavity, the space between the lungs and the chest wall. Air in this space causes the lung to collapse.

The most significant diagnostic test for emphysema uses a simple instrument, a spirometer, to measure the movement of air in and out of the lungs. X-rays do not show emphysema in the early stages. Physical exam reveals a chest wall permanently expanded, producing a characteristic "barrel" chest. A stethoscope placed on the chest detects abnormal respiratory sounds called rales. Because of right-sided heart failure and hypoxia, cyanosis is evident.

The cause of emphysema is not known, but it is strongly associated with heavy cigarette smoking. An inherited form involves a genetic deficiency in alpha-1-antitrypsin, which leaves the lungs susceptible to alveolar destruction. Other causes may include air pollution, long-term exposure to chemical irritants, and chronic bronchitis.

Progression of the disease can be controlled by eliminating smoking and avoiding polluted air containing smoke, fumes, irritating dust, and ozone, especially on days when the ozone level is high. Medications that clear mucus from the lungs help prevent infection. Some medica-

tions relieve difficult breathing. Physical therapy teaches how to use all the possible muscles for respiration in the abdomen and chest wall.

## Pneumonia

Pneumonia is an acute inflammation of the lung in which air spaces in the lungs become filled with an inflammatory exudate. Symptoms include dyspnea, fever, chest pain, and a productive cough. A chest x-ray and analysis of sputum can diagnose pneumonia and determine its cause. Pneumonia can be caused by a variety of microorganisms, and it may affect different areas within the lungs.

**Lobar Pneumonia** Lobar pneumonia is inflammation of a section, often an entire lobe, of the lung. Lobar pneumonia is caused by the pneumococcus bacterium *Streptococcus pneumoniae*. Many people carry this bacterium in their respiratory passages, and it can infect the lungs under optimal conditions (Figure 9–6). Influenza, chronic bronchitis, or weakened immune systems increase the risk of developing lobar pneumonia. Treatment includes antibiotics such as penicillin.

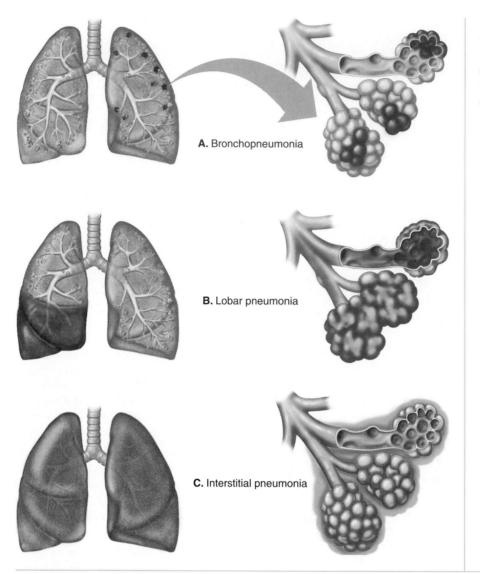

**A.** Bronchopneumonia

**B.** Lobar pneumonia

**C.** Interstitial pneumonia

**Figure 9–6**
(A) Bronchopneumonia with localized pattern. (B) Lobar pneumonia with a diffuse pattern within the lung lobe. (C) Interstial pneumonia is typically diffuse and bilateral.

**Bronchopneumonia**  Bronchopneumonia is a form of pneumonia focused in small bronchi. Because many foci of infection develop in the various bronchi, the chest x-ray will show a diffuse pattern of inflammation (Figure 9–6). This type of pneumonia is more common in debilitated patients who are bedridden from other diseases. Infection and aspiration of gastric contents are common causes. Major factors that increase the risk for bronchopneumonia include:

- Chronic bronchitis
- Measles or whooping cough
- Bronchiectasis
- Old age
- Cancer

**Primary Atypical Pneumonia**  Also known as walking pneumonia, primary atypical pneumonia is caused by a variety of pathogens, including viruses and atypical bacteria called *Mycoplasma pneumoniae*. Interstitial pneumonia, common in viral pneumonia, describes the diffuse pattern on x-ray (Figure 9–6). The disease is more common among adolescents and young adults.

**Secondary Pneumonia** Pneumonia can develop as a secondary disorder from other diseases that weaken the lungs or the body's immune system. Graft recipients and immunocompromised people, especially HIV/AIDS patients, are susceptible to pneumonia caused by unusual infectious agents like the fungi *Pneumocystis carini* and *Cryptococcus neoformans*. Postoperative patients, bedridden patients, and those with chronic respiratory illness may lack the ability to clear their lungs effectively and are at risk for developing pneumonia. Perhaps the most dangerous secondary pneumonia is the one acquired as a complication of influenza. It was responsible for most of the 20 million deaths in the influenza epidemic of 1918 to 1919. A devastating disease that apparently started in the United States, it was carried to (and from) Europe by American soldiers and always involved double pneumonia (both lungs). Today, influenza still causes many cases of pneumonia, therefore the flu vaccine is strongly recommended for persons at risk to prevent or reduce flu symptoms.

**Legionnaire's Disease** This lung infection is caused by the bacterium *Legionella pneumophila*. It is accompanied by flu-like symptoms, which sets it apart from other pneumonias. Because this is a serious and potentially fatal disease, it is important to differentiate it from other forms of pneumonia using sputum cultures and chest x-rays. The disease is acquired by inhaling small droplets contaminated with the bacteria from air conditioning cooling systems, humidifiers, and other equipment that produces aerosol water droplets. The antibiotic erythromycin is the treatment of choice.

## Pleurisy (Pleuritis)

Pleurisy is an inflammation of the pleural membranes and occurs as a complication of various lung diseases, such as pneumonia or tuberculosis. It may also develop from an injury or tumor formation. Pleurisy is extremely painful, with a sharp, stabbing pain accompanying each inspiration. The pain may stem from an excess or deficiency of pleural fluid, or from pus and blood in the pleural space. It is treated with antibiotics, heat applications, and bed rest.

## Pulmonary Tuberculosis

Pulmonary tuberculosis is a chronic infectious disease characterized by necrosis of vital lung tissue. Although it is most common in the respiratory system, it can affect other body systems as well.

The inhaled bacteria infect the lungs and induce a chronic inflammatory response that leads to necrosis. The tissue in this site becomes soft and cheese-like, which is why it is described as a caseous lesion. The tissue heals with fibrosis and calcification, walling off the bacteria for months or many years. These lesions are called tubercles. During this period, a person may have no symptoms. A secondary infection occurs when the person is infected again or when the bacteria escape the walled-off lesions in the lungs. The bacteria may spread this way when the person's resistance is reduced because of stress, infection, malnutrition, or immunodeficiency. During the secondary infection, leukocytes now recognize the bacteria and mount an attack that leads to greater necrosis and destruction of lung tissue. Necrotic tissue, blood, and bacteria may be coughed up. The bacteria may spread to other organs like the brain, kidney, and bones. Persons in the secondary stage of the disease also lose weight and become cachectic; this is the basis for the classic name for tuberculosis, *consumption*.

Tuberculosis is caused by the bacterium *Mycobacterium tuberculosis* and related bacteria. The bacteria are most commonly transmitted in contaminated sputum expelled in the coughs of infected persons, although tuberculosis can also be caused by contaminated milk from infected cattle. Expelled sputum may dry and settle in dust that can contain infective bacteria for a long time.

Antibiotics specially designed for *Mycobacterium* species include rifampin, isoniazid, ethambutol, and others. The drugs must be taken over an extended period of time for as long as 18 months to ensure that the bacteria are killed.

Screening for tuberculosis involves the Mantoux skin test in which antigens from the bacteria are injected beneath the skin. If previously exposed to tuberculosis, the skin swells with slight elevation at the injection site. A positive skin test should be followed up with a sputum culture and a chest x-ray to determine if there is an active infection.

Tuberculosis is relatively uncommon in much of the United States, but its incidence has increased since the 1980s and 1990s. The evolution of antibiotic-resistant bacteria and the increased numbers of HIV-infected people, homeless people, and immigrants contribute to this increase (Table 9–2).

Worldwide, however, the incidence of tuberculosis is rising rapidly, especially in Asia, Russia, and parts of Africa. In fact, tuberculosis remains the largest cause of death due to infectious disease, killing 3,000 people per day, and is a major cause of death among people infected with HIV. More than one-third of the world's population is exposed to *Mycobacterium tuberculosis*.

## Bronchogenic Carcinoma (Lung Cancer)

Bronchogenic carcinoma is the most common type of lung cancer, causing 28% of all cancer deaths, making it the leading cause of death from cancer among both men and women. In addition to primary carcinoma of the lungs, the lungs are a frequent site of metastases from the breast, GI tract, female reproductive system, and kidneys.

The great danger in bronchogenic carcinoma is blockage of the airway by the malignant tumor as it grows into the lumen of a bronchus, causing collapse of the affected part of the lung. A malignant lung tumor is shown in Figure 9–7. Few symptoms or signs accompany early stage lung cancer, but symptoms of later stages include a persistent cough and hemoptysis. The blood in the sputum results from the erosion of blood vessels by the growing malignancy. Anorexia, weight loss, and weakness accompany the disease, caused partly by poor oxygenation of the blood. Other symptoms include difficulty in breathing caused by the obstructed airway. Because these symptoms develop late in the disease, when metastasis is likely to have occurred, prevention and early detection are essential. At present, however, the average age at diagnosis is 60, and it is likely that many of these cancers began years earlier.

Approximately 80% of lung cancer is related to cigarette smoking, and it is 10 times more common in smokers than in nonsmokers. Other causes include inhalation of carcinogens, which may be an occupational hazard among workers who are constantly exposed to air pollution, exhaust gases, and industrial fumes.

Diagnosis of lung cancer is made from a biopsy of the tumor, detecting cancer cells in the sputum, or washings from the bronchoscopy examination.

| Table 9–2   Tuberculosis Increase in the United States | |
| --- | --- |
| Drug-resistant bacteria | More infections that cannot be treated with a single drug |
| | More infections resistant to multiple drugs |
| | Infections last longer and expose more people |
| Homeless/refugees/poverty | Reduced access to health care, screening, and treatment |
| | Living conditions, malnutrition, and other infections increase susceptibility |
| Immigration | Infected immigrants from areas where the disease is endemic, prevalent, drug-resistant |
| HIV/AIDS | Increased susceptibility to disease |

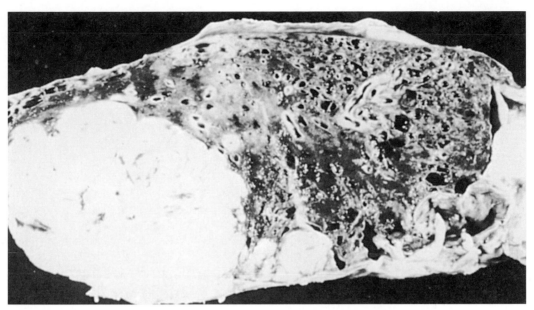

**Figure 9–7** Carcinoma of the lung (large white area). (Courtesy of Dr. David R. Duffell.)

Treatment includes surgery, radiation, or chemotherapy, depending on the particular tumor.

## Cystic Fibrosis

Cystic fibrosis is an inherited disease that affects the exocrine glands of the body, causing them to secrete excessively viscous mucus, which blocks ducts and prevents the glands from delivering their products. Exocrine glands secrete mucus, perspiration, and digestive enzymes.

The most serious manifestation of cystic fibrosis is in the respiratory system. The trachea and bronchi secrete thick mucus that accumulates and blocks the air passageway. Symptoms of cystic fibrosis are dyspnea, wheezing, persistent cough, and thick sputum. The abnormal mucosal surface increases susceptibility to recurrent bacterial infections. Bronchiectasis (weakened and dilated bronchial tubing) is a common complication of cystic fibrosis. Lung collapse can result from the inability to inflate them, and most deaths occur as a result of respiratory failure. Table 9–3 describes complications of cystic fibrosis.

Also exocrine glands, sweat glands are affected in cystic fibrosis. They excrete excessive perspiration and large amounts of salt, causing susceptibility to heat exhaustion.

Excessive mucus also blocks the ducts of the pancreas, preventing the release of digestive enzymes, resulting in weight loss and malnutrition. Lack of fat digestion results in large, bulky, foul-smelling stools. In the pancreas, the glands become dilated and develop into cysts containing thick mucus. Fibrous tissue then develops, which explains how cystic fibrosis gets its name.

Cystic fibrosis is a hereditary disease that first becomes manifested in young children. It is transmitted through a recessive gene carried by each parent (see Chapter 5). Before the disease was understood, the mortality rate of children was extremely high. Early diagnosis and treatment has greatly improved the prognosis.

Abnormal excretion of salt in sweat is the basis for the test that confirms cystic fibrosis. Treatment includes pancreatic enzyme supplements that can be given with food. Antibiotic treatment reduces the incidence of respiratory tract infection, and regular respiratory therapy relieves congestion in the respiratory tract.

| Table 9–3 Complications of Cystic Fibrosis | |
| --- | --- |
| Malnutrition | Blockage of pancreatic duct prevents secretion of digestive enzymes<br>Inability to digest and absorb nutrients |
| Dyspnea, lung collapse | Blocked airways, bronchiectasis |
| Recurrent respiratory infections | Abnormal mucosal lining<br>Inability to clear thick mucus |
| Electrolyte imbalance | Abnormal salt excretion |

## ▶ Age-Related Diseases

Because respiratory infections are generally highly contagious, they are common among infants and children. Historically, children have suffered a high mortality rate from diphtheria, pertussis, measles, and other contagious respiratory diseases. Vaccinations for these and other respiratory diseases have significantly reduced mortality in the United States. However, around the world where vaccines are unavailable these diseases continue to kill many children.

The onset of asthma may be early or later in life, and while some cases of early-onset asthma may resolve, later-onset asthma generally tends to persist.

In the elderly, elastic tissue of the lungs deteriorates and reduces lung capacity. This condition is exacerbated by weakening of respiratory muscles and arthritis in joints of the ribs and vertebrae.

Prescribed exercises performed regularly can help maintain or improve lung capacity and benefit the cardiovascular system as well.

Some degree of emphysema occurs in individuals age 50 to 70. On average, one square foot of the respiratory membrane is lost each year after age 30.

The incidence of lung cancer increases with age. However, the cancer probably begins earlier in life, and this incidence reflects the relatively late age at diagnosis.

## ▶ Diagnostic Procedures for Respiratory Diseases

Several important imaging procedures include bronchoscopy, chest x-rays, and fluoroscopy, which permits visualization of the lungs and diaphragm during respiration. Computerized tomography, or CT scans, augment chest x-rays.

Arterial blood analysis evaluates gas levels and blood pH, a key indication of respiratory function. Sputum examination is helpful in the evaluation of pneumonia and malignancies. Gram-stained smears and cultures are useful in identifying causative organisms, determining proper antibiotic treatment, and diagnosing tuberculosis and fungal lung infections. Spirometry measures changes in gas volume in the lungs and determines ventilation capacity and flow rate.

## CHAPTER SUMMARY

Viruses and bacteria can cause diseases of the upper respiratory system. Common viral infections include the common cold and influenza. Pyogenic bacteria cause pus formation as well as inflammation of the mucous membranes. Allergies affect the upper respiratory tract as well as the bronchi. Asthma and allergic rhinitis are caused by hypersensitivity to certain allergens. Excessive mucus production and narrowed airways are characteristics of these diseases. Airway obstruction causes other respiratory diseases. For example, chronic bronchitis can lead to pneumonia or emphysema. Pneumonia has a variety of causes, including viruses and bacteria. The elderly, chronically ill, and immunocompromised persons are especially susceptible and should consider receiving vaccines.

Tuberculosis is a chronic infection, typically affecting the lungs, and is increasing in incidence in the United States and throughout the world. HIV/AIDS and the development of resistant bacteria are two reasons for this increase.

Lung cancer is a malignancy with poor prognosis. Prevention and early diagnosis are key. This cancer is clearly linked to tobacco use. Since 1986, lung cancer has been the leading cause of cancer death in women and men.

Cystic fibrosis is an inherited disease that has its most serious manifestations in the respiratory system.

## RESOURCES

Frazier, M. S., & J. W. Drymkowski. *Essentials of Human Diseases and Conditions,* 2nd ed. Saunders, 2000.

Martini, F. H., E. F. Bartholomew, K. Welch, et. al. *The Human Body in Health and Disease.* Prentice Hall, 2000.

Cohen, B. J., & D. L. Wood. *Memmler's The Human Body in Health and Disease,* 9th ed. Lippincott Williams and Wilkins, 2000.

Tamparo, C. D. & M. A. Lewis, *Diseases of the Human Body, 3rd ed.* F.A. Davis, 2001.

Dacy, M. D. 1988. Nasal polyps, *Mayo Clinic Health Letter,* vol. 6, no. 8.

Haney, D. Q. 2004. Study discovers "bug" behind common cold, *Northwest Herald,* Feb. 29, 2004.

World Health Organization: www.who.org

# DISEASES AT A GLANCE

## Respiratory System

| DISEASE | ETIOLOGY | SIGNS AND SYMPTOMS |
| --- | --- | --- |
| Pharyngitis | Bacteria, viruses, irritants | Red, sore throat; pus; dysphagia |
| Laryngitis | Bacteria, viruses, irritants | Sore throat, difficulty speaking |
| Tonsillitis | Bacteria, viruses, irritants | Sore throat, swollen tonsils, dysphagia |
| Common cold | Paramyxoviruses | Nasal congestion, cough, sore throat |
| Seasonal allergic rhinitis (hay fever) | Airborne allergens, pollens | Nasal and sinus congestion; watery, itchy eyes |
| Influenza | Viruses | Fever, headache, weakness, body aches |
| Pulmonary tuberculosis | Mycobacterium | Primary may be asymptomatic, secondary with fever, weakness, weight loss/cachexia, cough producing blood, tissue, bacteria |
| Asthma | Allergies, fumes, heavy exertion, roaches | Dyspnea, difficulty exhaling, wheezing |
| Chronic bronchitis | Fumes, bacteria, viruses, smoking | Chest pains, dyspnea, chronic productive cough |
| Emphysema | Cigarette smoking, fumes, genetic | Difficulty exhaling, cyanosis, fatigue, barrel chest pneumonia as complication |
| Cystic fibrosis | Genetic | Recurrent lung infections, coughing and lung obstruction, weight loss due to poor absorption of nutrients |
| Pneumonia | Bacteria, viruses, fungi | Chest pain, fluid in lungs on x-ray, fever, productive cough |
| Bronchogenic carcinoma (lung cancer) | Smoking, fumes, air pollution | Obstruction of airways and associated complications, weight loss, weakness |

| DIAGNOSIS | TREATMENT |
| --- | --- |
| Physical exam, throat culture | If bacterial, antibiotics |
| Physical exam | Resting voice, steam inhalations, higher fluid intake |
| Physical exam, throat culture | Antibiotics if bacterial infections |
| Physical exam | Antihistamines, aspirin |
| Physical exam, allergy tests | Antihistamines |
| Physical exam | Bed rest, fluids, aspirin |
| Chest x-ray, skin test, sputum analysis | Antibiotics |
| Spirometry, physical exam | Ephedrine sprays, epinephrine, cortisone-like drugs, allergy shots |
| Patient history, physical exam | Vapors, sprays, cough medicine; if bacterial, antibiotics |
| Spirometry, physical exam | Elimination of inhaled irritants, mucus-thinning drugs |
| Sweat test for excess salt | Respiratory therapy, antibiotics, pancreatic enzyme supplements |
| Chest x-ray, sputum analysis | If bacterial, antibiotics |
| Bronchoscopy, x-ray, CT scan, biopsy, sputum evaluation | Radiation, chemotherapy, surgery |

# Interactive Activities

## Cases for Critical Thinking

1. A young man has chest pain, cough, difficulty breathing, and a fever. Obviously, these could be caused by a variety of diseases. What diagnostic procedures would be helpful in diagnosing the man's disease?

2. At age 62, Harry decided to retire from the grain mill where he had worked for 40 years. He was walking much slower and felt weaker even though he was walking less. He had enjoyed his smoke breaks and lunches with the guys, but now he had difficulty getting his breath, while his breathing rate had increased and his chest seemed inflated. What disease seems apparent here, and how may it be addressed?

3. Sara loved to run. She watched the track meets at school even as a first grader. An asthmatic, she occasionally had to use an inhaler, but seemed determined to be an athlete. Should Sara be discouraged from pursuing her goal? Why or why not?

## Multiple Choice

1. What COPD is primarily caused by smoking, may have a genetic link, and has no cure?
   a. bronchitis
   b. diphtheria
   c. tuberculosis
   d. emphysema

2. Inflammation of bronchial membranes, destruction of cilia, and excess thick mucus production are characteristics of _____.
   a. emphysema
   b. chronic bronchitis
   c. asthma
   d. tuberculosis

3. Antibiotics may be a part of the treatment for all of these diseases except _____.
   a. pneumonia
   b. Legionnaire's disease
   b. emphysema
   c. pharyngitis

4. The disease formerly known as consumption is _____.
   a. pneumonia
   b. asthma
   c. tuberculosis
   d. lung cancer

5. What disease of the young or old may be triggered by allergies and emotions or heavy exercise?
   a. bronchitis
   b. sinusitis
   c. asthma
   d. pharyngitis

6. Streptococci are one of the causes of _____.
   a. pneumonia
   b. tuberculosis
   c. Legionnaire's disease
   d. influenza

7. A "barrel chest" is often indicative of what respiratory disease?
   a. pneumonia
   b. emphysema
   c. cancer
   d. bronchitis

8. Legionnaire's disease is caused by _____
   a. fungi
   b. viruses
   c. low-humidity climates
   d. bacteria

9. What structures line respiratory epithelium and move mucus?
   a. cilia
   b. bronchi
   c. tonsils
   d. alveoli

10. Overuse of the voice can cause _____.
    a. pneumonia
    b. tonsillitis
    c. bronchitis
    d. laryngitis

## True or False

_____ 1. The flu can be prevented by vaccine.

_____ 2. The common cold is easily treated with antibiotics.

_____ 3. Laryngitis may be treated by removal of the tonsils.

_____ 4. Lungs are a common site for metastatic cancer.

_____ 5. Asthma and tuberculosis are declining because of new potent antibiotics.

_____ 6. Dyspnea is the coughing of blood.

_____ 7. Bronchiectasis is a collapse of lobes of the lung.

_____ 8. The body can survive only minutes without air.

_____ 9. COPD means Contagious Pulmonary Disorder.

_____ 10. Pharyngitis may include tonsillitis.

## Fill-Ins

1. The _____ test is used to screen for tuberculosis.

2. _____ is a complication of the cold and causes headache and nasal drainage.

3. The main cause of lung cancer is _____.

4. A simple breathing test for pulmonary functioning is _____.

5. The common cold, influenza, and atypical pneumonia are caused by _____.

6. Painful swelling of the membranes surrounding the lungs is called _____.

7. The most common form of pneumonia is _____.

8. Wheezing and difficulty in exhaling are symptoms of _____.

9. Nasal, tracheal, and bronchi linings are swept clean by tiny hairs called _____.

10. Mucus secretion is thick and excessive in the inherited disease called _____.

## MedMedia Wrap-Up

**www.prenhall.com/mulvihill**

Remember to visit this website for extra study practice, including exercises, Internet links, news updates, and an audio glossary.

**Activity CD-ROM**

Check out the CD-ROM in the back of this book. You will find games, exercises, puzzles, and videos to help enhance your understanding of this chapter.

# Diseases of the Digestive System

CHAPTER

10

## Learning Objectives

After studying this chapter, you should be able to

- Describe the normal structure and function of the digestive tract
- Describe the key characteristics of major diseases of the digestive tract
- Name key diagnostic tests for selected digestive tract diseases
- Explain the cause of digestive tract diseases
- Name the treatment of digestive tract diseases
- Describe the general disorders and symptoms associated with digestive tract diseases
- Describe the normal functions of the liver, gallbladder, and pancreas
- Describe the key characteristics of major diseases of the liver, gallbladder, and pancreas
- Name the causes of diseases of the liver, gallbladder, and pancreas
- Name the diagnostic procedures for diseases of the liver, gallbladder, and pancreas
- Describe the treatment options for diseases of the liver, gallbladder, and pancreas
- Describe age-related diseases of the digestive system

## Fact or Fiction?

Cancer of the colon or rectum is the second leading cause of cancer-related death in the United States.

*Fact:* The American Cancer Society estimates that each year 56,000 Americans will die of colorectal cancer, second only to lung cancer.

# Disease Chronicle

## Dysentery

Diseases of the digestive system include common ailments familiar to nearly everyone. Some are minor annoyances; others are serious, life-threatening diseases. The impact of digestive system diseases is undeniable. During the American Civil War, 81,360 soldiers died from dysentery, while 93,443 were killed in combat. Even today, 18,000 cases of bacillary dysentery occur annually in the United States. Despite modern medical diagnosis and treatment, cancer of the pancreas, colon, and liver remain deadly, and worldwide, dysentery remains a leading cause of death among children.

## MedMedia
www.prenhall.com/mulvihill

Use the web address to the left to access the free, interactive Companion Website created for this textbook. It features chapter-specific exercises, Internet links, news links, and an audio glossary. Additionally, explore the CD-ROM that accompanies this book to discover Disease Focus videos and a rich array of activities that accompany this chapter.

## ▶ The Digestive System

The digestive system consists of a digestive tract through which food passes and accessory organs that assist the digestive process. The digestive tract begins at the mouth and includes the pharynx, esophagus, stomach, small intestine, and large intestine. The accessory organs include the liver, gallbladder, and pancreas.

Digestion begins in the mouth with chewing, the mechanical breakdown of food. Salivation, the secretion of saliva, moistens the food and provides an enzyme for initial digestion of starch. The food is then swallowed and passes through the pharynx, or throat, and into the esophagus.

The moistened food moves down the esophagus to the stomach. A sphincter muscle at the juncture of the esophagus and stomach prevents regurgitation while digestion continues. The stomach secretes gastric juice that contains enzymes, biological catalysts that act on protein. Gastric juice also contains hydrochloric acid, which activates these enzymes. The acidic gastric contents would be very irritating to the stomach lining if the lining were not protected by a thick covering of mucus. A great deal of moistening and mixing occurs within the stomach. The moistened, mixed, and acidic food, is called chyme.

Chyme passes from the stomach into the small intestine through a sphincter muscle, the pyloric sphincter. This sphincter is closed until it receives nerve and hormonal signals to relax and open. Chyme is propelled along its course by rhythmical, smooth muscle contractions of the intestinal wall called peristalsis.

Most digestion occurs in the first part of the small intestine, the duodenum. Intestinal secretions contain mucus and digestive enzymes, which enter by means of the pancreatic duct from the pancreas. The pancreas secretes enzymes that digest protein, lipid, and carbohydrate. It also secretes an alkaline solution for the neutralization of acid carried into the small intestine from the stomach.

Bile, secreted by the liver and stored in the gallbladder, enters the duodenum through the common bile duct. Bile is not an enzyme but an emulsifier, a substance that reduces large fat droplets into much smaller fat droplets, enabling the lipid enzymes to digest fat into small, absorbable units.

When digestion is complete, nutrients such as sugars and amino acids are absorbed into blood capillaries and lymph vessels in the intestinal wall. The inner surface of the small intestine is arranged to provide the greatest amount of surface area possible for digestion and absorption. This mucosal surface contains numerous fingerlike projections called villi, each of which contains capillaries and lymph vessels for absorption (Figure 10–1).

Material not digested passes into the large intestine, or colon. The first part of the colon is a blind sac, the cecum, to which the appendix, a fingerlike mass of lymphatic tissue, is attached. Water and minerals are absorbed from the large intestine, and the remaining matter is excreted as feces. Figure 10–2 illustrates the complete digestive system.

In this chapter, the diseases of each part of the digestive system are described. These include diseases of the mouth, esophagus, stomach, small and large intestines, pancreas, liver, and gallbladder.

## ▶ Diseases of the Mouth

Complete coverage of oral pathology is beyond the scope of this book. This chapter discusses the major oral inflammatory diseases and neoplasms. Diseases of the mouth can adversely affect the ability to taste, chew, moisten, and swallow food.

### Oral Inflammation

Oral inflammation can be caused by local infection of the mouth with bacteria, viruses, or fungi, or it may be a sign of a systemic infection. Stomatitis refers to a widespread inflammation of oral tissue. Depending on the cause, inflammation may appear as patches, ulcers, redness, bleeding, or necrosis.

Streptococci, spread in salivary and respiratory droplets, are a common cause of oral bacterial infections, resulting in red, swollen mu-

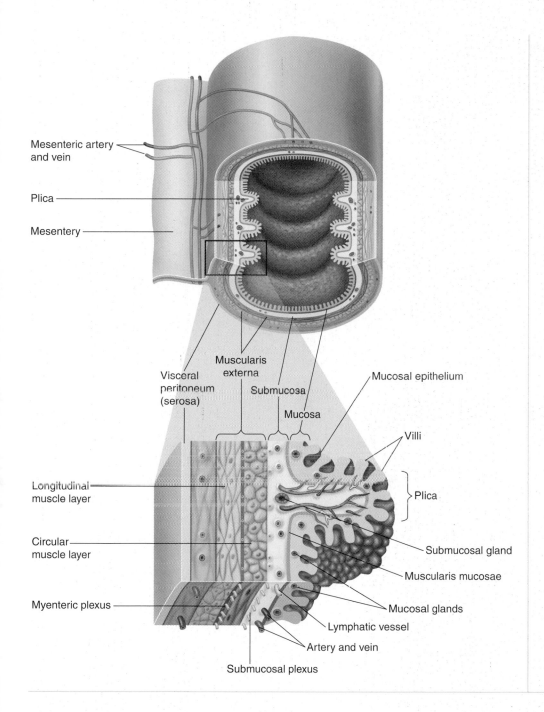

**Figure 10–1**
Mucosal surface of the
small intestine.

Mesenteric artery
and vein

Plica

Mesentery

Visceral
peritoneum
(serosa)

Muscularis
externa

Submucosa

Mucosa

Mucosal epithelium

Villi

Plica

Longitudinal
muscle layer

Circular
muscle layer

Submucosal gland

Muscularis mucosae

Mucosal glands

Myenteric plexus

Lymphatic vessel

Artery and vein

Submucosal plexus

cosa. Bacteria also cause canker sores, small circular lesions with a red border. These painful lesions heal without scars after a week. *Neisseria gonorrhea,* the cause of the sexually transmitted disease gonorrhea, causes painful ulcerations in the mouth and throat. Also sexually transmitted, *Treponema pallidum* causes syphilis, which causes oral chancres and ulcerations. These bacterial infections are treated with antibiotics.

Herpes simplex is a common cause of oral virus infections. Transmitted by oral–genital contact, herpes simplex type 2 causes vesicles that rupture to form ulcers. These lesions can

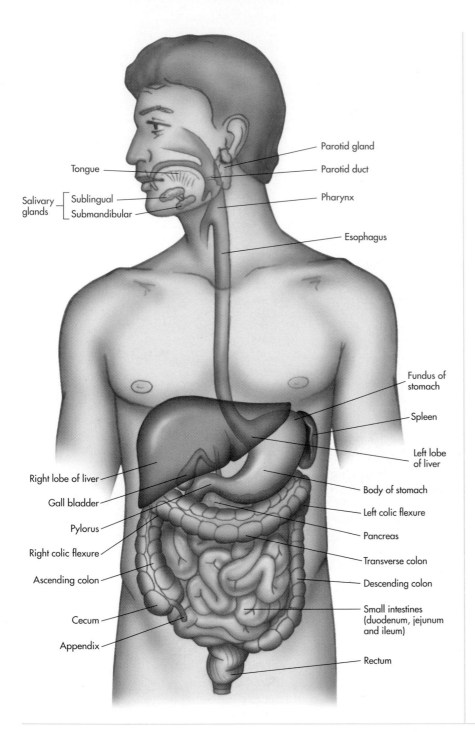

**Figure 10–2**
The digestive system.

appear inside and outside the mouth. Herpes simplex type 1 can also be acquired from salivary droplets. Pain makes eating, drinking, and swallowing difficult. The symptoms typically subside within two weeks when the viruses move from the area to nerve tissue known as ganglia. The infection can be reactivated following stressful events or suppression of immune function. Treatment is aimed at reducing inflammation and pain with systemic anti-inflammatory and analgesic medications or topical anesthetics.

The fungus *Candida albicans* is present in the mouth in low levels normally, but can overgrow in persons with immune deficiencies or following long courses of antibiotic or corticosteroid treatment. The fungal overgrowth, called candidiasis or thrush, resembles cheese curds, but if removed, leaves a raw, damaged mucosal surface. Antibiotics and antiviral medications are not effective treatments for fungal infections (see Chapter 3). Oral candidiasis is treated with oral antifungal agents like nystatin or fluconazole.

## Cancer of the Mouth

Mouth and throat cancer remains among the 10 leading causes of cancer death worldwide. The most common form of oral cancer is squamous cell carcinoma. Most of these cancers appear on the floor of the mouth, tongue, and lower lip. An aggressive form of the cancer occurs on the upper lip. Tobacco (including smokeless tobacco) and alcohol use are major risk factors. Use of both alcohol and tobacco increases the risk. Lip and tongue carcinoma may be removed surgically. Radiation therapy may be used to treat local carcinomas on the floor of the mouth.

## ▶ Diseases of the Esophagus

The function of the esophagus is the controlled passage of food to the stomach. Esophageal disease manifests itself as dysphagia, or difficult or painful swallowing.

## Cancer of the Esophagus

Relatively uncommon, cancer of the esophagus narrows the lumen, causing the principal symptom, dysphagia. The obstruction causes vomiting, and the person may experience a bad taste in his or her mouth or bad breath. There is accompanying weight loss because of the inability to eat.

The carcinoma spreads into adjacent organs and to remote sites through the lymph vessels. It frequently metastasizes before it is detected. Prognosis for cancer of the esophagus is poor. Like mouth cancer, tobacco and alcohol use are major risk factors.

## Esophageal Varices

Varicose veins that develop in the esophagus are called esophageal varices. They result from pressure within the veins, causing the veins to appear very dilated and knotty. Increased pressure develops when venous return to the liver is obstructed, as happens in cirrhosis. The most serious danger in esophageal varices is hemorrhage. Bleeding esophageal varices requires emergency treatment. Infusion of vasopressin may reduce bleeding, or bleeding can be stopped with pressure on the varices by inserting a Minnesota or Sengstaken-Blakemore tube. These are temporary measures. Surgical bypass of the portal vein to systemic flow may reduce pressure in the veins and thus stop bleeding, but will not repair liver damage and ultimately may not improve the prognosis.

## Esophagitis

Esophagitis, inflammation of the esophagus, causes burning chest pains, "heartburn," which can resemble the pain of heart disease. The pain may follow eating or drinking, and some vomiting of blood may occur. The most common cause of esophagitis is a reflux, a backflow of the acid contents of the stomach. The condition is known as gastroesophageal reflux disease. This may be caused by an incompetent cardiac sphincter, which normally prevents stomach contents from ascending the esophagus. The acid of the stomach irritates the lining of the esophagus and stimulates an inflammatory response. Treatment includes a nonirritating diet, antacids, and acid-reducing medications. Frequent, small meals are recommended. Alcohol is an irritant to the inflamed mucosal lining and should be avoided.

### Hiatal Hernia

A hernia is the protrusion of part of an organ through a muscular wall or body opening. A hiatal hernia is the protrusion of part of the stomach through the diaphragm at the point where the esophagus joins the stomach. Figure 10–3 shows this condition. The person experiences indigestion and heartburn after eating and may feel short of breath. Avoidance of irritants such as spicy foods and caffeine, and frequent small meals, may be adequate treatment. If the person is obese, weight loss is recommended. Surgery is often required to correct the defect.

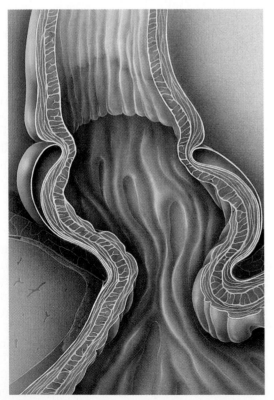

**Figure 10–3**   Hiatal hernia. (© K. Somerville/Custom Medical Stock Photo.)

## Diseases of the Stomach

The stomach is well adapted for storing and mixing food with acid and enzymes. Alterations in the stomach lining or malignancies can cause painful and sometimes serious disease.

### Gastritis

Acute gastritis is an inflammation of the stomach caused by irritants such as aspirin, excessive coffee, tobacco, alcohol, or infection. Vomiting of blood frequently occurs as the principal symptom. Gastroscopy is extremely valuable in diagnosing this disease. A camera may be attached to the gastroscope, and the entire inner stomach is photographed. Acute alcoholism is a major cause of hemorrhagic gastritis. Alcohol stimulates acid secretion, which irritates the mucosa. If the bleeding cannot be controlled, surgery may be required.

### Chronic Atrophic Gastritis

In cancer of the stomach, neither intrinsic factor nor hydrochloric acid is secreted. Intrinsic factor is required for the absorption of vitamin $B_{12}$, and hydrochloric acid aids digestion of proteins. This degenerative condition is described as chronic atrophic gastritis. Little can be done to treat the disease, as the name, atrophic (wasting), suggests. Irritants such as alcohol, aspirin, and certain foods should be avoided.

### Peptic Ulcers

Ulcers are lesions of any body surface where necrotic tissue forms as a result of inflammation and is sloughed off, leaving a hole. Ulcers of the stomach and small intestine are termed peptic ulcers. Ulcers of the stomach are called gastric ulcers, and those of the small intestine are called duodenal ulcers. Figure 10–4 shows common sites of peptic ulcers.

Peptic ulcers are caused, in part, by pepsin, a proteolytic enzyme secreted by the stomach. Hydrochloric acid of the stomach and intestinal juice, including bile, which is regurgitated through the pyloric sphincter, also irritate the gastric mucosa. Irritated and inflamed mucous

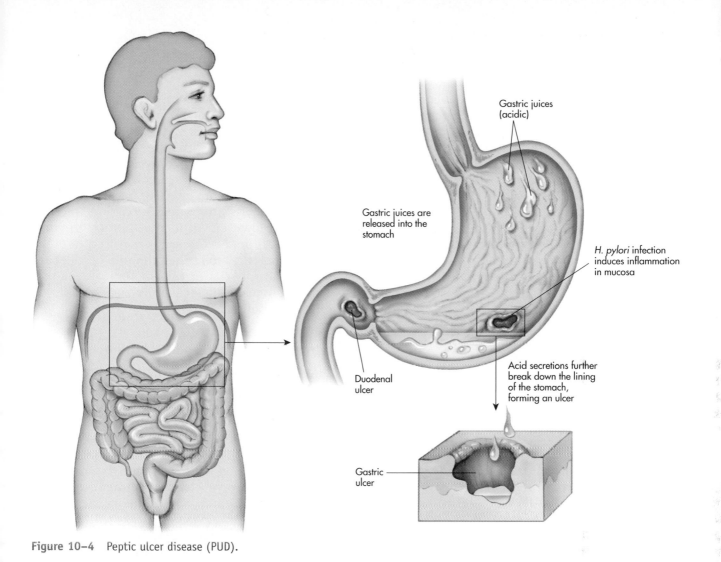

**Gastric juices (acidic)**

**Gastric juices are released into the stomach**

*H. pylori* infection induces inflammation in mucosa

**Duodenal ulcer**

Acid secretions further break down the lining of the stomach, forming an ulcer

**Gastric ulcer**

**Figure 10–4** Peptic ulcer disease (PUD).

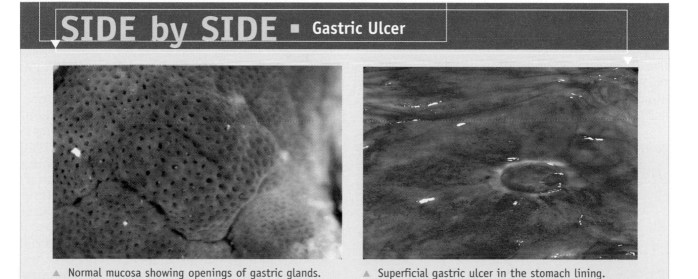

## SIDE by SIDE ■ Gastric Ulcer

▲ Normal mucosa showing openings of gastric glands.
(© C. Abrahams, M.D./Custom Medical Stock Photo.)

▲ Superficial gastric ulcer in the stomach lining.

membrane may become necrotic, leaving a hole. Infection with the bacterium *Helicobacter pylori* is associated with ulcers. The bacterial infection causes mucosal inflammation, exposing the surface to the effects of pepsin and acid. Because hydrochloric acid secretion is under nerve and hormonal control, stressful situations can trigger or exacerbate ulcers.

Ulcer pain is caused by the action of hydrochloric acid on the exposed surface of the lesion. The muscular contractions of peristalsis also intensify the pain. The person with a gastric ulcer experiences nausea, vomiting, and abdominal pain.

Several complications of a peptic ulcer are given in Table 10–1. A potential complication of any ulcer is hemorrhage; severe hemorrhage may lead to shock. It is possible for a large artery at the base of the ulcer to rupture as the lesion erodes deeper into underlying tissues. Bleeding from the ulcer may appear as **hematemesis** or bloody vomitus, or the blood may appear in stools, where it gives the stools a dark, tarry appearance, referred to as **melena**. A serious ulcer complication is **perforation**. If an ulcer perforates—that is, breaks through the intestinal or gastric wall—there is sudden and intense abdominal pain. **Peritonitis**, inflammation of the lining of the abdominal cavity, usually results when the digestive contents enter the cavity, because this material contains numerous bacteria. Surgical repair of the perforation is required immediately. Obstruction of the gastrointestinal tract can result from an ulcer and the scar tissue surrounding it. Obstruction occurs most frequently in a narrow area of the stomach, near the pyloric sphincter. Ulcer pain can cause the sphincter to go into spasm, also resulting in obstruction.

The main objectives of treatment for peptic ulcer disease are to promote healing, prevent complications and recurrences, and provide pain relief. Acid reducers, such as omeprazole or ranitidine, are more effective for peptic ulcers than are antacids and mucosal barriers such as sucraflate. However, antibiotic therapy in combination with acid reducers is required to eradicate *H. pylori* and to reduce the rate of ulcer relapse. If the ulcer is stress- or tension-related, certain changes in lifestyle or approach to stress might be beneficial.

## Gastroenteritis and Food Poisoning

Gastroenteritis is an inflammation of the stomach and intestines. Symptoms include anorexia, nausea, vomiting, and diarrhea. The onset may be abrupt and violent with rapid loss of fluid and electrolytes. Possible causes are bacterial or viral infection, chemical toxins, lactose intolerance, or other food allergy, although the actual cause is not always clear. Treatment replaces fluid and nutritional requirements, including the lost salts. Antispasmodic medications can control the vomiting and diarrhea.

Food contaminated with human or animal feces may carry microorganisms that cause gastroenteritis and food poisoning. *Escherichia coli* is a common normal inhabitant of human or animal intestines. Certain strains may cause disease, like traveler's diarrhea, or more serious diseases, like hemolytic uremic syndrome, in which toxins cause potentially fatal shut-down of the kidneys. To prevent infection, cook meat thoroughly and practice good hygiene in the kitchen.

One of the common forms of food poisoning is caused by the bacterium *Salmonella*. These bacteria invade the intestinal mucosa and cause sudden, colicky abdominal pain, nausea, vomiting, and sometimes bloody diarrhea and fever that begins approximately 6 to 48 hours after eating contaminated food and lasts up to 2 weeks. A stool culture can identify the bacteria. *Salmonella* food poisoning (salmonellosis) is associated with contaminated eggs and poultry, but most any food may harbor the bacteria. Treatment usually consists of replenishing

| Table 10–1 | Complications of Peptic Ulcers |
|---|---|
| Obstructions | |
| Peritonitis | |
| Hemorrhage/shock | |

water, electrolytes, and nutrients. Elderly individuals, young children, and immunocompromised people are at risk of developing serious infection, and they may require more intervention, including a short course of antibiotics and antidiarrheal medications.

## Cancer of the Stomach

Carcinoma of the stomach may be a large mass projecting into the lumen of the stomach, or it may invade the stomach wall, causing it to thicken. As the tumor grows, the lumen is narrowed to the point of obstruction. The remainder of the stomach becomes extremely dilated due to the blockage, and pain results from pressure on nerve endings. Infection frequently accompanies cancer, which causes additional pain. Because pain is not an early sign, carcinoma of the stomach may be very advanced before it is detected. It may even have spread to the liver and surrounding organs through the lymph and blood vessels. Early symptoms are vague and include loss of appetite, heartburn, and general stomach distress. Blood may be vomited or appear in the feces. Pernicious anemia generally accompanies cancer of the stomach, because the gastric mucosa fails to secrete intrinsic factor. Gastric analysis by means of a stomach tube demonstrates the absence of hydrochloric acid, or achlorhydria. Biopsy of any lesions seen through the gastroscope is an essential diagnostic procedure for carcinoma of the stomach.

The etiology of this malignancy is not known, but current research suggests an association with the consumption of preserved, salted, cured foods and a diet low in fresh fruits and vegetables. It is more common in men than women. *H. pylori* infection appears to increase the risk for stomach cancer, probably through its damaging effects on the mucosal cells. Good prognosis for this disease depends on early detection and treatment.

## ▶ Diseases of the Intestines

The small intestine is the site of most of the digestion and absorption that occurs in the digestive tract, while the large intestine absorbs remaining water and stores and concentrates the feces. Diseases in these areas may manifest themselves as diarrhea, constipation, changes in stool characteristics, or in secondary diseases that arise as a result of poor nutrition.

### Appendicitis

Appendicitis is an acute and painful inflammation of the appendix. The wormlike shape of the appendix and its location on the cecum make it a trap for fecal material, which contains bacteria, particularly *Escherichia coli*. Figure 10–5 illustrates this potential site of infection. Obstruction with fecal material and infections cause the appendix to become swollen, red, and covered with an inflammatory exudate. Because the swelling interferes with circulation to the appendix, it is possible for gangrene to develop. The appendix then becomes green and black. The wall of the appendix can become thin and rupture, spilling fecal material into the peritoneal cavity, causing peritonitis. Before antibiotic treatment, peritonitis was almost always fatal. Rupture of the appendix tends to give relief from the pain, which is very misleading. The

---

## Prevention ✚ PLUS!

### Bacteria, Coolers, and Food Poisoning

Refrigeration and freezing do not kill bacteria. The cold temperature inhibits their growth, which can resume at warmer temperatures. Bacteria can multiply rapidly; under optimum conditions, they may double their numbers every 30 minutes. A contaminated potato salad may be safe to eat right out of the refrigerator, but it may become the source of a serious infection if brought to a picnic and left to stand at air temperature for a couple of hours. In other words, it is a good idea to keep the potato salad in the cooler while you are playing softball at your next picnic!

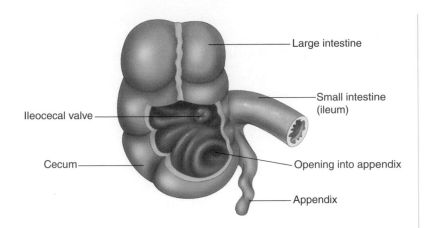

Large intestine

Small intestine (ileum)

Ileocecal valve

Cecum

Opening into appendix

Appendix

pain of appendicitis is not always typical, but it often begins in the middle of the abdomen and shifts to the lower right quadrant. Nausea, vomiting, and fever are common symptoms. Surgery should be performed before rupture occurs.

## Malabsorption Syndrome

A person unable to absorb fat or some other substance from the small intestine is said to have malabsorption syndrome. Signs and symptoms of malnutrition occur, including lack of energy and inability to maintain weight. Because fat cannot be absorbed from the intestine, it passes into the feces, and the result is unformed, fatty, pale stools that have a foul odor. The fat content causes the stools to float.

Although defective mucosal cells can cause the abnormal absorption, other diseases can result in secondary malabsorption syndrome. A diseased pancreas or blocked pancreatic duct deprives the small intestine of lipase. In the absence of lipase, fat is not digested and cannot be absorbed. Inadequate bile secretion, due to liver disease or a blocked bile duct, also prevents lipid digestion and causes secondary malabsorption. One of the complications of the malabsorption syndrome is a bleeding tendency. Vitamin K, a fat-soluble vitamin that is essential to the blood-clotting mechanism, cannot be absorbed. Treatment for malabsorption syndrome depends on its cause, and diet is carefully controlled. Supplements are administered, such as the fat-soluble vitamins A, D, E, and K.

## Diverticulitis

Diverticula are little pouches or sacs formed when the mucosal lining pushes through the underlying muscle layer of the intestinal wall. These may cause no harm themselves. Diverticulitis is an inflammation of the diverticula. This may occur in the colon or in the small intestines. Diverticulitis occurs when the sacs become impacted with fecal material and bacteria. The patient experiences low, cramplike pain, usually on the left side of the abdomen. As inflammation spreads, the lumen of the intestine is narrowed and an obstruction can develop. Abscesses frequently form. Antibiotic therapy, together with a controlled diet, is usually effective. Figure 10–6 shows an example of diverticulitis.

## Regional Enteritis (Crohn's Disease)

Regional enteritis is an inflammatory disease of the intestine that most frequently affects young adults, particularly females. The intestinal walls become thick and rigid. As the wall thickens with the formation of fibrous tissue, the lumen narrows and a chronic obstruction develops. The pain of regional enteritis resembles that of appendicitis, occurring in the lower right quadrant of the abdomen, where a tender mass may be felt. Diarrhea alternating with constipation, and melena, dark stools containing blood pigments, are common. Severe diarrhea can cause an electrolyte imbalance because of the large amount of water and salt lost in the stools.

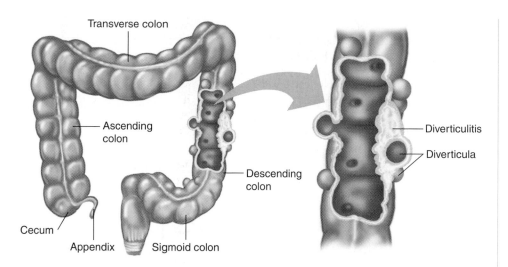

**Figure 10–6**
Diverticulitis.

Anorexia, nausea, and vomiting lead to weight loss. Periods of exacerbation, remission, and relapse are common. Severe cases entail a risk for hemorrhage or perforation. The cause of regional enteritis is not known, but a psychogenic element may be involved, because emotional stress can trigger relapses. Regional enteritis is usually treated with anti-inflammatory medications such as corticosteroids, aminosalicylates, immunosuppressive agents, and antibiotics. Surgery is not performed unless complications demand it.

## Chronic Ulcerative Colitis

Chronic ulcerative colitis is a serious inflammation of the colon characterized by extensive ulceration of the colon and rectum. Typical symptoms include diarrhea with pus, blood, and mucus in the stools, and cramplike pain in the lower abdomen. Periods of remission and exacerbation are common in ulcerative colitis. Anemia often accompanies ulcerative colitis because of the chronic blood loss through the rectum. The colon with chronic ulcerative colitis has a characteristic appearance on x-ray examination. The normal pouchlike markings of the colon, the *haustra*, are lacking. The colon appears straight and rigid, and it is referred to as a pipestem colon. Increased risk for colon malignancy is associated with long-standing ulcerative colitis.

The cause is unclear. A psychogenic factor may be involved, as the condition is often aggravated by stress. Hypersensitivity to certain foods may play a part in the course of the disease. Chronic ulcerative colitis may be an autoimmune disease in which the person's antibodies destroy the body's own tissue.

The symptoms of chronic ulcerative colitis may be alleviated if certain stressful conditions are removed. Foods found to aggravate the disease should be avoided. Mild sedation may reduce anxiety and stress. Corticosteroids are sometimes administered to control autoimmunity. If the person does not respond to these treatments, surgery may be necessary, occasionally requiring a colostomy. A colostomy is an artificial opening in the abdominal wall with a segment of the large intestine attached. Fecal waste is evacuated through this opening and collected in a bag. A colostomy may be temporary or permanent depending on the nature of the colon surgery.

## Carcinoma of the Colon and Rectum

Carcinoma of the colon and rectum is a leading cause of death from cancer in the United States, yet it can be diagnosed more easily than many other cancers. The mass is often felt by rectal examination or seen with the protoscope or colonoscope, endoscopes used for viewing the rectum and colon. If detected early, it responds well to surgical treatment.

The symptoms vary according to the site of the malignancy. A change in bowel habits, diarrhea, or constipation is symptomatic. As the tumor grows, there may be abdominal discomfort and pressure. Blood often appears in the stools, and continuous blood loss from the malignant tumor causes anemia. The mass can partially or completely obstruct the lumen of the colon. As the tumor invades underlying tissue, the cancer cells spread through the lymph vessels and veins.

Two diseases increase the risk for cancer of the colon: long-standing ulcerative colitis and familial polyposis of the colon. Familial polyposis is a hereditary disease in which numerous polyps develop in the intestinal tract. The polyps usually give no symptoms unless a malignancy develops. Another factor associated with risk for colon cancer is a diet high in red meat and low in food sources of fiber, such as vegetables, legumes, and whole-grain cereals.

As in all cancers, early detection and treatment are essential to prevent its spread. Most malignancies of the large intestine are in the rectum or the sigmoid colon. This makes their detection and removal easier than malignant tumors in other areas of the digestive tract. A colostomy may be necessary.

## Intestinal Obstructions

An obstruction can occur anywhere along the intestinal tract, preventing contents within the tract from moving forward. Obstructions are classed as organic when there is some material blockage, or as paralytic, in which case there is a decrease in peristalsis, preventing the propulsion of intestinal contents.

Tumors and hernias, both hiatal and inguinal, can cause organic obstructions. The intestine may be twisted on itself, a condition known as volvulus that may be unwound surgically (Figure 10–7). The intestine may be kinked, allowing nothing to pass. Adhesions, the linking together of two surfaces normally separate, can distort the tract. Abdominal adhesions sometimes follow surgery, when fibrous connective tissue grows around the incision. Adhesions also develop as a result of inflammation. Another type of organic obstruction is intussusception in which a segment of intestine telescopes into the part forward to it. This occurs more often in children than in adults. Figure 10–8 shows various types of organic obstructions. An acute organic obstruction causes severe pain. The abdomen is distended and vomiting occurs. There is complete constipation; not even gas, or flatus, is passed. Sometimes the obstruction can be relieved by means of a suction tube, but frequently surgery is required. If the obstruction is a strangulated hernia, a protrusion of intestine through the abdominal wall, surgery is required because the blood supply is cut off to the strangulated segment, and it can become gangrenous.

A paralytic obstruction can result from peritonitis. If a loop of small intestine is surrounded by pus from the infection, the smooth muscle of

## Prevention ✚ PLUS!

### Cancer Prevention through Detection

Early detection of colorectal cancer is the key to survival. Death rates are low for patients whose colorectal cancer is detected at an early localized stage: about 9% die within 5 years. Death rates are much higher, however, when the diagnosis occurs at an advanced stage: about 92% die within 5 years. Screening remains underused even though its benefits seem clear. Regular screening should be done for adults aged 50 years and over. This includes an annual fecal occult blood test, a flexible sigmoidoscopy every 5 years, and a colonoscopy every 10 years. These tests could identify precancerous polyps that can be removed, or they can detect cancer in the early localized stage, which can be treated before the cancer has a chance to spread.

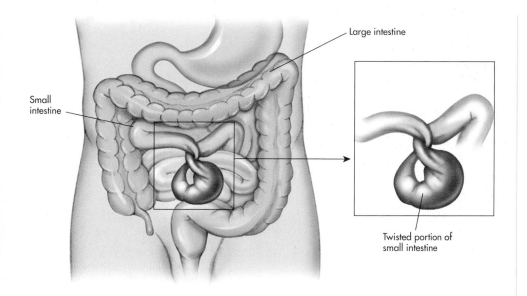

**Figure 10–7**
Volvulus.

Large intestine

Small intestine

Twisted portion of small intestine

the intestinal wall cannot contract. Sphincters can go into spasm and fail to open as a result of intense pain.

## Spastic Colon (Irritable Bowel Syndrome)

Many of the symptoms described for diseases of the lower intestinal tract are also characteristic of a spastic colon or irritable bowel. These symptoms include diarrhea, constipation, abdominal pain, and gas. The difference between a spastic or irritable colon and the diseases already discussed is that the spastic colon has no lesion. There is no tumor or ulceration. It is a functional disorder of motility, the movement of the colon. The pain is probably caused by muscle spasms in the wall of the intestine.

Abuse of laxatives and consumption of certain foods and beverages, particularly caffeine, alcohol, spicy foods, fatty foods, and concentrated orange juice, can irritate the bowel. Foods such as beans and cabbage, which contain carbohydrates fermented by colon bacteria, promote gas production and should be avoided. Laxatives should be avoided as well. Adding fiber to the diet helps prevent constipation. Emotional stress has an adverse effect on the digestive system, because the nerves of the au-

tonomic nervous system affect digestion. If stressful situations can be alleviated, the colon will function more normally. Tension-relieving activities, sports, hobbies, or regular exercise may help.

## Dysentery

People often use the terms dysentery and diarrhea interchangeably, which is not accurate. Dysentery is a disease; diarrhea is a symptom. Dysentery is an acute inflammation of the colon, a colitis. The major symptom of dysentery is diarrhea in which the stools contain pus, blood, and mucus. Severe abdominal pain accompanies the diarrhea. Bacteria, parasitic worms, and other microorganisms can cause dysentery. The protozoan *Entamoeba histolytica*, which is transmitted in feces-contaminated food and water, causes amoebic dysentery. *E. histolytica* invade the wall of the colon and cause numerous ulcerations, which account for the pus and blood in the stools. Bacillary dysentery is caused by various species of gram-negative bacteria in the genus *Shigella*. Antibiotics can be effective for bacillary dysentery, and amebicides are used for amoebic dysentery.

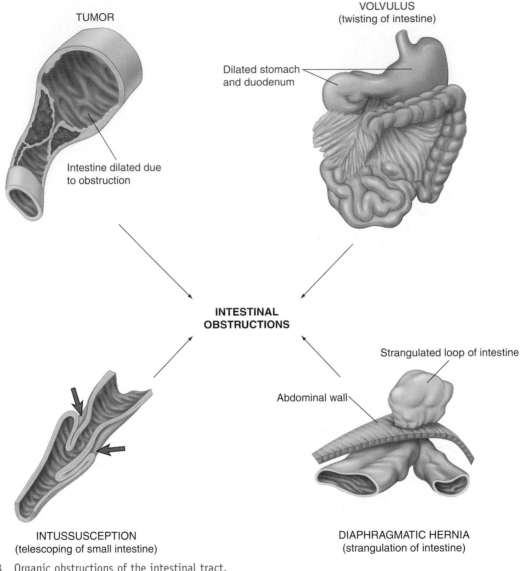

TUMOR

VOLVULUS
(twisting of intestine)

Dilated stomach
and duodenum

Intestine dilated due
to obstruction

**INTESTINAL
OBSTRUCTIONS**

Strangulated loop of intestine

Abdominal wall

INTUSSUSCEPTION
(telescoping of small intestine)

DIAPHRAGMATIC HERNIA
(strangulation of intestine)

**Figure 10–8** Organic obstructions of the intestinal tract.

## ▶ General Disorders of the Digestive Tract

The symptoms associated with the diseases of the digestive system are common phenomena. Vomiting, diarrhea, and constipation are some of these symptoms. The physiologic basis and significance of each symptom is described briefly.

## Vomiting

Vomiting is a protective mechanism, a response to the presence of an irritant, a distention, or a blockage. These stimulate sensory nerve fibers, and the message is conveyed to the vomiting center in the medulla of the brain. Motor impulses then stimulate the diaphragm and abdominal muscles. Contraction of these muscles squeezes the stomach. The sphincter at the base of the esophagus is opened, and the gastric contents are regurgitated. A feeling of nausea often precedes vomiting. The cause of the nausea may be factors other than a gastric or intestinal irritant. Motion sickness produces this effect. A very unpleasant smell or sight can cause nausea with possible subsequent vomiting.

## Diarrhea

Diarrhea results when the fluid contents of the small intestine are rushed through the large intestine, causing watery stools. It was stated earlier that the main function of the large intestine is to reabsorb water and minerals. In an attack of diarrhea, there is no time for this reabsorption. The smooth muscle in the walls of the intestine is so stimulated that peristalsis is intensified. Anxiety and stress can trigger this increased motility of the large intestine. An intestinal infection or food poisoning can cause diarrhea through toxins that increase intestinal motility or impair water absorption by mucosal cells.

## Constipation

Constipation results when feces remain in the colon too long, with excessive reabsorption of water; they then become hard and dry. Poor habits of elimination are a cause of constipation. Defecation should be allowed to occur when the defecation reflexes are strong. A diet that contains adequate amounts of fiber aids elimination. Fiber is obtained from fresh fruits, vegetables, and cereals. Various disorders of the digestive system cause constipation. Any obstruction of the lumen or interference with motility will result in this condition.

## Hemorrhoids

Hemorrhoids are varicose veins in the lining of the rectum near the anus. Hemorrhoids may be internal or external. A physician can observe internal hemorrhoids with a proctoscope, a hollow tube with a lighted end. External hemorrhoids can be seen with a handheld mirror and appear blue because of decreased circulation. They can become red and tender if inflamed.

Causes of hemorrhoids include heredity, poor dietary habits, inadequate fiber, overuse of laxatives, and lack of exercise. Straining to have a bowel movement can cause bleeding or cause the hemorrhoid to prolapse, or come through the anal opening. Hemorrhoids frequently develop during pregnancy because of pressure from an enlarged uterus. Treatment includes adding fiber and water to the diet and stool softeners to reduce straining and subsequent inflammation. Medicated suppositories and anorectal creams relieve pain and reduce inflammation.

## ▶ Diseases Indicated by Stool Characteristics

Microscopic examination of stool may identify the cause of food poisoning, gastroenteritis, or dysentery. Other information can also be obtained from stool samples. Signs of several of the diseases discussed include blood in the stools. Blood appears differently, however, depending upon the site of bleeding.

If the blood in the stools is bright red, the bleeding originated from the distal end of the colon, the rectum. Streaks of red blood can indicate bleeding hemorrhoids. This symptom can also indicate cancer of the rectum. Dark blood may appear in the stools, giving them a dark, tarry appearance, the condition of melena. This blood was altered as it passed through the digestive tract, so it originated from the stomach or duodenum. A bleeding ulcer or cancer of the stomach may be indicated by melena. Certain medications, those containing iron, for instance, can also give this tarry appearance to the stools. Blood may not be apparent to the naked eye, but a chemical test can show its presence. This is referred to as occult blood. It can indicate bleeding ulcers or a malignancy in the digestive tract.

If the stools are large and pale, appear greasy, and float on water, they contain fat. This is a symptom of malabsorption syndrome. It may also indicate a diseased liver, gallbladder, or pancreas. Diseases of these organs are discussed next.

## ► Functions of the Liver and the Gallbladder

The liver is located below the diaphragm, in the upper right quadrant of the abdominal region. The liver is the largest glandular organ of the body, and it is unique in that it has great powers of regeneration; it can replace damaged or diseased cells. Still, chronic liver disease may cause irreversible damage and loss of function.

The liver has a dual blood supply: It receives oxygenated blood from the hepatic artery and blood rich in nutrients from the portal vein. The blood reaching the liver through the portal vein comes from the stomach, intestines, spleen, and pancreas. Blood from the small intestines carries absorbed nutrients such as simple sugars and amino acids. One of the functions of the liver is to store any excess of these substances. The liver plays an important role in maintaining the proper level of glucose in the blood. It takes up excess glucose, storing it as glycogen. When the level of circulating glucose falls below normal, the liver converts glycogen into glucose, which is then released into the blood. The liver also stores iron and vitamins.

The liver synthesizes various proteins, including enzymes necessary for cellular activities. One means of evaluating liver function is to determine the level of these enzymes in the blood. The liver also synthesizes plasma proteins. Albumin is the plasma protein that has a water-holding power within the blood vessels. If the albumin level is too low, plasma seeps out of the blood vessels and into the tissue spaces, causing edema. Other essential plasma proteins synthesized by the liver are those required for blood clotting: fibrinogen and prothrombin. If the liver is seriously diseased or injured and cannot make these proteins, hemorrhaging may occur.

The liver can detoxify various substances; that is, it can make poisonous substances harmless. Ammonia, which results from amino acid metabolism, is converted to urea by the liver. The urea then enters the bloodstream and is excreted by the kidneys. Certain drugs and chemicals are also detoxified by the liver. Specialized cells called Kupffer cells line the blood spaces within the liver. These cells engulf and digest bacteria and other foreign substances, thus cleansing the blood.

Bile, necessary for fat digestion, is secreted by the liver. Bile is an emulsifier, acting on fat in such a way that the lipid enzymes can digest it. The products of lipid digestion are then absorbed by the walls of the small intestine. In the absence of bile, the fat-soluble vitamins A, D, E, and K cannot be absorbed. Various functions of the liver are shown in Table 10–2. Bile consists of water, bile salts, cholesterol, and bilirubin, which is a colored substance resulting from the breakdown of hemoglobin. It is bilirubin that gives bile its characteristic color of yellow or orange.

The gallbladder is a small, saclike structure on the underside of the liver. Bile is secreted continuously by the liver into the hepatic duct, which carries bile to the gallbladder for storage and concentration (Figure 10–9). The gallbladder releases the bile through the cystic duct to the common hepatic duct, which carries the bile to the duodenum. Release of bile is coordinated with the appearance of fats in the duodenum.

## ► Diseases of the Liver

Liver disease manifests itself when chronic damage to liver cells cannot be repaired. When fibrous tissue replaces liver cells, the normal functions of the liver become impaired.

| Table 10–2   Liver Functions |
| --- |
| Secrete bile |
| Store nutrients, glucose, amino acids, iron |
| Remove nitrogenous waste from blood |
| Inactivate ingested toxins |
| Remove dead blood cells, cell debris, and bacteria from blood |
| Synthesize enzymes and plasma proteins |

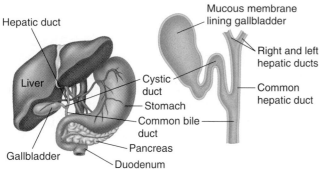

Hepatic duct

Liver

Gallbladder

Mucous membrane
lining gallbladder

Cystic
duct

Stomach

Common bile
duct

Pancreas

Duodenum

Right and left
hepatic ducts

Common
hepatic duct

**Figure 10–9**   Bile duct system of the liver and gallbladder.

## Jaundice

One sign frequently associated with liver disease is jaundice. Jaundice, or icterus, is a yellow or orange discoloration of the skin, tissues, and the whites of the eyes. It is caused by a build-up of bilirubin, a pigment that is normally secreted in the bile and removed from the body in the feces.

**Causes of Jaundice**   The normal flow of bile from the gallbladder to the duodenum may be obstructed by a tumor, a gallstone in the duct system, or a congenital defect. Because the bile cannot move forward, it leaks into the blood, with bilirubin coloring the plasma. When the blood reaches the kidneys, the bile appears in the urine, giving it a dark color. Because bile is unable to reach the duodenum, the stools are light in color. They are usually described as clay-colored. Complications can result from this blockage to bile flow. Infection or inflammation of the gallbladder or bile ducts could occur. Lack of bile interferes with fat digestion and absorption, which means that the fat-soluble vitamins are not being absorbed. In the absence of vitamin K, bleeding tendencies may develop. The obstruction can also cause liver damage. Jaundice can also indicate liver disease, such as hepatitis or cirrhosis.

Hemolytic jaundice has an entirely different etiology. This type of jaundice accompanies the hemolytic anemias explained in Chapter 7. In these anemias, the red blood cells hemolyze, and an excess of bilirubin results from the breakdown of released hemoglobin. Abnormal discoloration follows. Table 10–3 summarizes the causes of jaundice.

## Viral Hepatitis

Hepatitis, or inflammation of the liver, is caused by a number of factors, including several viruses. Important causes are hepatitis virus A, hepatitis virus B, hepatitis virus C, and hepatitis virus D. Hepatitis E is uncommon in the United States.

Hepatitis virus A, formerly called *infectious hepatitis,* is the least serious form and can develop as an isolated case or in an epidemic. The incubation period, the time from exposure to the development of symptoms, is from 2 to 6 weeks. The symptoms include anorexia, nausea, and mild fever. The urine becomes dark in color, and jaundice appears in some cases. On examination, the liver may be found to be enlarged and tender. Contaminated water or food is the usual source of the infection, which spreads under conditions of poor sanitation. The virus is excreted in the stools and urine, infecting soil and water. Hepatitis virus type A is usually mild in children; it is sometimes more severe in adults. Prognosis is usually good, with no permanent liver damage resulting. Immunoglobulin injections provide temporary protection against hepatitis virus type A for people exposed to it. Once a person has had either type of hepatitis, he or she is immune to that particular type for life.

Hepatitis virus B, formerly called *serum hepatitis,* is a more serious disease. It can lead to chronic hepatitis or cirrhosis of the liver. The symptoms are similar to those of hepatitis virus

| Table 10–3   Causes of Jaundice |
| --- |
| Obstruction of bile ducts |
| Hepatitis |
| Cirrhosis |
| Hemolytic anemia |

A but develop more slowly. The incubation period is long, lasting from 2 to 6 months. The severity of the disease varies greatly. A person with poor nutritional status, for example, will be more adversely affected by hepatitis. Occasionally, a *fulminating* form of hepatitis virus B develops, and it is fatal. This form has a sudden onset and progresses rapidly. The person becomes delirious, then becomes comatose, and dies. Hepatitis virus B can be transmitted by donated blood or serum transfusions that contain the virus. It also is transmitted through the use of contaminated needles or syringes used by drug addicts and as a sexually transmitted disease. A person's physical condition at the onset of the disease makes a difference in the seriousness of the infection. Blood and plasma are screened for hepatitis, but hospital personnel still must be well informed of the hazards that can lead to acquiring hepatitis. Precautions must be taken by nurses, laboratory technicians, dialysis workers, and blood bank personnel to prevent becoming infected. Vaccination provides immunity to the virus, and it should be administered to personnel who handle or come in close contact with blood or other bodily fluids. (See "Precautions for Health-Care Providers," Chapter 2, under "AIDS").

Hepatitis C is the leading viral cause of chronic liver disease and cirrhosis, and is now the most common reason for liver transplants. The initial symptoms are nonspecific and similar to those of hepatitis A or B, but the disease persists for months, even years. About 20% of infected persons develop cirrhosis, and a number of these can lead to end-stage liver disease. The virus is transmitted mostly through blood transfusions, although transmission has been traced to intravenous drug use, and epidemiologic studies show a risk associated with sexual contact with someone with hepatitis and with having had more than one sex partner in a year. Treatments of hepatitis C include interferon injections and oral ribavirin. Treatment for end-stage cirrhosis may include liver transplant.

Hepatitis D virus is a defective virus that cannot reproduce in a cell unless the cell is also infected with hepatitis B. The resulting disease is more serious and more frequently progresses to chronic liver disease. Although relatively uncommon, its transmission is similar to that of hepatitis B.

Hepatitis E is rare in the United States, but worldwide is the leading cause of epidemics of infectious hepatitis. Major epidemics occur in Africa, Asia, and Mexico, where it is transmitted primarily through fecal-contaminated drinking water. Nearly every case in the United States occurs in travelers to areas where the disease is endemic. No effective treatment or vaccine exists. Fortunately, there is no evidence that type E progresses to chronic disease.

## Cirrhosis of the Liver

*Cirrhosis* is chronic destruction of liver cells and tissues with a nodular, bumpy regeneration. Alcoholic cirrhosis, the most common type of cirrhosis, is described in detail. This disease is also called portal, Laennec, or fatty nutritional cirrhosis (an accumulation of fat often develops within the liver). The exact effect of excessive alcohol on the liver is not known, but it may be related to the malnutrition that frequently accom-

## Prevention PLUS!

### Know Your Viruses

The more you know about how a virus is transmitted, the better prepared you can be to prevent infection. Hepatitis A is transmitted primarily through contaminated food and water. Workers in the food-service industry must use sanitary procedures when handling food, including the simple task of washing their hands. You can protect yourself at home by thoroughly cooking meat and seafood. Hepatitis B and C are transmitted through blood transfusions, contaminated needles and syringes, and sexually. Health-care workers receive vaccination against hepatitis B, and blood is screened for contamination by hepatitis B and C.

## SIDE by SIDE ■ Cirrhosis

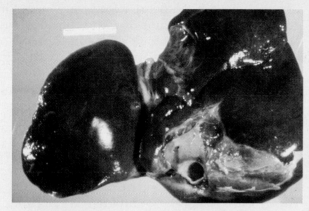

▲ Normal human liver.

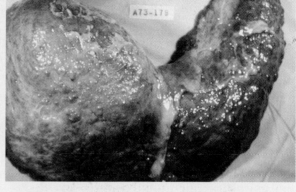

▲ Cirrhosis of the liver from chronic alcoholism.

panies chronic alcoholism, or the alcohol itself may be toxic. In the normal liver, there is a highly organized arrangement of cells, blood vessels, and bile ducts. A cirrhotic liver loses this organization and, as a result, the liver cannot function. Liver cells die and are replaced by fibrous connective tissue and scar tissue. This tissue has none of the liver cell functions. At first, the liver is generally enlarged due to regeneration but then becomes smaller as the fibrous connective tissue contracts. The surface acquires a nodular appearance. This is sometimes called a "hobnailed" liver.

In cirrhosis, circulation through the liver is impaired. As a result, high pressure builds in vessels of the abdomen and in other areas. The esophageal veins swell, forming esophageal varices. Abdominal organs like the spleen, pancreas, and stomach also swell. These organs and vessels may hemorrhage, causing hemorrhagic shock. Hemorrhage of vessels in the stomach or intestines may cause vomiting of blood, hematemesis. A characteristic symptom of cirrhosis is distention of the abdomen caused by the accumulation of fluid in the peritoneal cavity. This fluid is called ascites and develops as a result of liver failure. The pressure within the obstructed veins forces plasma into the ab-

dominal cavity. This fluid often has to be drained. When the liver fails to produce adequate amounts of albumin, an albumin deficiency, hypoalbuminemia, develops and fluid leaks out of the blood vessels, causing edema. Because the necrotic cells of the cirrhotic patient fail to produce albumin, ascitic fluid develops, as does edema, particularly in the ankles and legs.

Blockage of the bile ducts, like that of the blood vessels, follows the disorganization of the liver. Bile accumulates in the blood, leading to jaundice and, because bile is not secreted into the duodenum, stools are clay-colored. The excess of bile, carried by the blood to the kidneys, imparts a dark color to urine.

Other signs are related to the fact that the diseased liver cannot perform its usual biochemical activities. Normally, the liver inactivates small amounts of female sex hormones secreted by the adrenal glands in both males and females. Estrogens then have no effect on the male, but the cirrhotic liver does not inactivate estrogens. They accumulate and have a feminizing effect on males. The breasts enlarge, a condition known as gynecomastia, and the palms of the hands become red because of the estrogen level. Hair on the chest is lost, and a female-type distribution of hair develops. Atrophy of the testicles can also occur.

The damaged liver cells are unable to carry out their normal function of detoxification, so ammonia and other poisonous substances accumulate in the blood and affect the brain, causing various neurologic disorders. The person becomes confused and disoriented, even to the point of stupor, and a characteristic tremor or shaking develops. This shaking is called "liver flap." Somnolence or abnormal sleepiness are symptoms of cirrhosis. Hepatic coma is a possible cause of death in cirrhosis. The typical signs of cirrhosis are summarized in Table 10–4.

Although chronic alcoholism is the leading cause of cirrhosis, other disease can also cause cirrhosis. Severe chronic hepatitis, chronic inflammation of the bile ducts, and certain drugs and toxins can cause necrosis of the liver cells, which is the first step in the development of cirrhosis.

| Table 10–4    Signs of Advanced Cirrhosis |
| --- |
| Neurologic manifestations, somnolence, mental confusion, flapping tremor, coma |
| Loss of chest hair |
| Severe liver damage, hobnailed liver |
| Ascitic fluid |
| Red palms |
| Testicular atrophy |
| Tendency to hemorrhage |
| Edema in ankles |
| Female distribution of hair |
| Dilated abdominal veins |
| Enlarged spleen |
| Gynecomastia |
| Esophageal varices |

## Carcinoma of the Liver

Hepatocarcinoma, or cancer of the liver, is sometimes a complication of cirrhosis. This is a primary malignancy of the liver, which is rare. The symptoms of hepatocarcinoma vary according to the site of the tumor. If the tumor obstructs the portal vein, ascites develops in the abdominal cavity, as it does in cirrhosis. If the fluid contains blood, a malignancy is indicated. A tumor blocking the bile duct will cause jaundice. General symptoms may include loss of weight, an abdominal mass, and pain in the upper right quadrant of the abdomen.

More often, cancer detected in the liver is a result of metastasis from other organs, such as the breast, the colon, or the pancreas. Such liver tumors are secondary carcinomas. Because of the arrangement of blood and lymphatic vessels through the liver, it is a frequent site of metastases. A high percentage of people who die of cancer are found to have had liver metastases.

Prognosis for cancer of the liver is poor because usually the malignancy has developed elsewhere and has spread to the liver. Techniques such as the liver scan and needle biopsy are used in diagnosing the condition.

## ▶ Diseases of the Gallbladder

The gallbladder stores and concentrates bile. Gallbladder disease impairs the storage and delivery of bile to the duodenum.

## Cholecystitis

Cholecystitis is an inflammation of the gallbladder. The gallbladder becomes extremely swollen, causing pain under the right rib cage that radiates to the right shoulder. At this point, the gallbladder can usually be felt (palpated). The person experiences chills and fever, nausea and vomiting, belching and indigestion. A person with chronic cholecystitis experiences these symptoms especially after eating fatty foods. The presence of fat in the duodenum stimulates the gallbladder to contract and release bile, and the contraction of the inflamed gallbladder causes pain. Prolonged inflammation causes the gallbladder to lose its ability to concentrate bile. The walls of the gallbladder may thicken, making it impossible for the gallbladder to contract properly. Serious complications can result from cholecystitis. Lack of bloodflow because of the obstruction brought about by the swelling can cause an infarction. With the death of the tissues, gangrene can set in. The acutely inflamed gallbladder, like an inflamed appendix, may rupture, causing peritonitis. A complication of chronic cholecystitis is that bile accumulates in the bile ducts of the liver. This causes necrosis and fibrosis of the liver cells lining the ducts. This is another form of cirrhosis, biliary (bile) cirrhosis. Possible complications of bile duct obstruction are summarized in Table 10–5.

Cholecystitis is usually caused by an obstruction, a gallstone or tumor. Because of the blockage, bile cannot leave the gallbladder. The bile becomes more concentrated and irritates the walls of the gallbladder.

## Gallstones (Cholelithiasis)

Gallstones, also called biliary calculi, may be present in the gallbladder and give no symptoms. There may be one gallstone present or several hundred, which can be large or small (Figure 10–10). Small stones, referred to as gravel, can enter the cystic duct and cause an obstruction with excruciating pain. The danger of gallstones is obstruction of the bile ducts, which causes inflammation. The converse is also true; inflammation of the gallbladder causes gallstone formation. Gallstones form when substances that

are normally soluble precipitate out of solution. The stones consist principally of cholesterol, bilirubin, and calcium when in excess. Certain factors tend to stimulate gallstone formation, such as obesity and pregnancy (because of an increased cholesterol level). The incidence of gallstones is higher in women. Gallstones can be located by sonography and x-ray. The usual treatment for cholecystitis and cholelithiasis is surgical removal of the gallbladder, a cholecystectomy. The cystic duct is then ligated, and the common bile duct examined for stones. Occasionally, undetected cholesterol stones are retained in the common bile duct after surgery. Administering a solubilizing agent through a catheter into the bile duct may dissolve the remaining stones, preventing the necessity of repeated surgery.

## ▶ Structure and Function of the Pancreas

The pancreas is a fish-shaped organ extending across the abdomen behind the stomach. The head fits into the curve of the duodenum, where the pancreatic duct empties digestive enzymes from the pancreas. These enzymes include amylase, which breaks down carbohydrates, trypsin and chymotrypsin, which digest protein, and lipase, which breaks down lipid or fat.

Diseases of the pancreas severely interfere with the digestive process. The many digestive enzymes contained within the pancreas make it a threat to itself, as is explained shortly in a particular disease condition. Figure 10–11 shows the structure of the pancreas. Figure 10–12 shows the relationship between the pancreas and other digestive organs.

## ▶ Diseases of the Pancreas

### Pancreatitis

Acute pancreatitis is a serious, painful inflammation of the pancreas. Severe, steady abdominal pain of sudden onset is the first symptom. The

| Table 10–5 | Complications of Bile Duct Obstruction |
| --- | --- |
| Rupture and peritonitis | |
| Impaired lipid digestion and absorption | |
| Impaired circulation and necrosis | |
| Biliary cirrhosis | |

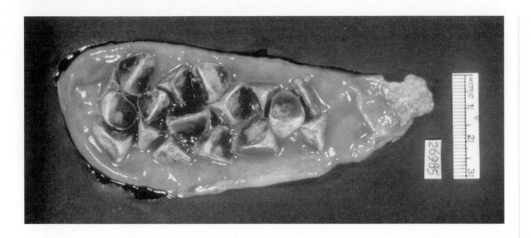

**Figure 10–10**
Gallbladder opening showing gallstones. (Martin Rotker/Phototake NYC.)

intense pain radiates to the back and resembles the sharp pain of a perforated ulcer. Drawing up the knees or assuming a sitting position may provide some relief. There may also be nausea and vomiting. Jaundice sometimes develops if the swelling blocks the common bile duct. If a large area of the pancreas is affected, both endocrine and digestive functions of the gland become impaired. In the absence of lipid enzymes from the pancreas, fat cannot be digested, resulting in greasy stools with a foul odor. Secondary malabsorption syndrome develops because fat that is not digested cannot be ab-

sorbed. In pancreatitis, the protein- and lipid-digesting enzymes become activated within the pancreas and begin to digest the organ itself. Severe necrosis and edema of the pancreas result. The digestion can extend into blood vessels, which causes severe internal bleeding and shock. When the condition becomes this severe, it is called acute hemorrhagic pancreatitis.

Several factors can cause pancreatitis, but the most common one is excessive alcohol consumption. Inflammation of pancreatic ducts caused by the presence of gallstones is another possible cause. Many cases of pancreatitis can-

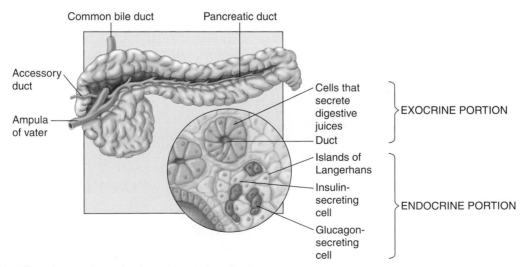

**Figure 10–11** The pancreas: An endocrine and exocrine gland.

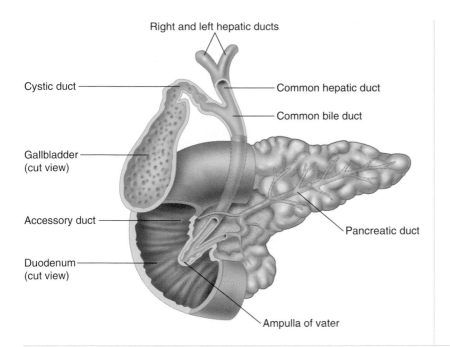

Right and left hepatic ducts

Cystic duct

Common hepatic duct

Common bile duct

Gallbladder
(cut view)

Accessory duct

Pancreatic duct

Duodenum
(cut view)

Ampulla of vater

**Figure 10–12**
Relationship between the pancreas and the digestive system.

not be attributed to either of these causes and are said to be idiopathic. Pancreatitis is more common in women than in men and usually occurs after age 40.

The most significant diagnostic procedures for pancreatitis are blood tests and urine tests. High levels of pancreatic enzymes, particularly amylase, confirm the diagnosis of pancreatitis.

## Cancer of the Pancreas

Cancer of the pancreas, adenocarcinoma, has a high mortality rate. A malignancy in the head of the pancreas can block the common bile duct (Figure 10–13). This gives earlier symptoms than does cancer in the body or tail of the pancreas, which can be very advanced before it is discovered. Obstruction of the bile duct causes jaundice and impairs digestion because the pancreatic enzymes and bile cannot enter the duodenum. This causes malabsorption of fat and clay-colored stools. The person cannot absorb sufficient nutrients and calories, and therefore loses weight. Great pain is experienced as the tumor grows, and the cancer usually metastasizes to the surrounding organs: the duodenum, stomach, and liver. Prognosis for

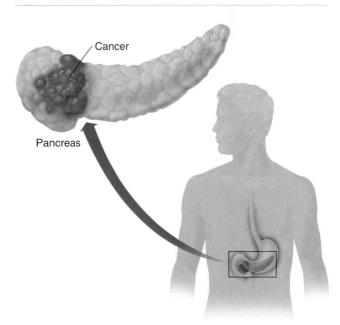

Cancer

Pancreas

**Figure 10–13** Pancreatic cancer. A common site of pancreatic cancer is within the pancreatic ducts.

cancer of the pancreas is poor, and death occurs in a relatively short time. Pancreatic cancer is linked to cigarette smoking, high protein and fat diets, food additives, and exposure to industrial chemicals like beta-naphthalene, benzidine, and urea. Chronic alcohol abuse, chronic pancreatitis, and diabetes mellitus increase the risk of developing pancreatic cancer. It occurs more frequently in males than in females.

## ▶ Age-Related Diseases

The digestive system functions fairly well in healthy elderly people, despite normal age-related changes like thinning mucosa and decreased muscle motility. However, some diseases occur with greater frequency with increasing age and thus significantly impact elderly populations.

### Mouth and Esophagus

Periodontal disease and osteoporosis contribute to tooth loss in elderly people. The number of taste buds decrease, and together with decreased saliva secretion, may lead to decreased appetite. Esophageal cancer incidence is highest in persons over 60. As stated earlier, this cancer is closely linked with the use of alcohol and tobacco.

### Gastrointestinal

Hiatal hernia is a common disorder in elderly people. Peptic ulcers are no more common in elderly than in middle age; however, the risk of hemorrhage is greater in old age. Carcinoma is also no more common among elderly than in middle age. Diarrhea poses greater risk of dehydration and malnutrition. Therefore, gastrointestinal infections like food poisoning and dysentery can be serious diseases. Overall, the function of the intestines remains fairly normal, although intestinal motility is slightly decreased. Thus, changes in diet or new medications that affect intestinal motility can more easily lead to constipation. Diverticula are most common in elderly, and therefore the incidence of diverticulitis rises. Colon cancer incidence increases after age 45, which emphasizes the importance of regular screening and early diagnosis.

### Liver and Gallbladder

Liver function diminishes, which results in the persistence of high blood levels of medications or toxins. Levels of clotting factors decline, leading to increased hemorrhage. Cholelithiasis incidence is highest in persons over age 80. Obstruction of the bile duct leads to jaundice.

### Pancreas

The incidence of pancreatic cancer peaks in the 60s and is most common among older men. Acute pancreatitis is common in elderly. However, unlike it is in younger people, acute pancreatitis in the elderly is more likely due to gallstones that block the pancreatic duct and less often associated with chronic alcoholism.

## CHAPTER SUMMARY

The structure and function of the digestive system was reviewed, emphasizing the normal digestive process. Diseases of the digestive tract were discussed, including malignancies (mouth, esophagus, stomach, colon), infections (oral, gastroenteritis, food poisoning, dysentery, ulcers), abnormal structure and function (herniations, obstructions), and inflammatory/immune disorders (gastritis, ulcerative colitis, Crohn's disease). General conditions like diarrhea, constipation, and vomiting were explained and related to diseases. Certain diagnostic tools such as endoscopy, barium x-rays, stool analysis, and biopsy were also discussed. The normal functions of the liver were reviewed and related to pathologic changes underlying symptoms of liver disease. Hepatitis and cirrhosis are the serious liver diseases that were considered. Alcoholism and its effects on the liver were discussed.

Cholecystitis, inflammation of the gallbladder, and its relationship to gallstone formation was discussed. Inflammation of the pancreas, pancreatitis, and carcinoma of the pancreas, a malignancy with a very poor prognosis, were discussed. Diseases of the endocrine pancreas are discussed in Chapter 14.

## RESOURCES

Beers, M. H. & R. Berkow, *The Merck Manual of Diagnosis and Therapy,* 17th ed., John Willey & Sons, 1999.

*Professional Guide to Diseases,* 6th ed., Springhouse 1998.

# DISEASES AT A GLANCE

## Digestive System

| DISEASE | ETIOLOGY | SIGNS AND SYMPTOMS |
| --- | --- | --- |
| Stomatitis | Bacteria, viruses, fungi | Redness, ulcers, patches, bleeding, depending on the cause |
| Cancer of the mouth | Use of tobacco products, especially in conjunction with consuming alcohol | Abnormal growths, sores, or lesions that don't heal |
| Cancer of the esophagus | Use of tobacco and alcohol | Dysphagia, vomiting, weight loss |
| Esophagitis | Acid reflux due to incompetent cardiac sphincter | Burning chest pain (heartburn), especially after eating or while lying down |
| Esophageal varices | Increased venous pressure; accompanies advanced cirrhosis | Dilated esophageal veins, hemorrhage |
| Hiatal hernia | Stomach protrudes through weakened diaphragm | Indigestion, heartburn following meals, acid reflux, and esophagitis |
| Gastritis | Aspirin, coffee, tobacco, alcohol, infection | Stomach pain, hematemesis |
| Chronic atrophic gastritis | Degeneration of stomach mucosa results in no HCl secretion and no intrinsic factor secretion | Gastritis, poor digestion and absorption of nutrients, weight loss |
| Peptic ulcer | Infection with *H. pylori* and erosion of mucosa by stomach acid | Upper abdominal pain, hemorrhage, blood in stool |
| Gastroenteritis | Food- and water-borne infection by bacteria, viruses, protozoa | Nausea, vomiting, diarrhea, abdominal discomfort or pain, and possibly fever, depending on the pathogen |
| Cancer of the stomach | Idiopathic; associated with salted, cured foods and diet low in vegetables and fruit; associated with prior infections with *H. pylori* | Appetite loss, stomach discomfort, hematemesis, blood in stool, late-stage pain |

| DIAGNOSIS | TREATMENT |
|---|---|
| Physical exam, immunodiagnostic tests, and pathogen culture | Antibiotics, antivirals, or antifungals, depending on the pathogen |
| Physical exam, biopsy | Surgical excision of tumor, radiation |
| Endoscopy and esophageal washings | Surgery, radiation, chemotherapy |
| Physical exam | Nonirritating diet, antacids, acid reducing medications |
| Endoscopy, physical exam, history of alcoholism | Hemorrhage requires infusion of vasopressin or insertion of inflatable tube to compress veins; surgical bypass of portal veins to reduce intravenous pressure |
| X-ray | Avoid irritating foods, eat frequent small meals, surgery to repair diaphragm |
| Gastroscopy | Avoid irritants, drink ice water, antacid medications, surgery to control bleeding |
| Analysis of stomach content reveals low levels of HCl and intrinsic factor | Avoid stomach irritants, vitamin $B_{12}$ supplements |
| Gastroscopy, gastric washings, barium x-ray | Antibiotics |
| Stool culture, history | Fluid and electrolyte replacement; antidiarrheal medication; self-limiting in healthy people |
| Gastroscopy, biopsy, gastric fluid analysis (low HCl), barium x-ray | Surgery, chemotherapy |

# DISEASES AT A GLANCE

## Digestive System

| DISEASE | ETIOLOGY | SIGNS AND SYMPTOMS |
|---------|----------|--------------------|
| Appendicitis | Obstruction with fecal material leads to infection, inflammation, and necrosis | Acute lower right quadrant abdominal pain, nausea, fever |
| Malabsorption syndrome | Congenitally abnormal intestinal mucosa or malabsorption secondary to diseases of pancreas or gallbladder | Malnutrition, failure to absorb fats and fat-soluble vitamins, failure to grow in children and weight loss in adults |
| Diverticulitis | Diverticula of colon become impacted with fecal material and infected or inflamed | Cramping and pain in lower abdomen |
| Regional enteritis (Crohn's disease) | Idiopathic; possible link to autoimmune disease | Lower right pain, diarrhea and constipation, emission and exacerbation, weight loss, melena |
| Chronic ulcerative colitis | Idiopathic; may be autoimmune, stress-related, food allergy | Diarrhea; pus, blood, mucus in stool; cramping in lower abdomen |
| Carcinoma of colon and rectum | Genetic; associated with familial polyposis and chronic ulcerative colitis | Change in bowel habits, diarrhea or constipation, blood in stool |
| Spastic colon/irritable bowel syndrome | Abuse of laxatives; irritating foods; stress | Diarrhea, pain, gas, constipation |
| Dysentery | Food- or water-borne intestinal infection by bacteria or protozoa | Abdominal pain, bloody diarrhea with pus and mucus |
| Viral hepatitis A (infectious hepatitis) | Food- or water-borne infection with hepatitis A virus | Anorexia, nausea, mild fever, jaundice, enlarged tender liver |
| Hepatitis B (serum hepatitis) | Blood-borne or sexually transmitted infection with hepatitis B virus | 2–6 month incubation period followed by anorexia, nausea, mild fever, jaundice, enlarged tender liver; may lead to chronic hepatitis and cirrhosis |

| DIAGNOSIS | TREATMENT |
| --- | --- |
| Blood count, physical exam | Surgery |
| Stool analysis and history | Manage diet and vitamin supplements |
| Endoscopy | Antibiotics, manage diet |
| Stool analysis, endoscopy, patchy thickening of intestinal wall | Corticosteroids, occasionally surgery |
| Stool analysis, endoscopy, diffuse thickening of colon (pipestem colon) | Corticosteroids, stress reduction, diet management, colostomy |
| Endoscopy, biopsy, barium x-ray, stool analysis | Surgery, radiation, chemotherapy |
| History and physical exam; no lesions present | Avoid caffeine, alcohol, spicy food, fat, increase fiber in diet, reduce stress |
| Stool culture and history | Antibiotics if bacterial and amebicides if caused by protozoa |
| Physical exam, stool analysis, immunodiagnostics | Immunoglobulin injections |
| Physical exam, stool analysis, immunodiagnostics | Immunoglobulin injections, antiviral medications, vaccine for prevention |

# DISEASES AT A GLANCE

## Digestive System

| DISEASE | ETIOLOGY | SIGNS AND SYMPTOMS |
|---|---|---|
| Hepatitis C | Blood-borne or sexually transmitted infection with hepatitis C virus | Symptoms as for hepatitis A and hepatitis B following incubation period of months to decades; commonly results in cirrhosis and end-stage liver disease |
| Hepatitis D | Rare blood-borne or sexually transmitted co-infection with hepatitis D virus and hepatitis B virus | Same as for hepatitis B; more serious and frequently progresses to chronic liver diseases |
| Hepatitis E | Water-borne infection with hepatitis E virus rare in United States | As for hepatitis A |
| Cirrhosis | Alcohol-induced damage to liver; hepatitis | Jaundice, abdominal distension, ascites, bleeding tendencies, edema, malabsorption of fats, gynecosmastia, delerium tremens, hepatic coma |
| Carcinoma of the liver | Primary carcinoma is complication of cirrhosis; more common is secondary or metastatic | Bile duct obstruction, jaundice, impaired clotting, ascites, weight loss |
| Cholecystitis | Obstruction by infection/ inflammation or by tumor | Upper right abdominal pain especially following a meal of fatty food, nausea, indigestion, belching |
| Cholelithiasis | Related to obesity; higher incidence in pregnancy and among women | None, or upper right abdominal pain especially following a meal |
| Pancreatitis | Idiopathic, commonly associated with excessive alcohol consumption or with gallstones | Acute, severe, sharp, radiating abdominal pain; risk of hemorrhage; jaundice; vomiting; malabsorption |
| Cancer of the pancreas | Linked to cigarette smoking, alcohol abuse, chemical carcinogens, chronic pancreatitis, diabetes mellitus | Malabsorption, jaundice, upper abdominal pain |

| DIAGNOSIS | TREATMENT |
|---|---|
| Physical exam, stool analysis, immunodiagnostics | Ribavarin, interferon, liver transplant |
| Physical exam, stool analysis, immunodiagnostics | Immunoglobulin injections, antiviral |
| Physical exam, stool analysis, immunodiagnostics | No treatment, no vaccine |
| Patient history, physical exam, serum liver enzyme levels | No specific treatment; improved diet, liver transplant |
| Ultrasound, CT scan, needle biopsy | Chemotherapy (prognosis poor) |
| Ultrasound, CT scan, fecal fat test | Cholecystectomy |
| Ultrasound, CT scan, fecal fat test | Cholecystectomy, administration of solubilizing agent into bile duct |
| Ultrasound, CT scan, serum pancreatic enzymes | No specific treatment; analgesics, fluid replacement, IV nutrients |
| Ultrasound, CT scan, needle biopsy | Chemotherapy (prognosis poor) |

# Interactive Activities

## Cases for Critical Thinking

1. A 45-year-old woman experiences frequent heartburn, occasional swallowing difficulty, and sharp pains below her sternum. Sometimes at night, she experiences gastric reflux, or a regurgitation of stomach acid into the esophagus, a condition that is extremely painful. What could produce these symptoms? What diagnostic procedures could be used? How should she be treated?

2. T. W. experiences sharp pain in his upper right abdomen after eating a high-fat meal. Also, he has noted that his feces are grayish white instead of brown. What disease is the likely cause of his symptoms? Explain why each of these symptoms occurs with this disease.

3. Explain how cirrhosis leads to each of these signs and symptoms: jaundice, malnutrition, hemorrhage, esophageal varices.

## Multiple Choice

1. Which of the following is a sign of gastritis?
   a. constipation
   b. inflammation of stomach mucosa
   c. achlorhydria
   d. diarrhea

2. Recurrent bloody diarrhea may be a symptom of _____.
   a. gastric ulcer
   b. ulcerative colitis
   c. hiatal hernia
   d. esophagitis

3. Which disease is characterized by the destruction of intestinal villi, leading to inability to absorb fats and other nutrients?
   a. ulcerative colitis
   b. celiac disease/malabsorption syndrome
   c. Crohn's disease
   d. peptic ulcer

4. Small pouches of the large intestine become inflamed during which disease?
   a. Crohn's disease
   b. gastritis
   c. hemorrhoids
   d. diverticulitis

5. Which is FALSE about pancreatic cancer?
   a. characterized by abdominal pain, weakness, weight loss
   b. higher incidence with age
   c. most are diagnosed after the cancer has metastasized
   d. prognosis is good with an 85% cure rate

6. Which is FALSE about cirrhosis?
   a. irreversible degenerative changes in liver
   b. normal liver replaced with fibrous scar tissue
   c. most often caused by diabetes
   d. esophageal varices

7. Acute pancreatitis is most closely associated with _____.
   a. hepatitis C virus infection
   b. chronic alcoholism
   c. bile duct obstruction
   d. complication of cirrhosis

8. Esophageal varices arise in which disease?
   a. cirrhosis
   b. pancreatic cancer
   c. cholecystitis
   d. cholelithiasis

9. Oral thrush is caused by _____.
   a. *Candida albicans*
   b. herpes simplex virus type 1
   c. *Treponema pallidum*
   d. *Streptococcus pyogenes*

10. Pain in the upper right quadrant, especially after eating, could be a sign of _____.
   a. appendicitis
   b. pancreatitis
   c. cholecystitis
   d. colitis

## True or False

_____ 1. Hemorrhoids are caused by infection with *E. coli*.

_____ 2. Oral and esophageal cancers are linked to tobacco and alcohol use.

_____ 3. Drinking too much water causes diarrhea.

_____ 4. Dark stools are known as melena.

_____ 5. Neurologic disorders can accompany liver disease.

_____ 6. Hepatitis A is acquired through blood products.

_____ 7. Most cancer in the liver is primary liver cancer.

_____ 8. Gallstones are made of undigested food particles too large to pass.

_____ 9. There is no vaccine for hepatitis B.

_____ 10. Gastric ulcers are caused by infection with *Helicobacter pylori*.

## Fill-Ins

1. *Entamoeba histolytica* is the cause of _____ _____.

2. Thickened intestinal walls, leading to obstruction and abdominal pain, are found in

_____ _____.

3. An abdominal _____ is protrusion of an organ through abdominal wall muscles.

4. An instrument called a(n) _____ is used to view the lining of the esophagus or other organs of the digestive tract.

5. Hepatitis type _____ is the major viral cause of cirrhosis.

6. Cholecystectomy is used to treat _____.

7. Biliary cirrhosis arises if there is obstruction of the _____ _____.

8. Accumulation of fluid in the abdomen is called _____.

9. Stomatitis refers to inflammation of the _____.

10. The primary function of the _____ _____ is to absorb water.

# MedMedia Wrap-Up

**www.prenhall.com/mulvihill**
Remember to visit this website for extra study practice, including exercises, Internet links, news updates, and an audio glossary.

**Activity CD-ROM**
Check out the CD-ROM in the back of this book. You will find games, exercises, puzzles, and videos to help enhance your understanding of this chapter.

# Diseases of the Urinary System

CHAPTER

# 11

## Learning Objectives

After studying this chapter, you should be able to

- Name the primary kidney functions
- Identify major diseases of the kidney
- Describe common signs and symptoms of urinary tract infections
- Name diagnostic procedures to analyze urinary tract infections
- Differentiate between ascending and descending modes of urinary tract infections
- Describe how urinary tract infections affect other organ systems
- Name the causes, signs and symptoms, and treatments of pyelonephritis and glomerulonephritis
- Identify causes, signs and symptoms, and treatments of kidney stones
- Describe urinary bladder diseases and treatments
- Describe age-related changes of the urinary system

## Fact or Fiction?

Renal calculi, or kidney stones, form only in the kidneys. They also form in the population equally throughout all regions of the United States.

*Fiction: Renal calculi may form anywhere within the urinary system, but they usually form in the renal pelvis or calyces of the kidney. Within the United States, there is an area considered the "stone belt." The southeastern region of the country tends to have a greater proportion of persons with renal calculi, but the exact cause is unknown.*

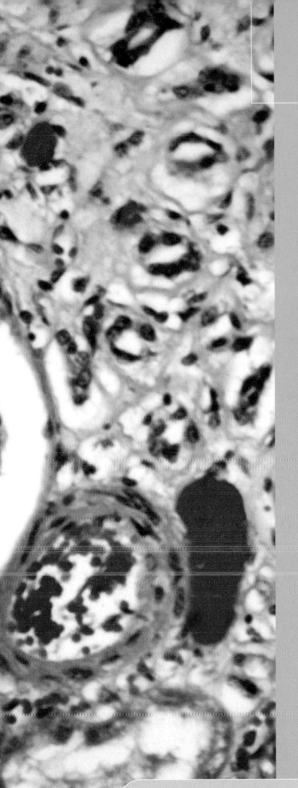

# History

## The Kidney Transplant

In 1854, Anne Belle was very ill from accidental poisoning. After two painful weeks, the 25-year-old mother died of apparent kidney failure. In those days, no renal dialysis or kidney transplantation could save her. The concept of transplantation was not new, having been proposed in ancient Greek myths and by cultures before them. One hundred years later, in 1954 at the Peter Bent Brigham Hospital in Boston, the first successful kidney transplant was performed between two identical twins. In this case, no immune-mediated rejection occurred because the twins shared identical tissue types, but rejection remained the primary barrier to successful transplantation. In 1959, doctors discovered that the drug Imuran, which was used to fight leukemia, could be used to block transplant rejection by suppressing the immune system. In 1962, tissue typing as well as immune suppression with drugs increased the success of kidney transplantation. From 1954 to 1973, some 10,000 kidney transplants were performed. In the 1980s, the drug cyclosporine was introduced, and in 1986 alone, nearly 9,000 successful kidney transplants were performed in the United States.

## MedMedia
www.prenhall.com/mulvihill

Use the web address to the left to access the free, interactive Companion Website created for this textbook. It features chapter-specific exercises, Internet links, news links, and an audio glossary. Additionally, explore the CD-ROM that accompanies this book to discover Disease Focus videos and a rich array of activities that accompany this chapter.

# ▶ Functions of the Kidney

The kidneys filter the blood, producing approximately 1 milliliter of urine per minute. In fact, between 20% and 25% of the body's blood volume is contained within them at any given time. As they filter the blood, the kidneys maintain water and electrolyte balance, correct the pH levels, produce erythropoietin, which stimulates red blood cell production, and secrete renin, which raises blood pressure.

## The Nephron

The functional unit of the kidney is the nephron. Approximately 1 million nephrons reside in each kidney. As blood passes through the nephrons, these minute structures filter metabolic waste products from the blood. Water and nutrients such as glucose and amino acids are resorbed. Then extra water, ions, drugs, and metabolic wastes are excreted. The product at the end of the nephron is urine.

Each nephron consists of a pair of arterioles, a glomerulus, a glomerular capsule, a proximal convoluted tubule, a loop of Henle, and a distal convoluted tubule that leads to a collecting duct. Figure 11–1 illustrates the parts of the nephron.

## Formation of Urine

Blood in the renal arteries enters a tuft of capillaries called the glomerulus, which is situated inside the glomerular capsule. These capillary walls are very thin and porous, and the blood pressure within them is higher than the pressure in the surrounding capsule. When blood enters these capillaries, fluid filters into the glomerular capsule. This blood filtrate is equivalent to protein-free plasma. In a healthy nephron, neither protein nor red blood cells pass through the filter into the glomerular capsule.

In the proximal convoluted tubule, most of the nutrients and a large amount of water are reabsorbed and taken back into blood capillaries surrounding the tubules. Salts, particularly sodium and chloride, are selectively reabsorbed according to the body's needs. Eventually, about 99% of the water is also reabsorbed along with the salts.

The nitrogen-containing waste products of protein metabolism, urea and creatinine, pass on through the tubules to be excreted in the urine. Those substances that are in excess in the body fluids, such as hydrogen ions when the fluid is too acidic, are secreted into the distal tubules to be excreted.

The Aldosterone and antidiuretic hormone play very important roles in the regulation of salt and water reabsorption. These hormones are discussed in detail in Chapter 13.

Urine from all the collecting ducts eventually empties into the renal pelvis, the juncture between the kidneys and the ureters, and moves down the ureters to be stored in the urinary bladder, which empties to the outside through a single tube called the urethra. Figure 11–2 illustrates the urinary system.

# ▶ Diseases of the Kidney

## Glomerulonephritis

Glomerulonephritis is an inflammatory disease of the glomeruli. It is nonsuppurative; that is, no pus formation is associated with it, nor are any bacteria found in the urine. Glomerulonephritis is caused by an antigen-antibody reaction that occurs approximately 1 to 4 weeks following skin or throat infection with β-hemolytic streptococci. Antigens of the streptococci and antibodies form complexes in the circulatory system and become trapped within the glomeruli, causing the inflammatory response. Numerous neutrophils crowd into the inflamed glomeruli, bloodflow to the nephrons is reduced, and filtration is reduced, resulting in decreased urine formation. Many glomeruli degenerate, and the remaining glomeruli become extremely permeable, allowing albumin and red blood cells to appear in the urine (Figure 11–3). Signs of glomerulonephritis thus include proteinuria, edema, and hypertension.

Acute glomerulonephritis is most common in young children, but can occur at any age, and usually follows a streptococcal infection of the throat or skin. The symptoms include chills and

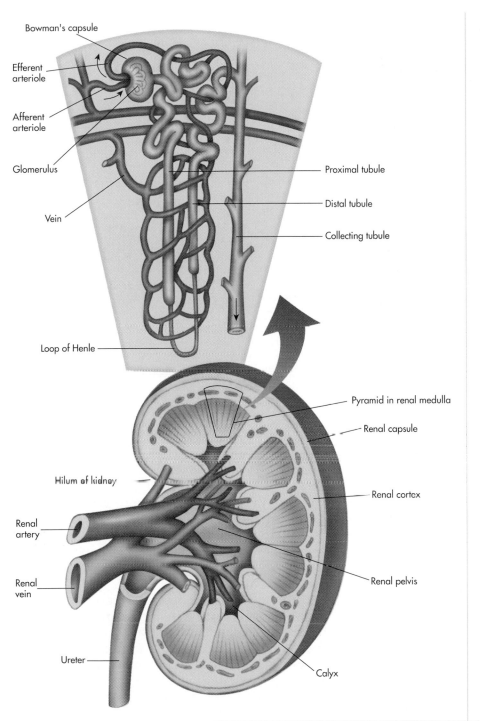

Bowman's capsule

Efferent arteriole

Afferent arteriole

Glomerulus

Vein

Loop of Henle

Proximal tubule

Distal tubule

Collecting tubule

Pyramid in renal medulla

Renal capsule

Hilum of kidney

Renal cortex

Renal artery

Renal vein

Renal pelvis

Ureter

Calyx

**Figure 11–1**
The kidney with an expanded view of the nephron.

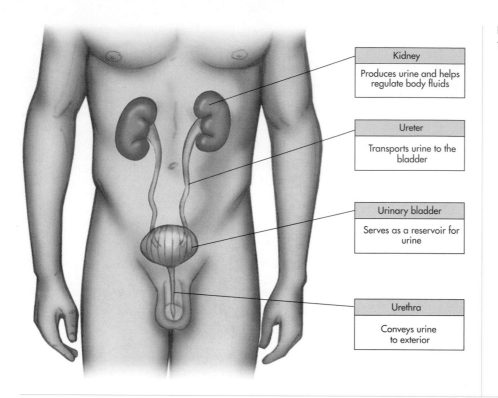

**Figure 11–2**
The urinary system.

| Kidney |
| --- |
| Produces urine and helps regulate body fluids |

| Ureter |
| --- |
| Transports urine to the bladder |

| Urinary bladder |
| --- |
| Serves as a reservoir for urine |

| Urethra |
| --- |
| Conveys urine to exterior |

fever, loss of appetite, and a general feeling of weakness. There may be edema, or puffiness, particularly in the face and ankles. A urinalysis shows albuminuria, the presence of the plasma protein albumin in the urine. Hematuria, blood in the urine, is also commonly found. Casts, which are the structural elements or molds of kidney tubules consisting of coagulated protein and blood, are present. The signs and symptoms of acute glomerulonephritis are presented in Figure 11–4.

The prognosis for acute glomerulonephritis is good. Normal kidney function is restored after following bed rest and dietary salt restrictions. Repeated attacks of acute glomerulonephritis, however, can lead to a chronic condition.

## Chronic Glomerulonephritis

Chronic glomerulonephritis may persist for many years with periods of remission and relapse. Hypertension generally accompanies this disease. As more glomeruli are destroyed, blood filtration becomes increasingly impaired.

A test to determine the extent of kidney function is the specific gravity of a urine specimen. Specific gravity indicates the amount of dissolved substances in a sample compared with distilled water. Distilled water has a specific gravity of 1.000, and the normal specific gravity of urine is 1.015 to 1.025. In advanced chronic glomerulonephritis, the specific gravity is low and fixed, indicating that the kidney tubules are unable to concentrate the urine.

Chronic glomerulonephritis causes the kidneys to shrink, and they gradually atrophy and cease to function. Uremia, a buildup of metabolic toxins in the blood, results from kidney failure. Chief among these waste products is urea, a small molecule that easily penetrates red blood cells and causes their destruction (hemolysis). Therefore, uremia often is associated with gastrointestinal, neuromuscular, and cardiovascular insufficiencies.

Individuals suffering uremic toxicity experience nausea, headache, dizziness, and faint vision. Left unchecked, this condition may result in convulsions and coma. Dialysis treatment is

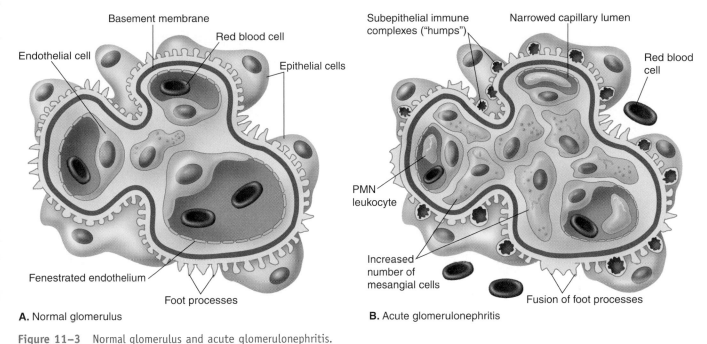

**A.** Normal glomerulus

**B.** Acute glomerulonephritis

**Figure 11–3** Normal glomerulus and acute glomerulonephritis.

quickly needed to restore blood nitrogen and electrolyte balance.

A less common form of glomerulonephritis is caused by autoantibodies directed against the basement membranes of the glomerular capillaries. This form is called antiglomerular basement membrane glomerulonephritis. In this case, the inflammatory disease results in scar-ring and fibrosis of the glomerular structure. (Figure 11–4).

## Renal Failure

Ischemia, hemorrhage, poisons, and severe kidney disease may cause renal failure. In renal failure, the kidneys are unable to clear the blood of urea and creatinine, which are nitrogen-containing waste products of protein metabolism and are toxic if they accumulate in the blood. Uremia signifies the terminal stage of renal insufficiency.

The level of blood urea nitrogen, or BUN, reflects the degree of renal failure. Measurement of the glomerular filtration rate (GFR) also can assess the severity of renal disease or follow its progress. GFR is evaluated through tests of the ability of the kidney to clear the waste product creatinine. Serum creatinine level rises and creatinine clearance rate falls when the GFR is impaired. As may be expected, creatinine clearance levels decline in renal insufficiency and with aging. The test for creatinine is the most specific for kidney functioning and therefore a crucial diagnostic measurement (Box 11–1).

**Figure 11–4** Signs and symptoms of acute glomerulonephritis.

SIGNS AND SYMPTOMS OF ACUTE GLOMERULONEPHRITIS

- Chills, fever, and weakness
- Edema in face and ankles
- Hematuria
- Albuminuria
- Casts

> ### Box 11–1    Calculating Creatinine Clearance as a Measurement of Kidney Function
>
> Creatinine is a nitrogenous waste product normally found in the blood. Healthy kidneys remove creatinine from the blood, and the rate of removal from the blood is called creatinine clearance. Normal levels for creatinine clearance are 88 to 128 ml/min in women and 97 to 137 ml/min in men.
>
> $$\text{Creatinine clearance for men} = \frac{140 - \text{age(yr)} \times \text{body weight (kg)}}{(72) \times \text{serum creatinine (mg/dl)}}$$
>
> $$\text{Creatine clearance for women} = \frac{140 - \text{age(yr)} \times \text{body weight (kg)}}{(72) \times \text{serum creatinine (mg/dl)}} \times 0.85$$

## Acute Renal Failure

Acute renal failure develops suddenly but has a better prognosis than chronic renal failure. Acute renal failure is caused by decreased bloodflow to the kidneys resulting from surgical shock, shock after an incompatible blood transfusion, or severe dehydration. Kidney disease, trauma, or poisons can also cause acute renal failure.

Acute renal failure is a characterized by a sudden drop in urine volume, called oliguria, or complete cessation of urine production, called anuria. Symptoms include headache, gastrointestinal distress, and the odor of ammonia on the breath caused by accumulation in the blood of nitrogen-containing compounds. Of special concern is hyperkalemia, excess blood potassium, which causes muscle weakness and can slow the heart to the point of cardiac arrest. Treatment includes restoration of the blood volume to normal, restricted fluid intake, and dialysis.

## Chronic Renal Failure

Chronic renal failure is life-threatening and has a much poorer prognosis than acute renal failure. Chronic renal failure results from long-standing kidney disease such as chronic glomerulonephritis, hypertension, or diabetic nephropathy, a kidney disease resulting from diabetes mellitus.

The condition develops slowly, with urinary output dropping slowly over time. Metabolic wastes accumulate in the blood with adverse effects on all the systems. For example, urea builds up to toxic levels, and some is converted to ammonia, which acts as an irritant in the gastrointestinal tract, producing nausea, vomiting, and diarrhea. Vision becomes dim, cognitive functions decrease, and convulsions or coma may ensue. Manifestations of chronic renal failure are summarized in Figure 11–5. These cases are now often considered end-stage kidney disease.

Renal failure is treated with kidney dialysis, a technique that removes toxic substances from the blood. In hemodialysis, blood is removed from the body, toxic substances are removed from the blood, and the blood is returned to the body (Figure 11–6). For hemodialysis, a patient typically must visit a clinic for dialysis and stay during the process. However, residential dialysis units are available that allow patients more convenient and private treatment. Small portable dialysis units have further reduced cost and increased access to treatment. In peritoneal dialysis (PD), dialyzing fluid is introduced into the abdominal cavity, where the peritoneum (cavity lining) acts as a filter membrane. The fluid draws toxic materials out of capillaries surrounding the body cavity, and after a suitable amount of time, the peritoneal fluid is removed, along with its dissolved toxins. A bag may be attached externally to collect the fluid, permitting the patient to remain mobile and providing more freedom and flexibility during treatment. Dialysis may be required for years, but may not be sufficient in advanced chronic renal failure.

Another alternative treatment for advanced kidney failure is kidney transplant. Advances in

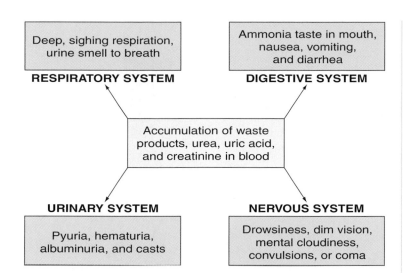

**Figure 11–5**
Manifestations of chronic renal failure.

antirejection medications have reduced complications and allowed kidney transplants to prolong and save thousands of lives (Figure 11–7).

## Pyelonephritis

Pyelonephritis is a suppurative urinary tract infection of the kidney and renal pelvis, caused by pyogenic (pus-forming) bacteria including, *Escherichia coli*, streptococci, and staphylococci. Obstruction of the urinary tract, such as a congenital defect, a kidney stone, or an enlarged prostate gland slows urine flow and increases the risk for infection. The infection may originate in the bladder and spread up into the kidneys, or it may originate in blood or lymph. Figure 11–8 shows the possible routes of infection.

In pyelonephritis, abscesses form and rupture, draining pus into the renal pelvis and the urine. Pus in the urine is called pyuria and may be discovered during urinalysis. The abscesses can fuse, filling the entire kidney with pus. Left untreated, pyelonephritis may lead to renal failure and uremia. In less severe infections, healing occurs but scar tissue forms. Because fibrous scar tissue tends to contract, the kidney shrinks and becomes what is described as a granular contracted kidney.

Symptoms of pyelonephritis include chills, high fever, sudden back pain that spreads over the abdomen, dysuria, and hematuria. Micro- scopic examination of the urine reveals numerous pus cells and bacteria. Treatment includes antibiotics for the infection.

## Pyelitis

Pyelitis is an inflammation of the renal pelvis, the juncture between the ureter and the kidney. Pyelitis is caused by *E. coli* and other pyogenic bacteria. The bacteria may originate from a urinary bladder infection or the blood. Pyelitis occurs commonly in young children, particularly girls, because the urethra in females is much shorter than that of males. Microorganisms from fecal contamination can enter from the outside and travel easily to the bladder. The infection can then spread up the ureter to the renal pelvis. Dysuria as well as increased frequency and urgency are common symptoms of pyelitis. A urinalysis will reveal numerous pus cells.

This disease responds well to treatment with antibiotics. Early diagnosis and treatment are important in preventing the spread of the infection into the kidney tissue, thus becoming pyelonephritis.

## Renal Carcinoma

Kidney cancer, also called hypernephroma, causes enlargement of the kidney and destroys the organ. Renal carcinoma is a relatively rare type

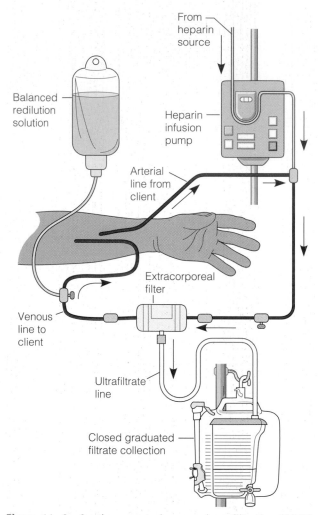

**Figure 11–6** Continuous arteriovenous hemofiltration (CAVH).

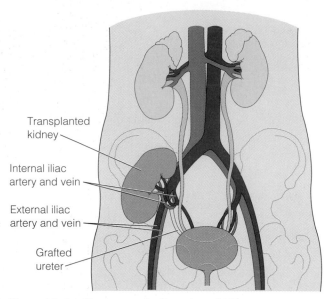

**Figure 11–7** Placement of a transplanted kidney.

of kidney cancer, comprising only 3% of all adult cancers, but causes 85% of all kidney cancers. Two other types, transitional cell carcinoma and sarcoma make up the remaining 15% of kidney cancers. The incidence of kidney cancer in men is twice that for women, and it normally occurs between ages 50 and 60. Smokers are twice as likely as nonsmokers to develop kidney cancer.

The tumor may not manifest itself for a long time. Painless hematuria eventually becomes the chief sign. When the tumor becomes large, an abdominal mass may be felt. This mass can then be detected on an x-ray as a tumor of the kidney. Metastasis to other organs often occurs before the presence of the kidney tumor is known. The malignancy frequently spreads to the lungs, liver, bones, and brain. Besides pain, typical signs include loss of appetite, weight loss, anemia, and an elevated white blood cell count (leucocytosis). Surgical removal is the best treatment.

A malignant tumor of the kidney pelvis that develops in very young children (1 in 10,000) is **Wilms' tumor**, an adenosarcoma. A fast-growing tumor, it metastasizes through the blood and lymph vessels. Symptoms and signs include hematuria, pain, vomiting, and hypertension similar to symptoms of renal carcinoma in an adult. In recent years, without metastasis, surgery and radiation and chemotherapy offer a good prognosis.

Wilms' tumor has a genetic connection. It appears that at least three different genes influence the occurrence of this disease. The Wilms' tumor gene 1 (WT-1), whose actual function is unknown, seems to play an important role in embryonic development. When this particular gene is missing or mutated, congenital defects appear, and this abnormal tissue later becomes the site of cancer.

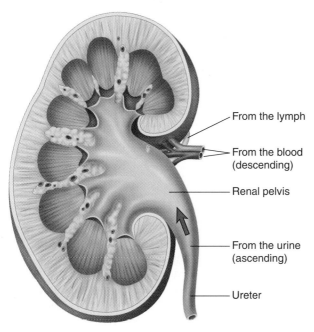

**Figure 11–8**  Routes of infection for pyelonephritis.

- From the lymph
- From the blood (descending)
- Renal pelvis
- From the urine (ascending)
- Ureter

## Kidney Stones

Kidney stones, known as urinary calculi, predominantly form in the kidney. The prevalence of urinary calculi is approximately 10%, and by age 70, 5% to 15% of all U.S. citizens experience kidney stones. Men are four times more likely than women to produce renal calculi, with the first episodes occurring between age 20 and 40.

Urinary calculi may be present and cause no symptoms, even when passed through the urinary tract, unless they are larger than a quarter inch in diameter, in which case they become lodged in the ureter. The stones then cause intense pain that radiates from the kidney area to the groin. In addition to intense pain, signs and symptoms include hematuria, nausea, vomiting, and diarrhea.

Kidney stones may cause urinary tract infections by blocking urine flow and permitting bacterial growth in the urinary tract. Conversely, a urinary tract infection that blocks urine flow can trigger kidney stone formation because of urine stasis in the renal pelvis. Calculi are formed when certain minerals in the urine form a precipitate, that is, come out of solution and grow in size. Bacteria in urine can serve as sites for calcium deposition. The resulting stones, if small enough, can be passed in the urine, but larger stones may require surgery or other treatment.

Four renal calculi formations are recognized. Calcium stones comprise 80% of all kidney stones and consist mainly of calcium salts, calcium oxalate, and calcium phosphate. Calcium excess often leads to stone formation. Hyperactive parathyroid glands can cause the excess of circulating calcium, promoting formation of urinary calculi. No evidence suggests that "hard water" influences kidney stone formation. Men are four to five times more likely than women to form these stones. Uric acid stones comprise 10% of stones and occur especially in men subject to gout. Colon surgery increases the risk for uric acid stones. When portions of the colon are removed, the urine becomes more acidic, which enhances the formation of uric acid stones. Struvite stones, also called infection stones, comprise nearly 10% of stone formations. Bacterial growth in these kidney stones produces ammonia, making the urine alkaline, which also triggers stone precipitation. When bacteria become encased in minerals, antibiotics are ineffective, and the stones tend to enlarge and require surgical removal. A stone may become so large that it fills the renal pelvis completely, blocking the flow of urine. A stone of this type, named for its shape, is the staghorn calculus illustrated in Figure 11–9. A kidney containing numerous small calculi is also shown. Cysteine stones account for the remaining 1% of the renal calculi. These stones are aggregates of the amino acid cysteine, which does not dissolve easily in water. Cysteine stones result from a hereditary disorder in which the kidneys fail to reabsorb cysteine, which builds up in urine, precipitates, and eventually forms stones.

Stones can also form in the urinary bladder. The presence of bladder stones causes urinary tract infections because they frequently obstruct the flow of urine.

Diagnostic tools include CT, intravenous pyelogram (IVP), renal ultrasound/scan, and a KUB (kidney, ureter, bladder) exam that consists of a single x-ray without dye to view the abdominopelvic region.

Urinary calculi may be treated with medication that partially dissolves the stone, permitting it to be passed in the urine. Lithotripsy, the crushing of kidney stones, is necessary for the 20% of kidney stones that do not pass on their own. In lithotripsy, sonic vibrations are applied externally to crush the stones. If performed while the patient is immersed in a tank of water, the procedure is called hydrolithotripsy (Figure 11–10). In this technique, the patient is the sonic waves shatter the hard stones into sand-sized particles that can be eliminated within the urine stream. Because recovery is rapid, the patient usually requires only 0-1 day of hospitalization.

Recurrence of stones is not uncommon. To avoid recurrence, fluid intake should be increased to keep the urine dilute, and dietary calcium and protein should be reduced.

## Hydronephrosis

As a result of urinary calculi, a tumor, an enlarged prostate gland, a congenital defect, or other obstruction of the renal pelvis, the kidney can become extremely dilated with urine. This condition is called hydronephrosis. The ureters dilate above the obstruction from the pressure of urine that is unable to pass and are called hydroureters. Figure 11–11 shows this dilated condition. A ureterocele can cause hydronephrosis. Here, the terminal portion of the ureter prolapses, or slips into the urinary bladder. When detected (see "Diagnostic Tests and Procedures"), it can be corrected surgically.

The degree of pain accompanying hydronephrosis depends on the nature of the blockage. Hematuria is generally present. If an infection develops because of the stagnation of urine, pyuria and fever occur. Figure 11–12 depicts hydronephrosis of the kidney.

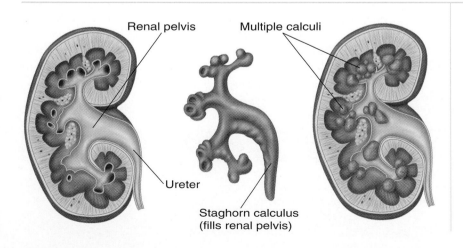

Renal pelvis    Multiple calculi

Ureter

Staghorn calculus
(fills renal pelvis)

**Figure 11–9**
Urinary calculi.

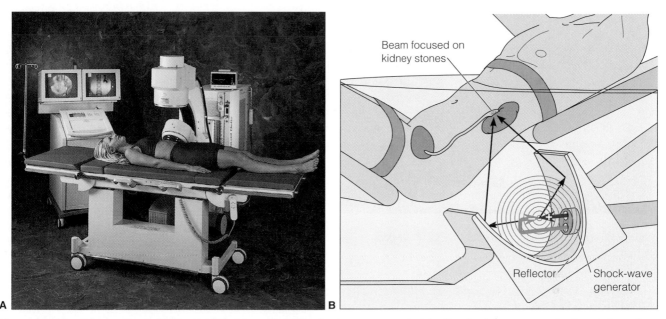

**Figure 11–10** Extracorporeal shock-wave lithotripsy. Acoustic shock waves generated by the shock-wave generator travel through soft tissue to shatter the renal stone into fragments, which are then eliminated in the urine. (A) A shock-wave generator that does not require water immersion. (B) An illustration of water immersion lithotripsy procedure.

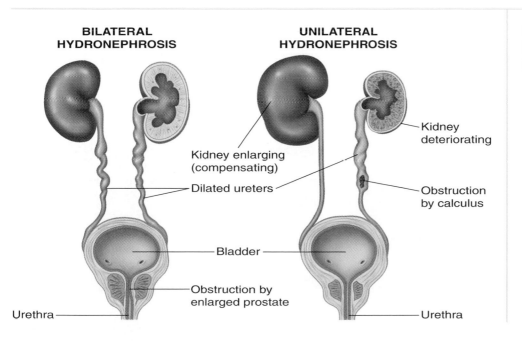

**Figure 11–11**
Hydronephrosis: bilateral (left), unilateral (right).

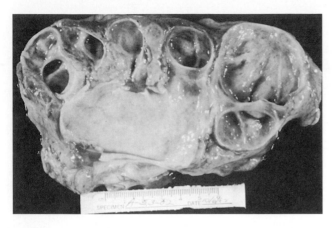

**Figure 11–12**    Hydronephrosis. (Courtesy of Dr. David R. Duffell.)

## Polycystic Kidney

Solitary renal cysts are relatively common, with sizes varying from a few millimeters to 15 mm, having little effect on kidney function. However, the polycystic kidney is a congenital defect, an error in development that usually involves both kidneys. An autosomal recessive gene causes polycystic kidney in children, while in adults it is caused by an autosomal dominant gene.

Adult polycystic kidney disease affects 1 of 500 to 1000 individuals.

The cysts are dilated kidney tubules that do not open into the renal pelvis as they should. Instead, the cysts enlarge, fuse, and usually become infected. As the cysts enlarge, they compress the surrounding kidney tissue. The Side by Side illustrates the polycystic kidney of an adult. By middle age, signs and symptoms appear, including pain, hematuria, polyuria, renal calculi, and hypertension. This disease may be diagnosed with a combination of a physical exam, a renal ultrasound or CT, or an IVP (see "Diagnostic Tests and Procedures").

No specific treatment is available. Renal failure eventually occurs, requiring dialysis or kidney transplant.

## ▶ Diseases of Urinary Bladder and Urethra

### Cystitis

Cystitis is an inflammation of the urinary bladder usually caused by an infection. It is more common in women than in men because of

## SIDE by SIDE ■ Polycystic Kidney

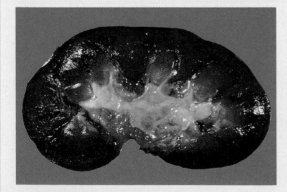

▲ Normal kidney (© Logical Images/Custom Medical Stock Photo.)

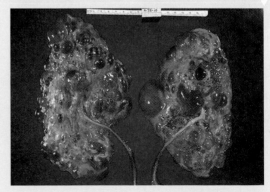

▲ Polycystic kidney. (Courtesy of the CDC/Dr. Edwin P. Ewing, Jr., 1972.)

women's shorter urethra. The chief cause is *E. coli*, which resides in the colon and can reach the urethra and travel upward to the bladder. Cystitis can also develop following sexual intercourse if bacteria around the vaginal opening spread to the urinary opening. Occasionally, pressure from coughing or exertion squeezes the bladder, which pushes some urine into the urethra, and then draws it back to the bladder. This action contaminates the normally sterile fluid within the urinary bladder.

The symptoms of cystitis include increased urinary frequency and urgency, and a burning sensation during urination. Microscopic examination of the urine reveals bacteria, pus, casts, and leukocytes. Treatment depends on the type of bacteria and may include a type of penicillin, such as ampicillin or amoxicillin.

## Carcinoma of the Bladder

Certain industrial chemicals and cigarette smoking have been linked to carcinoma of the urinary bladder. The tumor grows by sending fingerlike projections into the lumen of the bladder. Although these tumors can be seen with a cystoscope and removed, they tend to recur. A more invasive pattern of growth involves infiltration of the bladder wall, which cannot be surgically removed without destroying the bladder.

One treatment involves an infusion of BCG solution (Bacillus Calmette Guerin), a weakened tuberculosis bacillus, that coats the bladder's internal epithelial surface, which causes it to "peel off" and be replaced by new surface cells. This treatment lasts from months to years, depending on the status of the patient. If this procedure is not appropriate or is ineffective, then surgical removal of the cancer is required.

If the entire urinary bladder is surgically removed (radical cystectomy), an ileal conduit (see Figure 11–13) is constructed surgically to store and evacuate urine.

## Urethritis

Any part of the urinary tract can become inflamed, and the urethra is no exception. This inflammation is called urethritis. In men, the cause may be a gonococcus or other bacteria, viruses, or noxious chemicals. In women, urethritis frequently accompanies cystitis. An obstruction at the urinary opening may cause the inflammation in women. The symptoms of urethritis include a discharge of pus from the urethra, an itching sensation at the opening of the urethra, and a burning sensation during urination. Treatment includes antibiotics for bacteria infections.

## ▶ Age-Related Diseases

Several changes accompany the aging urinary system. With aging comes less control over urination (the micturition reflex) because the urethral sphincter muscles lose tone, allowing urine to leak, a condition called urinary incontinence. Brain and spinal cord damage may lead to a weak micturition urination reflex. Dehydration due to water loss via the aging kidneys is possible, because the total number of functioning nephrons declines with age, perhaps as much as 30% to 40% between ages 25 and 85, and the kidney loses sensitivity to antidiuretic hormone. Urinary retention occurs because bladders lose muscle tone and are unable

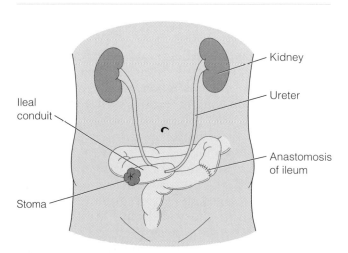

**Figure 11–13** Ileal conduit. A segment of ileum is separated from the small intestine and formed into a tubular pouch with the open end brought to the skin surface to form a stoma. The ureters are connected to the pouch.

to empty completely. Obstruction exacerbates urine retention and is common in men because of prostate enlargement. Urinary retention, in turn, increases the risk for urinary tract infections.

## ▶ Diagnostic Tests and Procedures

Pain, dysuria (painful urination), blood or pus in urine, or edema indicate kidney disease, but specific diagnostic tests are required to determine the nature of the disease. Edema is caused by the loss of protein from the blood. These blood proteins have a water-holding power within the blood vessels. With their depletion, fluid moves out of the capillaries and into the tissues, causing swelling or puffiness.

Significant information can be obtained by a simple diagnostic procedure, a urinalysis, in which a urine specimen is studied physically, chemically, and microscopically. Physical observation gives the color, pH, and specific gravity of a urine specimen. Chemical tests reveal the presence of abnormal substances such as protein—specifically albumin—glucose, and blood. A centrifuged urine sample is examined microscopically for solids such as crystals, epithelial cells, or blood cells.

Urine is normally yellow or amber, but hematuria (blood in the urine) can darken the color to a reddish brown. The degree of color depends on the amount of water the urine contains. Urine is pale in the case of diabetics, whose water output is large. In long-standing kidney diseases, the ability of the tubules to concentrate the urine is lost. As a result, the urine is dilute and pale, and the specific gravity is low.

The pH of urine has a broad range. The ability of the kidneys to excrete acidic or alkaline urine permits the kidney to regulate the pH of the blood within narrow limits. Urine specimens should be examined when fresh because they tend to become alkaline on standing due to bacterial contamination. Urine from a cystitis patient tends to be alkaline for the same reason.

Albuminuria indicates inflammation of the urinary tract, particularly of the glomeruli. The inflammation increases the permeability of blood vessels, allowing the protein albumin to enter the nephrons and appear in the urine. This loss reduces the level of protein in the blood, causing the condition called hypoproteinemia. Therefore, there is a tendency to lose fluids to the surrounding tissues, causing edema.

The presence of sugar (glucose) in the urine usually indicates diabetes mellitus. This is not a sign of a disease of the kidneys but of the endocrine areas of the pancreas. Diabetes over an extended period of time adversely affects the kidneys (see Chapter 13).

Hematuria may be obvious to the naked eye or require microscopic determination. Hematuria is associated with many serious diseases of the urinary tract, including glomerulonephritis, kidney stones, tuberculosis, cystitis, and tumors. If the passage of urine is accompanied by pain, a stone or tuberculosis may be the cause. Painless hematuria indicates the possibility of a malignant tumor in the urinary system.

Pyuria results from a suppurative inflammation caused by pyogenic bacteria, and pus causes the urine to appear cloudy. Microscopic examination of the urine reveals numerous leukocytes. Diseases such as pyelonephritis, pyelitis, tuberculosis, and cystitis show pus in the urine.

Casts are shaped like cylindrical rods because they form within kidney tubules. They consist of coagulated protein, a substance not normally present in kidney tubules. Casts can include various kinds of blood cells as well as epithelial cells from the lining of the urinary tract. Casts always indicate inflammation. Microscopic examination determines the presence or absence of bacteria. Bacteria are found in tuberculosis of the kidney, pyelonephritis, and frequently in cystitis. For microscopic examinations, a urine sample may be removed from the bladder by catheterization to ensure that no external contamination occurs.

A cystoscopic examination enables the physician to view the inside of the bladder and urethra. The cystoscope is a long, lighted instrument resembling a hollow tube. Tumors, stones, and inflammations may be identified with this device. Using an additional instrument, small tumors or polyps may be removed or biopsied. Stones in the bladder can be crushed and removed.

The intravenous pyelogram (IVP) allows the visualization of the urinary system by means of contrast dyes injected into the veins followed by x-ray examination. When these dyes concentrate in the urinary system, it is possible to note tumors, obstructions, and other deformities. The kidney may be viewed by renal ultrasound, and the whole urinary system may be surveyed by CT or KUB exams.

which left untreated causes renal failure. Various other urinary tract infections were considered: cystitis, pyelitis, and urethritis. These infections frequently follow some obstruction of the flow of urine. Urinary calculi, tumors, and congenital anomalies can cause such blockages. Symptoms and signs of kidney disease may include pain, painful urination, and blood or pus in the urine. Edema is also a sign of certain kidney diseases. A mass may be felt when a tumor of the kidney or bladder is large, but this is a late sign of malignancy, and metastases have probably already occurred. Interpretations of abnormal conditions of the urine were also discussed along with certain diagnostic procedures.

## CHAPTER SUMMARY

Although acute glomerulonephritis generally has a good prognosis, repeated attacks can lead to chronic glomerulonephritis, which may end with kidney failure. Kidney failure can be acute, and if treated, renal function is restored. Chronic renal failure does not respond to treatment and generally ends with uremia. Pyelonephritis is a destructive, suppurative inflammation of the kidney,

## RESOURCES

Cohen, B. J., & D. L. Wood, *Memmler's The Human Body in Health and Disease,* 9th ed., Lippincott, Williams, & Wilkens, 2000.

Cotran, R. S., V. Kumar, & T. Collins, *Robbins' Pathologic Basis of Disease,* 6th ed. Saunders, 1999.

Seal, G. M. *The Patient's Guide to Urology.* High Oaks Publisher, 1995.

Kidney Alert. *Saturday Evening Post,* Sep/Oct 2003, vol. 275, no. 5 p. 56.

# DISEASES AT A GLANCE

## Urinary System

| DISEASE | ETIOLOGY | SIGNS AND SYMPTOMS |
|---------|----------|--------------------|
| Hydronephroma | Idiopathic, radiation | Painless hematuria, later pain, loss of appetite, weight loss, anemia, elevated white blood count |
| Wilms' tumor | Idiopathic, possibly genetic | In young children, signs and symptoms similar to hydronephroma in adults |
| Pyelonephritis | Pyogenic bacteria | Pyuria, chills, high fever, sudden back pain, dysuria, bematuria, eventual renal failure, uremia |
| Pyelitis | Pyogenic bacteria | Dysuria, frequency, urgency |
| Acute glomerulonephritis | Prior bacterial infection, antigen-antibody complex | Follow strep infection: chills, fever, loss of appetite, weakness, edema, albuminuria, hematuria, casts |
| Chronic glomerulonephritis | Hypertension and glomerular destruction | Remission and exacerbation of glomerulonephritis; may end with granular contracted kidneys and uremia; specific gravity low and fixed in advanced cases |
| Acute renal failure | Incompatible blood transfusion, severe dehydration | Sudden oliguria, may become anuria, headache, GI distress, odor of ammonia in breath, muscle weakness |
| Chronic renal failure | Hypertension, chronic glomeru-lonephritis, diabetic nephropathy | Slow development, urinary wastes increase in blood, nausea, vomiting, diarrhea, dim vision, central nervous system affected, convulsions, coma |
| Urinary calculi (kidney stones) | Hyperparathyroidism, excess calcium | No symptoms until they block ureter, then intense pain radiating to groin |
| Hydronephrosis | Renal obstruction, congenital defect | Pain, hematuria, pyuria, and fever if infection present |
| Polycystic kidney | Genetic | Hypertension, eventual renal failure, uremia |
| Carcinoma | Idiopathic, radiation, smoking | Early asymptomatic, hematuria may occur, later pelvic pain and frequent urination |

| DIAGNOSIS | TREATMENT |
|---|---|
| X-ray | Surgery |
| X-ray | Surgery |
| Urinalysis, pus and blood in urine | Antibiotics |
| Urinalysis, numerous pus cells in urine | Antibiotics |
| Urinalysis, patient history | Antibiotics, steroids, immune suppression |
| Urinalysis, urine specific gravity low, patient history | Antibiotics, steroids, immune suppression |
| Patient history, blood and urinalysis | Drugs, fluid control, antibiotics, dialysis |
| Patient history, urinalysis, blood analysis | Dialysis, kidney transplant |
| Patient history, blood and urinalysis, x-ray | Lithotripsy, surgery |
| Urinalysis, IVP cystoscopic exam | Relief of obstruction, surgery |
| Urinalysis, IVP cystoscopic exam | Kidney transplant |
| Cystoscopy | Surgery |

# DISEASES AT A GLANCE *(continued)*

## Urinary System

| DISEASE | ETIOLOGY | SIGNS AND SYMPTOMS |
| --- | --- | --- |
| Cystitis | Usually bacteria infection | Urinary frequency, urgency, burning sensation during urination, blood in urine |
| Urethritis | Microbial agents, viruses, some chemicals | Burning sensation during urination, itching, pus discharge; in females, accompanies cystitis |
| Incontinence | Neurological injury, aging | Involuntary loss of urine |

| DIAGNOSIS | TREATMENT |
|---|---|
| Microscopic exam of urine, may be diagnosed by patient's description of typical signs and symptoms | Antibiotics |
| Microscopic exam of urine | Antibiotics |
| Patient history | Exercises for muscles of pelvic floor, antibiotics for infection |

# Interactive Activities

## Cases for Critical Thinking

1. Jane, a college sophomore, experienced painful urination and noticed blood in the urine. What can explain her symptoms and hematuria?

2. Britany, a relatively thin fourth grader, experienced a significant weight gain within two weeks' time. Just before holiday break, she had a bad sore throat, but after a visit to the doctor, those symptoms subsided. Her abdomen was distended and she had edema of the extremities. She complained of abdominal discomfort and general aches. Urinalysis indicated proteinuria and hematuria. A follow-up blood screen found antibodies to streptococcal toxins. What may explain Britany's symptoms?

3. A mother of a 4-month-old infant, while giving a bath, noticed and palpated a mass on the right side of the child's abdomen. The child was irritable and somewhat lethargic. What might explain this mass, and what diagnostic techniques can help determine the nature of the disease?

4. A 52-year-old grandfather's urinalysis revealed blood (hematuria). X-ray showed a renal mass on the right side. What is the probable cause for the hematuria, and what treatment would be recommended?

## Multiple Choice

1. Which of the following can cause chronic uremia?
   a. surgical shock
   b. severe dehydration
   c. complications of pregnancy
   d. diabetes mellitus

2. An inflammation of the tissue of the kidney is _____.
   a. pyelonephritis
   b. polycystic kidney
   c. hydronephrosis
   d. diabetic nephropathy

3. Inflammation of the renal pelvis is _____.
   a. pyelonephritis
   b. glomerulonephritis
   c. pyelitis
   d. congenital cystic kidney

4. Breath has an ammonia-like odor of urine in _____.
   a. glomerulonephritis
   b. pyelonephritis
   c. tuberculosis
   d. uremia

5. Urinary tract infections _____.
   a. are more common in males
   b. usually exhibit dysuria, urgency, and frequency
   c. are commonly caused by virus
   d. do not respond to antibiotic

6. The form of kidney dialysis that permits a patient to retain mobility is _____.
   a. peritoneal dialysis
   b. hemodialysis
   c. hemolysis
   d. ileal shunt

7. The inability to control urination is called _____.
   a. micturition
   b. incontinence
   c. anuria
   d. nocturia

8. To prevent uric acid calculi, diet should restrict _____.
   a. protein
   b. dairy products
   c. pasta and citrus
   d. spinach, cabbage, and tomatoes

9. The edema associated with nephritic syndrome primarily results from _____.
   a. hypertension
   b. hyperalbuminuria
   c. decreased plasma protein
   d. lower GFR

10. Reduced sensitivity to ADH, incontinence, and increased urination frequency are associated with _____.
    a. overhydration
    b. aging
    c. stress
    d. excess nitrogen intake

## True or False

_____ 1. A sudden drop in urine volume indicates chronic renal failure.

_____ 2. Cystitis is often an ascending infection.

_____ 3. In acute uremia, fluid intake should be decreased.

_____ 4. Albuminuria leads to hypoproteinemia.

_____ 5. Painful and frequent urination accompanies tuberculosis of the bladder.

_____ 6. Bacteria are not found in acute glomerulonephritis.

_____ 7. Pyelonephritis is a suppurative disease.

_____ 8. The urinary bladder stores urine that may be reused.

_____ 9. Leukocytes in urine indicate anemia.

_____ 10. Calcium (oxalate, phosphate) is the most common form of renal calculus.

## Fill-Ins

1. _____ is pus in the urine.

2. _____ _____ is a kidney disease resulting from diabetes mellitus.

3. Urinary calculi, or _____ _____, may be present and cause no symptoms until they become lodged in the ureter.

4. _____, the external crushing of kidney stones, is now the preferable procedure to remove kidney stones, replacing the need for surgery.

5. _____ _____ is a congenital anomaly that usually involves both kidneys.

6. Scanty urine or _____ is low urine volume (or formation).

7. Loss of urine at night is _____.

8. Struvite stones are associated with _____.

9. Urinary tract infections in males are usually caused by some form of _____ or STD.

10. An x-ray outline of the urinary system following an injection solution is the diagnostic technique called _____.

# MedMedia Wrap-Up

**www.prenhall.com/mulvihill**

Remember to visit this website for extra study practice, including exercises, Internet links, news updates, and an audio glossary.

**Activity CD-ROM**

Check out the CD-ROM in the back of this book. You will find games, exercises, puzzles, and videos to help enhance your understanding of this chapter.

*N. gonorrhoeae* gonococci (inside leukocytes) from a patient diagnosed with acute gonococcal urethritis. (Courtesy of the CDC/Joe Miller, 1979.)

CHAPTER

# 12

# Diseases of the Reproductive Systems

## Learning Objectives

After studying this chapter, you should be able to

- Describe the normal structure and function of the reproductive tract
- Describe the key characteristics of major diseases of the female reproductive tract
- Describe the key characteristics of major diseases of the male reproductive tract
- Explain the cause of reproductive tract diseases
- Name the diagnostic procedures for diseases of the reproductive tract
- Describe the treatment options for diseases of the reproductive system

## Fact or Fiction?

All sexually transmitted diseases (STDs) can be cured.

*Fiction: STDs caused by viruses cannot be cured. Medications can manage the symptoms but cannot cure the infection.*

# History

## Tuskegee Institute Experiment

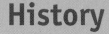

I n 1932, the U.S. Public Health Service with the assistance of the Tuskegee Institute recruited 600 African-American men to participate in an experiment involving the effects of untreated syphilis. Of this group, 399 men had been diagnosed with syphilis but were never informed that they had syphilis or that their disease was sexually transmitted. Originally meant to last 6 to 9 months, the study instead lasted 40 years until the men died. When the story broke in 1972, Congress convened hearings about the Tuskegee study. The hearings resulted in the rewriting of the Department of Health, Education, and Welfare's regulations on the use of human subjects in scientific experiments. A $1.8 billion class-action suit was filed on behalf of the Tuskegee participants and their heirs. A settlement for $10 million was made out of court.

## MedMedia

www.prenhall.com/mulvihill

Use the web address to the left to access the free, interactive Companion Website created for this textbook. It features chapter-specific exercises, Internet links, news links, and an audio glossary. Additionally, explore the CD-ROM that accompanies this book to discover Disease Focus videos and a rich array of activities that accompany this chapter.

## ► Anatomy of the Female Reproductive System

The female reproductive system consists of the vagina, the uterus, the fallopian tubes, and the ovaries. The vagina is a tubular structure extending backward and upward to the cervix, the lowest part of the uterus. The expanded, upper portion of the uterus tapers down to form the narrow cervix, giving the organ a pear-shaped appearance. The uterine wall is very strong, comprised of smooth muscle and lined with a mucosal membrane, the endometrium, and is responsive to hormonal changes. Figure 12–1 shows the female reproductive system.

The fallopian tubes extend laterally from each side of the uterus. The outer ends of the tubes are open to receive a released ovum. Fringelike projections at the outer ends, the fimbriae, propel the ova into the tube.

The ovaries, small, oval-shaped organs, are anchored near the open end of the fallopian tubes by ligaments. The ovaries contain hundreds of thousands of ova, which are present at birth. Surrounding each ovum is a single layer of cells, a primary follicle. The relationship between the ovaries and the fallopian tubes is shown in Figure 12–2.

The external genitalia, the vulva, include the mons pubis, the labia majora and labia minora, the clitoris, and the vaginal opening. The urinary meatus is between the clitoris and the vaginal opening. The mons pubis, a pad of fat tissue over the pubic symphysis, becomes covered with hair at puberty. Extending back from the mons pubis to the anus are two pairs of folds, the labia majora and the labia minora. The clitoris, a tuft of erectile tissue similar to that of the penis, is located at the anterior junction of the minor lips. A membranous fold, the hymen, partly or completely closes the vaginal opening. Occasionally, this membrane is imperforate or abnormally closed and requires a minor surgical procedure to open it. Bartholin's glands, a pair of mucus-secreting glands, are sit-

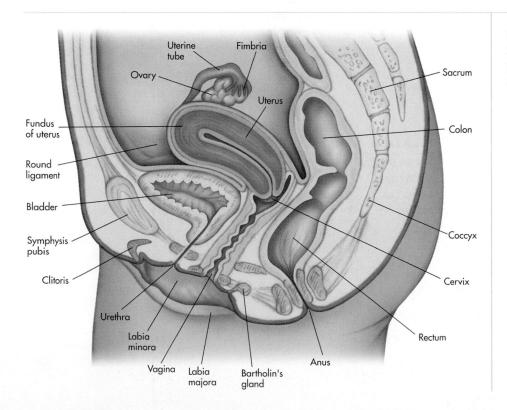

**Figure 12–1**
Sagittal section of the female pelvis, showing organs of the reproductive system.

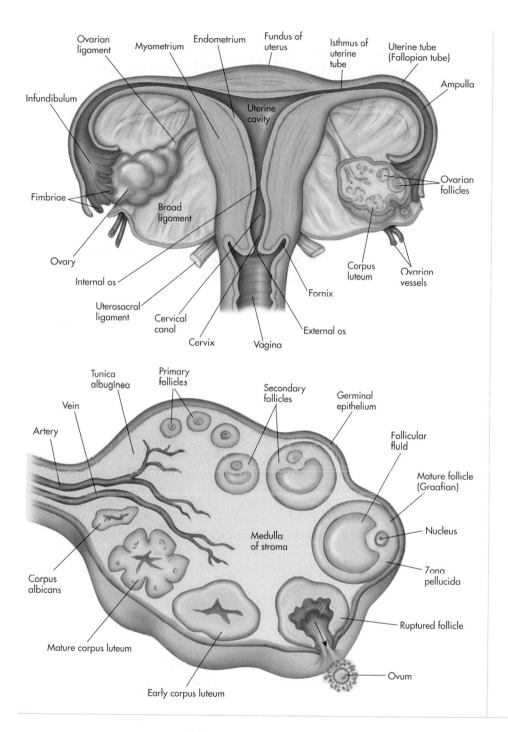

**Figure 12–2**
The uterus, ovaries, and associated structures.

uated at the vaginal entrance. These glands produce a lubricating secretion during sexual intercourse.

The breasts, accessory organs of reproduction, consist of milk glands supported by connective tissue covered with fatty tissue and skin. Ducts of the milk glands converge at the nipple, which is surrounded by a darkly pigmented area, the areola. The breasts overlie the pectoral muscles of the chest.

## ▶ Physiology of the Female Reproductive System

The cyclic hormonal changes in the life of a woman prepare the uterus monthly for a possible pregnancy. The secretion of female hormones, estrogen and progesterone, is governed by two gonadotropic hormones—follicle-stimulating hormone (FSH) and luteinizing hormone (LH)—of the anterior pituitary gland, which is controlled by the hypothalamus of the brain. Failure of the ovary to secrete sex hormones or to ovulate may result from pituitary disease or disturbances in the central nervous system.

A woman's reproductive life begins with the onset of menstruation, the menarche, occurring generally between ages 10 and 15. The reproductive years terminate with the cessation of menstrual periods, menopause, which usually begins in the late 40s or early 50s. At the beginning of each monthly cycle, pituitary gonadotropic hormone stimulates ovarian follicles to develop. The stimulated follicles begin to grow and develop into Graafian follicles. One of these matures first and is released at the midpoint of the cycle, which is the process of ovulation.

As the follicles grow during the first half of the cycle, the ovary secretes estrogen, which is carried by the blood to the uterus. Estrogen stimulates the endometrium of the uterus to enter the proliferative phase in which it thickens and becomes more vascular in preparation for pregnancy.

Once the ovum has been released from the ovary, the empty follicle is converted into the corpus luteum. which begins to secrete progesterone. Progesterone stimulates endometrial growth and promotes the storage of nutrients for nourishing a fertilized ovum. This is the secretory phase of the uterus.

If no fertilization occurs, the corpus luteum ceases to secrete hormones approximately 8 to 12 days after ovulation. At the end of the monthly cycle, the level of estrogen and progesterone drops, and menstruation, the sloughing of the endometrial lining, occurs. If pregnancy occurs, the corpus luteum greatly enlarges and continues to secrete high levels of progesterone. The placenta gradually assumes the role of the corpus luteum in secreting these hormones.

The placenta is formed from both maternal and embryonic tissue. Near the site of implantation in the uterus, the endometrium greatly thickens, becomes highly vascular, and develops large blood sinuses. An embryonic membrane, the chorion, develops fingerlike projections called villi, which dip into the maternal blood sinuses. This interdigitation of embryonic and maternal tissue constitutes the placenta. Human chorionic gonadotropin hormone (HCG) is secreted by the chorionic villi after implantation of the fertilized ovum in the uterus. Laboratory diagnosis of pregnancy is based on the presence of HCG in the mother's blood or urine.

The umbilical arteries extend into the chorionic villi, where carbon dioxide and waste are exchanged for oxygen and nutrients. Maternal and fetal bloods do not mix; the exchange of these substances is by diffusion across the blood vessel walls. Oxygen and nutrients return to the fetus through the umbilical vein.

## ▶ Diseases of the Female Reproductive Tract

Diseases include infections, tumors, and cysts in the reproductive organs and in the breasts. Abnormalities of the menstrual cycle and of pregnancy also occur.

### Pelvic Inflammatory Disease (PID)

The pelvic reproductive organs become inflamed as a result of bacterial, viral, fungal, or parasitic invasion. The infection can ascend to the cervix (cervicitis), the endometrium (endometritis), fallopian tubes (salpingitis), and ovaries (oophoritis). The most common cause of PID is sexually transmitted diseases, including gonorrhea and chlamydia. Streptococcal and staphylococcal organisms can enter the female reproductive tract after an abortion or delivery in which sterile procedures were not carefully followed.

The symptoms of pelvic inflammatory disease are lower abdominal pain, fever resulting from the infection, chills, and leukorrhea, a white foul-smelling vaginal discharge. Antibiotics, aspirin, bedrest, and fluids are the usual treatments. If the infection is not treated, abscesses form. Untreated PID increases the risk of ectopic pregnancy and infertility.

## Puerperal Sepsis

Puerperal sepsis is an infection of the endometrium after childbirth or an abortion. The puerperium is the period after childbirth when the endometrium is open and particularly susceptible to infection. The trauma and blood that occurs during puerperium provide a portal of entry for microorganisms through the birth canal. Streptococci are the principal causative organisms, but staphylococci and *E. coli* can also enter the uterus.

The infection leads to necrosis of the endometrium. Infected blood clots may leave the uterus and travel as septic emboli, resulting in a systemic infection of the blood, septicemia. The deep veins of the leg are frequently affected, resulting in thrombophlebitis, a condition described in Chapter 7. The symptoms of puerperal sepsis are fever, chills, profuse bleeding, foul-smelling vaginal discharge, and pain in the lower abdomen and pelvis. Puerperal sepsis responds well to antibiotic treatment.

## ▶ Neoplasms of the Female Organs

Early detection, diagnosis, and treatment of any abnormal mass or lump are extremely important in preventing the growth and spread of cancer. Many tumors and cysts are harmless, but tests are required to differentiate between malignant and benign growths.

## Carcinoma of the Cervix

Carcinoma of the cervix is one of the cancers most easily diagnosed in the early stages. Incidence of this malignancy has decreased significantly since the development of the Pap smear. The Pap smear, explained in Chapter 4, enables physicians to obtain cell samples from the cervix. These scrapings are examined microscopically, and biopsies of suspected lesions are taken if cell abnormalities indicate precursors of cancer.

Carcinoma in situ is the earliest stage of cervical cancer in which the underlying tissue has not yet been invaded. Progression from carcinoma in situ to an invasive malignancy may be slow. Ulceration then occurs, causing vaginal discharge and bleeding. The cancer spreads to surrounding organs: the vagina, bladder, rectum, and pelvic wall. Widespread cancer becomes inoperable, and radiation therapy is the usual treatment. Carcinoma of the cervix is strongly associated with infection by human papilloma virus. Early sexual activity and promiscuity are also related to the incidence of this cancer.

## Carcinoma of the Endometrium

Carcinoma of the endometrium occurs most often in postmenopausal women who have had no children. The malignant tumor may grow into the cavity of the uterus or invade the wall itself. Ulcerations develop, and erosion of blood vessels causes vaginal bleeding. Surgery and radiation are the usual treatments.

## Fibroid Tumor

Benign tumors of the smooth muscle of the uterus, leiomyomas or fibroid tumors, are the most common tumors of the female reproductive system and frequently cause no symptoms. Fibroids are often multiple and vary greatly in size. Fibroid tumors, some of which are stalked or pedunculated, are shown in Figure 12–3. The cause of fibroid tumors is unknown, although

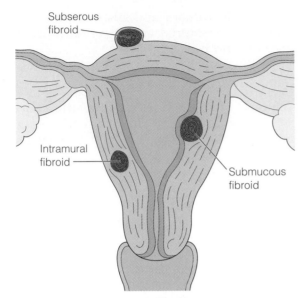

**Figure 12–3** Types of uterine fibroid tumors.

their growth is stimulated by estrogen. Symptoms include abnormal bleeding between periods or excessively heavy menstrual flow and pelvic pain. Fibroid tumors can also interfere with delivery of the newborn. Treatment for fibroid tumors depends on severity and child-bearing plans. Myolyosis, a laparoscopic technique, may be used to destroy the blood vessels of the tumor, causing it to starve and die, or, magnetic resonance imaging can guide a high energy ultrasound beam to kill the fibroid tissue, a technique called ultrasound ablation. The tumor may also be removed surgically, and a hysterectomy may be necessary.

## Ovarian Neoplasm

The ovaries are a common site for cancer to develop. The ovaries' position deep in the pelvis makes early detection of the tumor difficult. Extensive metastasis often occurs before there are noticeable symptoms. Symptoms include abdominal and pelvic pain, weight loss, general malaise, and digestive disturbances. The cause of ovarian cancer is not known. Routine screening for ovarian cancer is part of a pelvic examination. Diagnosis requires visualization of the

ovaries via laparoscopy. Treatment options include surgical removal of the mass, hysterectomy, radiation, and chemotherapy.

## Hydatidiform Mole

The hydatidiform mole is a benign tumor of the placenta. A hydatidiform mole is a developmental anomaly that occurs when the chorionic villi develop into a mass of grapelike vesicles. The mass secretes HCG, the hormone that indicates a positive pregnancy test. The uterus enlarges greatly, but there are no fetal heart tones because no fetus develops. A sonogram may be used to verify the absence of a fetus. Bleeding usually occurs, and the mole is expelled. Scraping of the uterus, the procedure of dilatation of the cervix and curettage (D&C), removes any fragments of the mass or placenta.

## Choriocarcinoma

Choriocarcinoma is a highly malignant tumor of the placenta. A part of the placenta is formed by the embryonic membrane called the chorion. This tumor may develop after a hydatidiform mole, a normal delivery, or an abortion. The tumor is highly invasive and metastasizes rapidly, causing abdominal pelvic pain. A choriocarcinoma, like a hydatidiform mole, secretes large amounts of HCG. Since there is no fetus, fetal heart tones are absent. Laparoscopy is used to visualize the tumor. Chemotherapy rather than surgery is the usual treatment.

## Adenocarcinoma of the Vagina

Adenocarcinoma of the vagina has been linked to the synthetic hormone diethylstilbestrol (DES), which was used to prevent spontaneous abortion. This rather rare cancer has developed in some young girls whose mothers were given diethylstilbestrol during pregnancy. Daughters of women who received diethylstilbestrol therapy should be checked for possible cancer development, but the incidence is low. Diethylstilbestrol appears to have only slight effects in sons born to these women. Symptoms include leukorrhea and a bloody vaginal discharge. Treatment may include surgical removal of the tumor, radiation, and chemotherapy.

## Malignant Neoplasms of the Breast

Breast cancer, an adenocarcinoma, is the leading cause of cancer death in U.S. women. Regular screening and early diagnosis are critical to identify and treat this cancer. Women are strongly urged to examine their breasts monthly for signs of cancer. The American Cancer Society and the National Cancer Institute have done a great deal to encourage this practice, and they provide valuable information on the procedure. A genetic screen for breast cancer is also available. The breast cancer gene known as Brc increases the risk for the development of breast cancer. Results should be interpreted cautiously, because having Brc does not mean a woman will definitely develop cancer.

A hard, fixed lump in the upper, outer quadrant is the most common site for malignant tumors, but malignant tumors can appear anywhere in the breast. Benign tumors, because they are encapsulated (Chapter 4), are not fixed to underlying structures. The nipple often retracts, and the skin dimples due to contraction of dense, fibrous connective tissue that extends to the chest muscle and skin.

The lymph nodes of the axillary region may be swollen. This carcinoma spreads principally through the lymph system, and metastases are frequently found in the lungs, liver, brain, and bone. Mammography can detect small, early cancers and should be performed on the recommended schedule according to age. A biopsy of the suspected malignancy confirms the diagnosis or shows the tumor to be benign. Biopsy of the first lymph node draining a tumor (the sentinel lymph node) is an alternative to removing several lymph nodes in women with small, spreading breast cancers. Sentinel biopsy can predict the status of the regional lymph nodes, and it eliminates general anesthesia and decreases pain and discomfort common with regular biopsy of lymph nodes.

The cause of breast adenocarcinoma is not known. Risk factors include family history, exposure to radiation or carcinogens, age, never being pregnant, having your first child after age 35, early menarche, and menopause after age 50.

Treatment of breast cancer varies. In a simple mastectomy, only the breast is removed. The breast, chest muscles, and axillary lymph nodes

## SIDE by SIDE ◼ Adenocarcinoma

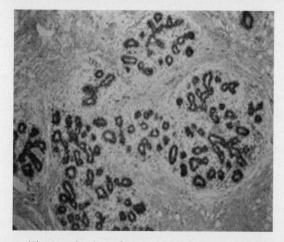

▲ Microscopic view of normal breast tissue. (© Nancy Kedersha Science Photo Library/Custom Medical Stock Photo.)

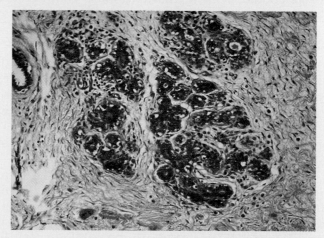

▲ Microscopic view of adenocarcinoma. (© J.L. Carson/Custom Medical Stock Photo.)

are removed in a radical mastectomy. Some studies indicate that prognosis after a radical mastectomy is not necessarily better than that after a less mutilating procedure. Less mutilating procedures involve removal of the tumor only, a lumpectomy, and radiation therapy. The ovaries are often removed to prevent the stimulating effect of estrogen on tumor growth when disease is metastatic. Hormonal therapy may also be used in breast cancer treatment. Hormonal therapy blocks or prevents cancer cells with receptors for estrogen from being exposed to estrogen, ultimately removing the growth stimulus of the cancer.

Paget's disease of the nipple is a rare cancer involving inflammatory changes that affect the nipple and the areola. The nipple becomes granular and crusted with lesions resembling eczema. In advanced Paget's disease, ulceration develops and there is a discharge from the nipple. The breast becomes edematous and is characterized as having a "pigskin" appearance. The cause of Paget's disease is unknown. A significant feature in Paget's disease is an accompanying underlying infiltrating duct cancer. Treatment depends on the extent of the disease and may include removal of the breast.

## Benign Tumors of the Breast

The most common benign tumor of the breast is a fibroadenoma, a firm, movable mass that is easily removed by surgery. The fibroadenoma does not become malignant. Cystic hyperplasia or fibrocystic disease (Figure 12–4) is very common and not serious. Development occurs at any age with the formation of numerous fluid-filled lumps in the breast. They tend to be painful at the time of the menstrual period as the breasts themselves respond to hormonal changes, enlarging and regressing. These cysts can be aspirated by inserting a needle to remove the fluid. The finding of fluid confirms that the lump is a cyst and not a solid tumor. There is a higher incidence of breast cancer in women who have cystic hyperplasia. These women should be examined regularly to prevent mistaking a tumor for a cyst. The etiology of cystic hyperplasia is unknown. Treatment may include surgical removal of the tumor.

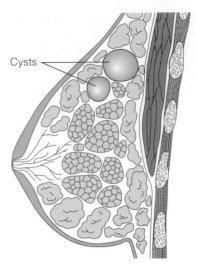

**Figure 12–4** Cystic hyperplasia of the breast.

## Menstrual Abnormalities

Amenorrhea is the absence of menstrual periods and is known as primary amenorrhea if menstruation fails to begin. Lack of gonadotropic hormones from the pituitary gland or a diseased ovary can cause the abnormality, and administration of hormones may be effective treatment. The cessation of menstrual periods for more than a year is termed secondary amenorrhea. This can result from an ovarian or uterine disease, hormonal imbalance, pituitary failure, and thyroid disease. Treatment includes hormone therapy.

Certain psychological states such as severe depression, anxiety, and continuous stress can cause cessation of menstruation. Certain eating disorders and/or excessive exercise, both of which deplete body fat, can cause amenorrhea. The condition of amenorrhea may resolve if the stressful conditions are eliminated.

Dysmenorrhea is painful or difficult menses and is one of the most common gynecologic disorders. Symptoms include dull to severe pelvic and lower back pain that may radiate to other areas. Causes of dysmenorrhea include pelvic infections and endometriosis, as well as unknown causes. Diagnosis is made based on pelvic examination and may be confirmed by laparoscopy and D&C. Treatment options include oral contraceptive therapy to regulate and decrease menstrual flow, nonsteroidal anti-inflammatory medications to reduce pain, and heat application to the pelvic area.

Menorrhagia is excessive or prolonged bleeding during menstruation. It can result from tumors of the uterus, pelvic inflammatory disease, endocrine imbalance, or failure to ovulate. If a corpus luteum is not formed following ovulation, progesterone is not secreted, but estrogen continues to stimulate endometrial thickening. Treatment varies according to the cause of the disease. Tumors should be removed surgically, pelvic inflammatory disease should be treated with antibiotics, and endocrine insufficiency should be treated with hormonal therapy.

If no specific anatomical cause is identified or if hormonal disturbances do not improve with hormone therapy, endometrial ablation or destruction of the uterine lining may be an alternative to hysterectomy for treatment of menorrhagia. Because both endometrial ablation and hysterectomy preclude childbearing, they are not options for patients who want to retain fertility.

Metrorrhagia is bleeding between menstrual periods or extreme irregularity of the cycle. It results from an abnormal buildup and sloughing of endometrial tissue. Hormonal imbalance or abnormal endometrial response to hormones may be the cause of metrorrhagia. A D&C will return the endometrium to normal.

## Toxic Shock Syndrome

Toxic shock syndrome (TSS) is caused by *Staphylococcus aureus* infection. The signs include high fever, rash, skin peeling, and decreased blood pressure. Other systemic involvements may include gastrointestinal disturbances, elevated liver enzymes, and neuromuscular disturbances. Treatment includes fluid replacement to counteract shock and administration of selected antibiotics.

Use of certain tampons was found to increase the risk of developing toxic shock syndrome. The synthetic fibers in "super-absorbent" tampons create an environment that favors growth of toxin-producing bacteria, apparently by removing magnesium from the vagina. These fibers are no longer used. It was found that some surgical dressings also contained the same fibers, a finding that may explain some cases of toxic shock syndrome in non-tampon users. Women who use tampons should use them only during the day, change them frequently, and avoid the super-absorbent type.

## Premenstrual Syndrome

Most women experience some mild premenstrual symptoms during their reproductive years, but when symptoms become temporarily disabling and disrupt family, business, and social relationships, premenstrual syndrome (PMS) is indicated. PMS consists of groups of severe emotional, physical, and behavioral symptoms that are associated with the luteal phase of the menstrual cycle and remit at or shortly after the onset of menstrual bleeding.

Physical symptoms include lower abdominal bloating, breast swelling and soreness, headache, and constipation. Women experience episodes of depression, anxiety, irritability, and hostility. Typical behavioral symptoms include crying, binge eating, and clumsiness. A daily diary that shows the relationship of the monthly cycle and the symptoms can assist in the diagnosis.

The cause of PMS is unknown, but research suggests that the cyclic production of ovarian hormones affect the levels of neurotransmitters. These chemicals may cause the symptoms, but it is not understood why some women are affected and others are not. Whereas in the past it was thought that PMS was emotional in origin or caused by stress, it is now known to have a physical cause (Figure 12–5).

Treatment is highly individualized because women respond differently to various suggestions. For some women, dietary changes during the week before the onset of menstruation are helpful. These changes might include the avoidance of salt, sugar, caffeine, and alcohol. Aerobic exercise, brisk walking, or swimming is helpful for others. Support groups and stress management techniques can be positive means of coping with the condition. To normalize the levels of neurotransmitters, antidepressant therapy may also be prescribed.

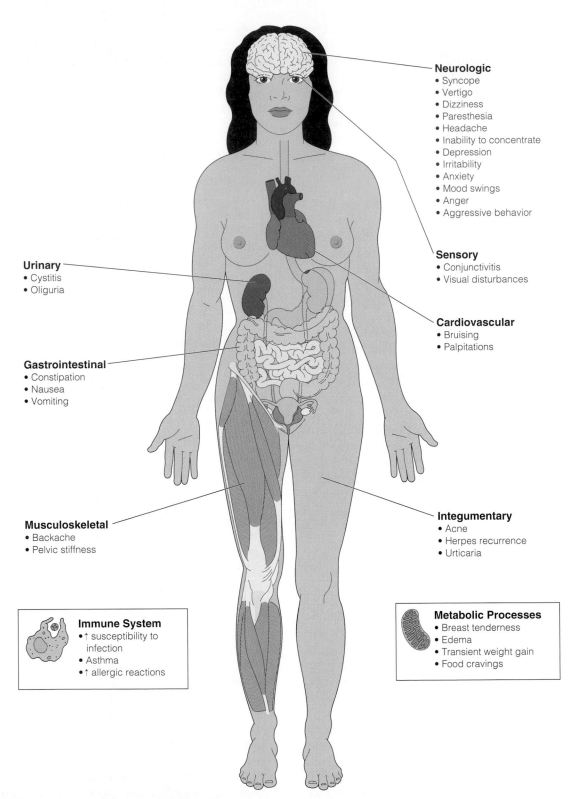

**Neurologic**
- Syncope
- Vertigo
- Dizziness
- Paresthesia
- Headache
- Inability to concentrate
- Depression
- Irritability
- Anxiety
- Mood swings
- Anger
- Aggressive behavior

**Sensory**
- Conjunctivitis
- Visual disturbances

**Cardiovascular**
- Bruising
- Palpitations

**Integumentary**
- Acne
- Herpes recurrence
- Urticaria

**Metabolic Processes**
- Breast tenderness
- Edema
- Transient weight gain
- Food cravings

**Urinary**
- Cystitis
- Oliguria

**Gastrointestinal**
- Constipation
- Nausea
- Vomiting

**Musculoskeletal**
- Backache
- Pelvic stiffness

**Immune System**
- ↑ susceptibility to infection
- Asthma
- ↑ allergic reactions

**Figure 12–5** Multisystem effects of premenstrual syndrome.

## Endometriosis

**Endometriosis** is a condition in which endometrial tissue from the uterus becomes embedded outside the normal location in the uterus. During menstruation, the tissue may be pushed through the fallopian tubes or carried by blood or lymph. It can embed on the ovaries, the outer surface of the uterus, bowels, or other abdominal organs (Figure 12–6), and appears rarely on other body structures and organs.

The endometrial tissue by nature responds to hormonal changes even when outside the uterus. This tissue goes through proliferative and secretory phases, along with the sloughing with subsequent bleeding. Endometriosis causes pelvic pain, abnormal bleeding, and dysmenorrhea. Infertility and pain during sexual intercourse (**dyspareunia**) can result. The etiology of endometriosis is unknown. The only certain means of diagnosing endometriosis is by seeing it with laparoscopy, which also enables a tissue biopsy.

Treatment of endometriosis depends on the extent of the abnormal growth and the age of the patient. Hormonal therapy is generally used for the young patient. Pregnancy, with the absence of menstruation, tends to hold the condition in check. Extensive proliferation of endometrial tissue requires surgery, and cysts filled with blood are usually found at this time.

## ▶ Abnormalities of Pregnancy

A most important factor during pregnancy is good prenatal health. The pregnant woman should be checked regularly for weight gain, blood pressure, and urine abnormalities. She should be instructed on the importance of proper diet and exercise. Most pregnancies progress normally, but occasionally complications arise.

### Ectopic Pregnancy

An **ectopic pregnancy** is a pregnancy in which the fertilized ovum implants in a tissue other than the uterus. The most common site of an ectopic

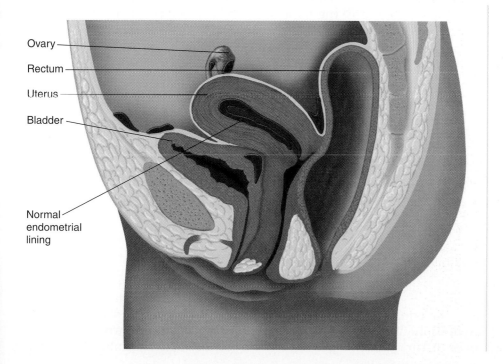

Ovary

Rectum

Uterus

Bladder

Normal endometrial lining

**Figure 12–6**
Locations of endometriosis outside the uterus are shown in red.

pregnancy is in the fallopian tubes. The fertilized ovum becomes trapped within the fallopian tube because of an obstruction such as a tumor or because scarring from infections has narrowed the tube lumen. Salpingitis is a predisposing condition for a tubal pregnancy due to the inflammatory effect on the mucosal lining.

Embryonic development proceeds for about 2 months, at which time the pregnancy terminates. The tube often ruptures, causing severe internal hemorrhage into the abdominal cavity. Intense pain and bleeding from the uterus result, and the embryo is usually destroyed by the trauma. Once the diagnosis has been made, the ruptured tube and embryo must be removed surgically.

## Spontaneous Abortion

A spontaneous abortion, commonly called a miscarriage, usually results from a genetic abnormality. The fetus is expelled before it is able to live outside of the uterus, usually in the second or third month of pregnancy. The first sign is vaginal bleeding with cramping. The woman who has aborted should receive medical attention at once to reduce the hazards of hemorrhage and infection. A D&C is usually performed to remove any tissue that remains in the uterus.

A woman who has repeated spontaneous abortions should be examined comprehensively to determine the cause. Hormonal imbalances can be corrected by hormone replacement. Repeated miscarriages can cause emotional and psychological trauma, in which case professional counseling should be sought.

## Morning Sickness

Morning sickness is transient nausea or vomiting associated with the first trimester of pregnancy. The cause of morning sickness is not known, but it is thought to be due to hormonal changes related to pregnancy. Treatment is not necessary unless there is excessive vomiting that causes dehydration and weight loss.

## Hyperemesis Gravidarum

Hyperemesis gravidarum is excessive vomiting during pregnancy leading to dehydration, weight loss, and electrolyte and acid-base disturbances in the mother and baby. The cause is not known, but is thought to be due to an increased production of chorionic gonadotropin by the fetus. This hypothesis is supported by hyperemesis gravidarum occurring more often in multiple fetus pregnancies. Diagnosis is made on the basis of symptoms, weight loss, and signs of dehydration. In severe cases, the patient is treated with intravenous fluids and electrolyte replacement, but all other fluids and food are withheld. Sedatives are given to control nausea and vomiting. Hyperemesis gravidarum usually subsides in the second trimester.

## Abruptio Placentae

Abruptio placentae is the sudden separation of the placenta from the uterus prior to or during labor. Usually the cause is unknown, but trauma, multiple births, convulsions, and chronic hypertension are known causes. Symptoms depend on the degree of separation. A partial separation during labor may be asymptomatic, while a complete separation prior to labor may be life-threatening to the mother and baby. Symptoms of a complete separation may include severe abdominal pain, vaginal hemorrhage, shock, and decrease in fetal movement. Treatment is prompt delivery of the baby and blood transfusions if necessary.

## Placenta Previa

Placenta previa is the abnormal positioning of the placenta in the lower uterus, often near the cervical opening. The cause is unknown, but risk factors include maternal age over 35 and previous uterine surgery. Symptoms include painless, bright red vaginal bleeding during the third trimester of pregnancy. Placenta previa may be life-threatening to the mother due to hemorrhage and to the baby due to anoxia. Treatment is prompt delivery of the baby and blood transfusion if necessary.

## Toxemia of Pregnancy

Toxemia of pregnancy sometimes develops during the last trimester. The condition is poorly named because no toxin appears to cause the disease and the cause is not known. The principal signs are hypertension, albuminuria, edema (particularly in the face and arms), and a significant weight gain. These signs are presented in Table 12–1. The first phase of toxemia is called pre-eclampsia, or pregnancy-induced hypertension (PIH), and symptoms include headache, visual disturbances, abdominal pain, and vomiting. A spasm of blood vessels apparently causes the headache and visual disturbances. If this condition is not treated, eclampsia develops and seizures and coma occur. The etiology of this condition is unknown. Diagnosis is made based on electrolyte levels, increase in blood pressure, and elevated blood albumin.

Preventive treatment for toxemia includes early prenatal care in which blood pressure is regularly checked, urine is analyzed for albumin, and weight gain is controlled. Pre-eclampsia, diagnosed early and treated, responds well. Restriction of salt (which tends to increase blood pressure), a nutritious low-calorie diet, and diuretics may be prescribed. This must be done with great care to prevent injury to the fetus. Anticonvulsant medications can be prescribed for eclampsia.

## Puerperal Mastitis

Mastitis is inflammation of the breast tissue. Puerperal mastitis occurs when bacteria from the nursing baby's mouth or mother's hands enter the breast tissue through the nipple and cause infection. Symptoms include redness, heat, swelling, pain, and bloody discharge from the nipple. Treatment includes antibiotics and analgesics, and should be started as soon as the infection is suspected.

## Gestational Diabetes Mellitus

Gestational diabetes is diabetes mellitus associated with pregnancy. It occurs in approximately 1% to 2% of all pregnancies, with an incidence that increases with maternal age (diabetes mellitus is discussed in detail in Chapter 13).

Increased metabolic demands during pregnancy require higher insulin levels, but certain normal, maternal, physiological changes during pregnancy can result in insufficient insulin levels, which, if uncorrected, result in diabetes. These changes include increased levels of estrogen and progesterone, which interfere with insulin action. In addition, the placenta normally inactivates insulin. Moreover, the normal pregnancy-induced elevation of stress hormones, such as cortisol, epinephrine, and glucagon, raises blood glucose. Insulin requirements continue to rise as pregnancy approaches term. In a normal pregnancy, more insulin is secreted to compensate for these changes, but in some women, insulin levels remain low as blood glucose continues to rise. Signs and symptoms of gestational diabetes are similar to insulin-dependent diabetes mellitus (Chapter 13), but include maternal hypertension, polyhydroamnios (excessive amniotic fluid), excessive weight gain during the last 6 months of pregnancy, and a fetus large for gestational age.

Women at risk for developing gestational diabetes should be screened early and monitored throughout their pregnancy. Table 12–2 lists risk factors for gestational diabetes. Screening requires a 50-gram, 1-hour glucose tolerance test in which a woman drinks a glucose solution and has her blood glucose measured over a period of time. This test typically is performed at 24 to 26 weeks of gestation, but it may be performed at her first prenatal visit and repeated at regular intervals if the woman exhibits risk factors for gestational diabetes.

The prognosis for gestational diabetes is good if diagnosed and treated early. Treatment consists of regular blood glucose monitoring, dietary control of blood glucose levels, weight control, and possibly insulin injections. Untreated

| Table 12–1 | Signs and Symptons of Toxemia | |
|---|---|
| **Signs** | **Symptoms** |
| Hypertension | Headache |
| Albuminuria | Visual disturbances |
| Edema of face and extremities | Abdominal pain |
| Significant weight gain | Vomiting |

| Table 12–2 | Risk Factors for Gestational Diabetes Mellitus |
|---|---|

Obesity

Excessive weight gain during pregnancy

Over age 35

Previous delivery of infant large for gestational age

Family history of diabetes

gestational diabetes mellitus entails many risks to mother and fetus. The fetus risks stillbirth, premature delivery, as well as high or low birth weight. Infants may experience severe hypoglycemia shortly after birth.

## Anatomy of the Male Reproductive System

The male reproductive system consists of a pair of testes that produce sperm and hormones, a system of tubules that convey sperm to the outside, and the penis, which transmits the sperm into the female tract. Accessory glands contribute to the formation of semen.

The testes are suspended in the scrotum, a saclike structure outside the body wall. The testes contain highly coiled tubules called the seminiferous tubules, which are the site of sperm development. When the sperm reach a certain maturity, they enter the epididymis, a coiled tube that lies along the outer wall of the testis. The epididymis leads into another duct, the vas deferens, which passes through the inguinal canal into the abdominal cavity.

Near the base of the urinary bladder, the vas deferens joins a duct of the seminal vesicle, an accessory gland, to form the ejaculatory duct. The ejaculatory ducts from each side penetrate the prostate gland to enter the urethra. Ducts of the prostate open into the first part of the male

urethra. Another pair of glands, the bulbourethral glands, secrete into the urethra as it enters the penis. The male reproductive system is illustrated in Figure 12–7.

The penis contains erectile tissue composed of three cylindrical bodies filled with sinuses that become engorged with blood during sexual excitement. The urethra passes through one of these cylindrical bodies as it extends to the outside, and connective tissue supports the erectile structures. The distal, expanded end of the penis is the glans penis. A flap of loosely attached skin covering the glans, the prepuce or foreskin, is sometimes removed shortly after birth, a procedure called circumcision.

## Physiology of the Male Reproductive System

Spermatogenesis, the formation of sperm, begins in the male at puberty and continues through life. The development of sperm and the secretion of the male hormone, testosterone, are processes stimulated by gonadotropic hormones of the anterior pituitary gland. Maturation of sperm continues in the epididymis, where they acquire motility. Sperm are stored in both the epididymis and vas deferens, where they can live for several

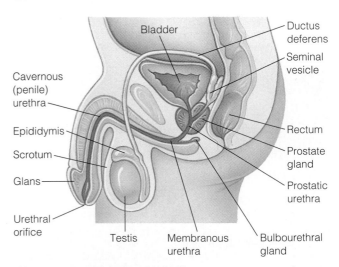

Figure 12–7 The male reproductive system.

weeks. Once ejaculated, they live for only 24 to 72 hours in the female reproductive tract.

The accessory glands produce a mucoid secretion, called semen, that nourishes and protects sperm. The seminal vesicles provide fructose, other nutrients, and prostaglandin, which increase uterine contractions, propelling the sperm toward the fallopian tubes. The seminal vesicles release their secretions into the ejaculatory ducts at the same time the vas deferens empty the sperm. The muscular prostate gland, which surrounds the first part of the urethra, contracts during ejaculation, releasing its secretions. The seminal fluid is alkaline, which buffers the highly acidic vaginal secretions that can inhibit sperm motility.

Sexual stimulation of the male transmits impulses into the central nervous system, which initiates the male response. Erection of the penis is the first effect. Nerve impulses cause the dilation of penile arteries, allowing blood to flow under high pressure into the erectile tissue. The high pressure temporarily impedes the emptying of the penile veins and causes the penis to become hard, elongated, and erect.

Intense sexual stimulation causes peristaltic contractions in the walls of the epididymis and vas deferens, propelling sperm into the urethra. The seminal vesicles and prostate gland simultaneously release their secretions, which mix with the mucous secretion of the bulbourethral glands forming the semen, the process of emission. Ejaculation of the semen, the culmination of the sexual act, occurs when contraction of this musculature increases pressure on the erectile tissue, and the semen is expressed through the urethral opening.

## ▶ Diseases of the Male Reproductive System

### Diseases of the Prostate Gland

Diseases of the prostate gland are the most common diseases in the male reproductive system and include inflammation and cancer.

**Prostatitis**  The cause of prostatitis, inflammation of the prostate, is not always known (Figure 12–8). Gonnococci from gonorrhea and *E. coli* from a urinary tract infection can infect the prostate. Signs and symptoms of prostatitis include pain and a burning sensation during urination, a tender prostate, pus emerging from the tip of the penis, and incomplete emptying of the bladder. Penicillin is the usual treatment unless hypersensitivity to the drug necessitates the use of other antibiotics.

**Carcinoma of the Prostate Gland**  Carcinoma of the prostate is common in old age, but the tumor may be small and asymptomatic. Rectal examination may reveal an enlarged prostate that is very hard, harder than a benign enlargement. Prostatic carcinoma tends to metastasize before it is discovered. Symptoms may include weak urine flow, difficulty starting or stopping urine flow, pain and burning during urination, need to urinate at night, urinary incontinence, and urinary infection. Etiology of carcinoma of the

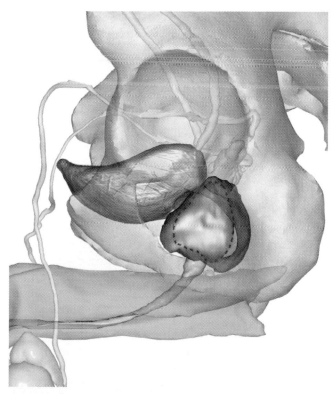

**Figure 12–8**  Enlarged prostate gland. Dashed line indicates the normal size.

prostate is unknown, although risk increases with age. Prognosis for this carcinoma is poor, as the malignancy spreads rapidly to nearby organs like the bladder and rectum, and metastasizes to the bone and other organs.

Early diagnosis is key to a favorable outcome (Table 12–3). Generally, men over age 50 should be screened for prostate cancer. Early diagnosis includes digital rectal examination and blood testing. In a digital rectal exam, the physician inserts a gloved, lubricated finger into the rectum and palpates for any growths. The prostate-specific antigen (PSA) blood test is used to screen for and monitor prostate cancer. PSA is a protein produced by prostate cells and is present in all men, but increasing levels are associated with infection, prostate enlargement, or cancer. The normal value of PSA is less than 4.0 ng/ml. Total PSA greater than 10.0 ng/ml may indicate cancer, but the total PSA level is not as significant as the change in PSA level over time.

Treatment depends on the extent of the cancer. If extensive and inoperable, hormonal therapy is generally prescribed. Because testosterone stimulates growth of the tumor, removal of the testes, the source of the hormone, may reduce its size. Estrogen, which has an inhibitory effect on the tumor's growth, is administered.

## Diseases of the Testes and Epididymis

The testes and epididymis can become inflamed from injury, infection, or some rare tumors that develop in the testes.

**Epididymitis**  Inflammation of the epididymis (epididymitis) is frequently caused by gonococci, but a urinary tract infection or prostatitis can also be the source of the epididymitis. Abscesses can form, and scar tissue develops that can cause sterility if both sides are affected. Symptoms include severe pain in the testes, swelling, and tenderness in the scrotum. Men should receive antibiotics, rest, and avoid alcohol and spicy foods.

**Orchitis**  Orchitis, a painful inflammation of the testes, can follow an injury or viral infection. The most common cause of orchitis is mumps, a viral infection of the parotid salivary glands. Swelling of the testes and severe pain usually develops about

| Table 12–3 | Clinical Manifestations of Prostate Cancer |
|---|---|
| **Genitourinary** | |
| Dysuria | Hematuria |
| Frequency of urination | Abnormal prostate |
| Reduction in urinary | on digital rectal |
| stream | examination |
| Nocturia | |
| **Musculoskeletal** | |
| Bone or joint pain | Back pain |
| Migratory bone pain | |
| **Neurologic** | |
| Nerve pain | Bowel or bladder |
| Bilateral lower | dysfunction |
| extremity weakness | Muscle spasms |
| **Systemic** | |
| Weight loss | Fatigue |

a week after mumps. In severe cases, atrophy of the testes can occur, and if both sides are affected, sterility results. Treatment is bedrest.

**Cryptorchidism**  Cyrptorchidism is not a disease but a failure of the testes to descend from the abdominal cavity, where they develop during fetal life, to the scrotum. Left uncorrected, this condition leads to sterility because maturation of the sperm cannot occur in the abdominal cavity, where the temperature is slightly higher than in the scrotum. Also, undescended testes atrophy and may become the site of cancer. The testes do not descend spontaneously later, and this condition should be corrected through surgery or hormonal therapy. Surgery usually takes place at one year of age, but can occur earlier. Evidence suggests that earlier intervention is associated with decreased incidence of infertility.

**Testicular Tumors**  Tumors of the testes are rare, with the highest incidence in young men between the ages of 18 and 35. These highly malignant tumors may be detected early as a painless lump in the testicle. Etiology is unknown, but predisposing factors include cryptorchidism, inguinal hernia during childhood, and history of mumps. Monthly testicular self-examinations are key to early detection. Treatment may include surgical removal of the testis, radiation, and chemotherapy.

## ▶ Sexually Transmitted Diseases

The incidence of sexually transmitted diseases (STDs) has increased dramatically in recent years, especially among women and teenagers. Left untreated, serious conditions may develop that can gravely affect a person's life. An estimated 1 million women contract pelvic infections each year as a result of undetected STDs. Infected individuals are often asymptomatic and spread the diseases to other sexual partners. Infected women may spread STDs to their offspring during pregnancy and childbirth. Sterility and life-threatening ectopic pregnancies are common complications of sexually transmitted diseases.

### HIV/AIDS

HIV is not only transmitted sexually but can also be acquired as a blood-borne infection. Because HIV destroys the immune system, the disease is covered in the discussion of immunity in Chapter 2.

### Gonorrhea

Gonorrhea, also known as "clap," is one of the most common and widespread of sexually transmitted diseases. It is caused by the bacterium *Neiserria gonorrhoeae*, the gonococcus, and is transmitted through sexual contact and during childbirth.

Gonococci cause inflammation of mucous membranes of the genital and urinary systems in males and females. In males, acute urethritis develops, causing difficult and painful urination. A copious discharge of pus ensues, and prostatitis frequently develops with abscess formation. In females, cervicitis with pus, vaginal discharge, pain and burning during urination, and dysuria occur.

Gonorrhea usually responds rapidly to penicillin, but early detection and treatment are extremely important. If untreated, a chronic condition develops, and the infection spreads from the initial site of infection. The inflammation causes fibrosis, which can produce a stricture in the male urethra or in the vas deferens. If both vas deferens become stenotic, sterility results. The fallopian tubes are frequenty affected in untreated gonorrhea, and salpingitis results. The pus-filled tubes can empty into the peritoneal cavity, causing peritonitis.

One of the most common causes of pelvic inflammatory disease (PID) is untreated gonorrhea. Symptoms include chills, fever, weakness, and intestinal disturbances. Chronic pelvic inflammatory disease causes abscesses to develop in the fallopian tubes, with fibrous scarring that can lead to sterility or ectopic pregnancies. Blood-borne gonococci can cause arthritis and life-threatening systemic infections such as meningitis and endocarditis.

The baby of an infected mother can be born with acute purulent conjunctivitis, inflammation of the conjunctiva. The gonococci enter the eye during delivery, and if the cornea becomes ulcerated, blindness results. To prevent this infection from developing, a drop of erythromycin is routinely placed in the eyes of newborn babies.

Although penicillin can control gonorrhea, resistant gonococci have evolved. Thus, prevention is key to controlling the spread of gonorrhea.

## Syphilis

Syphilis, commonly called "lues," is a serious STD. The causative bacterium is a spirochete, *Treponema pallidum*, transmitted by sexual intercourse or intimate contact with an infectious lesion. The baby of an infected mother may be born syphilitic.

A chancre, or ulceration, develops on the genitals in the primary stage of infection. This lesion, which may range from a small erosion to a deep ulcer, appears within a few days to a few weeks after sexual contact. The chancre usually develops on the vulva of the female and on the penis of the male, as shown in Figure 12–9. The chancre may develop on the lips, the tongue, or anus. The disease is highly contagious at this stage.

The lesion, which sometimes goes unnoticed, heals after a few weeks. If untreated with penicillin, the secondary phase of the disease occurs

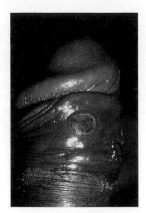

**Figure 12–9** Chancre of primary syphilis on the penis.

in a matter of weeks. The principal sign of the secondary phase is a nonitching rash that affects any part of the body: the trunk, soles of the feet, palms, mouth, vulva, or rectum. The individual is highly contagious during this stage, but he or she can be treated with penicillin.

An untreated case of syphilis may remain dormant for many years, but the organisms persist in the blood and eventually cause a systemic infection known as tertiary syphilis. The appearance of symptoms, years after the primary infection, marks the tertiary and most serious phase of syphilis.

The cardiovascular system is severely damaged at the tertiary stage. The inflammatory response to the spirochetes in the blood causes fibrosis, scarring, and obstruction of blood vessels, particularly of the aorta. Lesions develop on the cerebral cortex, causing mental disorders, deafness, and blindness. Loss of sensation in the legs and feet due to spinal cord damage causes a characteristic gait to develop. Paresis, a general paralysis associated with organic loss of brain function, results in death if untreated. The tertiary lesions of the syphilitic infection are irreversible.

Congenital defects are numerous in an infant born to an infectious mother and include mental retardation, physical deformities, deafness, and blindness. The syphilitic infection can cause death of the fetus and spontaneous abortion.

The severe consequences of syphilis point out the urgent need for early detection and treatment. Treatment with penicillin is successful except in reversing tertiary lesions. Development of antibiotic-resistant strains is a serious threat.

## Genital Herpes

Genital herpes is an extremely painful, viral disease that tends to recur periodically and for which there is no cure. Herpes virus is transmitted by intimate contact between mucous membrane surfaces. There are two types of herpes simplex virus: type I, causing "fever blisters" or "cold sores," and type II, involving the mucous membranes of the genital tracts.

Symptoms generally appear within 3 weeks after exposure to the virus. The symptoms intensify from a burning, itching sensation to severe pain. Multiple blisters appear on the genitalia and at times on the buttocks or thighs. As the blisters rupture, they become secondarily infected and ulcerate. Painful urination and vaginal discharge are common (Figure 12–10). Females with genital herpes should have Pap smears every six months because they are more likely to develop cervical cancer.

The active phase subsides as the lesions heal, but the virus remains dormant in ganglia until reactivated, perhaps at a time of stress or low resistance, when the painful lesions recur.

The disease is transmitted by contact with an active sore that is releasing the infectious virus. The virus can be spread from a cold sore on the lips to the genitals; the reverse is also true. Great caution should be used to avoid self-infection of the mucous membrane of the eye.

There is no cure for a herpes infection, but secondary infections can be prevented and healing promoted by keeping the lesions clean and dry. Ice-cold compresses may be used to relieve the pain. Prescription medications such as acyclovir, valacyclovir, and famcyclovir can be used for episodic treatment and suppressive therapy.

Active genital herpes has very serious consequences during pregnancy, causing spontaneous abortion or premature delivery, and infection of the newborn.

## Genital Warts

Genital warts can develop in both men and women and are caused by a virus in the group called HPV (human papilloma virus), which also causes other types of warts. The warts may appear within weeks after sexual relations with an infected partner, or they might not develop for several months. In men, the warts occur on the penis or scrotum. In women, they may occur on the vulva, vaginal opening, skin of the thighs, or even within the vagina and on the cervix (Figure 12–11). Warts can also develop in the mouth and around the anus.

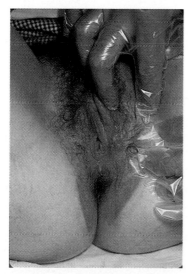

**Figure 12–10** Genital herpes blisters as they appear on the labia.

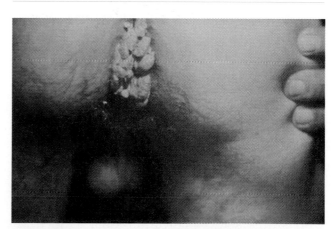

**Figure 12–11** Genital warts. (Courtesy of the CDC/Dr. Wiesner, 1972.)

Genital warts may cause symptoms such as itching or bleeding, but they may remain unnoticed until they are first detected during a physical exam. An abnormal Pap smear might be an indication of human papilloma virus infection. The types of human papilloma virus that cause genital warts are considered risk factors for cervical cancer when combined with other factors such as multiple sex partners, first intercourse at an early age, and other sexually transmitted infections. Treatment of genital warts depends on their size and number. Some are treated with medication applied by a health-care provider, but the procedure is very painful. Electrocautery (burning), cryosurgery (freezing), and laser surgery are alternative treatments. Surgical removal is not necessarily curative, and recurrence of genital warts is common.

## Chlamydial Infections

Chlamydial infections are now the most prevalent STD in the United States. *Chlamydia trachomatis* is the bacterium that causes sexually transmitted genitourinary infections in both men and women, as well as in newborns of infected mothers. The disease is a leading cause of PID in women, infertility, and severe urethritis. Women are often asymptomatic carriers of the infection and unknowingly continue to infect partners and offspring. Symptomatic females experience vaginal discharge with burning and itching of the genital area. Males with chlamydial infection are usually symptomatic with penile discharge, burning and itching with urination, and epididymitis. The disease responds to certain antibiotics but not to penicillin. The infection often coexists with gonorrhea.

## Trichomoniasis

Trichomoniasis is caused by the protozoan *Trichomonas vaginalis.* Symptomatic males experience urethritis, epididymitis, and prostatitis. Female symptoms include itching and burning in the genital area and a green, frothy vaginal discharge with a fishy odor. Treatment with antiparasitic medication such as metronidazole is effective.

## ▶ Male and Female Infertility

Infertility is failure to conceive a child after one year of regular, unprotected intercourse. Approximately 10% of couples are infertile, and 50% of couples that are treated for infertility become pregnant. The inability of a couple to conceive can originate in the male, female, or both.

Causes of infertility in males include low sperm count or decreased sperm mobility, the presence of an STD or other infections of the reproductive system, blockage in the reproductive tract, structural anomalies, and endocrine disorders. Causes of infertility in females include STDs or other infections of the reproductive system, hormonal problems, structural anomalies, blockage of the reproductive tract, and tumors.

Treatment of infertility may include STD treatment if applicable, surgery to remove reproductive tract blockages, surgical correction of any anomalies, hormone therapy, artificial insemination, and in vitro fertilization.

## ▶ Sexual Dysfunction

Sexual dysfunction, whether due to physical or psychological conditions, may limit the development of sexual relationships. The human sexual response cycle progresses from arousal to orgasm to resolution. Any disorder that interrupts this cycle may be considered a sexual dysfunction.

### Impotence

Impotence is the inability of the male to achieve and maintain an erection sufficient for sexual intercourse. Impotence is said to be primary if the man has never been able to complete intercourse successfully. Impotence is secondary if intercourse has been achieved successfully at least once.

Impotence may be caused by psychological factors. The dilation of penile arteries that leads to engorgement of the erectile tissue of the penis and then erection is under the control of the autonomic nervous system, which is affected by stress, anxiety, and fear.

Impotence may also be physiologic in nature. Arteriosclerosis, inadequate blood flow, diabetes mellitus, surgical complications, urologic disorders, medications, and premature ejaculation are all possible causes. Physiological causes can also be related to drug abuse or alcoholism.

Whether the cause is psychological or physiological in nature, treatment should be directed toward the source of the problem, which requires openness on the part of the patient with the physician or therapist. The man must be helped to overcome his personal insecurity and frustration, and his partner should also be supported and instructed about the problem. With correct treatment, impotence can usually be overcome. The medication sildenafil citrate (Viagra®) improves sexual function in some men. Those with heart conditions or other cardiovascular diseases should discuss use of this medication with their physician because of potentially dangerous side effects.

## Dyspareunia

Men and women can experience dyspareunia, painful sexual intercourse, although it is more common in women. In women, physical causes may include an intact hymen, insufficient lubrication, STD, endometriosis, PID, and cysts or tumors. In men, physiological causes may include anatomic abnormalities, prostatitis, or STD. Psychological causes may include guilt, trauma, sexual abuse, and anxiety. Treatment of dyspareunia depends on the cause. Treatments may include the use of lubricants during intercourse or a gentle stretching of the vaginal opening, treatment of underlying infections, surgery, and counseling.

## Female Arousal-Orgasmic Dysfunction

Female arousal-orgasmic dysfunction, also known as frigidity, is the lack of sexual desire or response in a woman. Frigidity is seldom caused by physical conditions, although medical problems that cause nerve damage can result in frigidity. Frigidity is usually due to a psychological con-

dition such as stress, fatigue, depression, sexual abuse, guilt, anxiety, and medications. Treatment may include therapy and arousal devices.

## Premature Ejaculation

Premature ejaculation is regularly ejaculating during foreplay or immediately after beginning sexual intercourse. This disorder can prevent the male from satisfying his partner or impregnating a woman. Premature ejaculation may have a psychological cause such as guilt or anxiety. Physical causes are rare but may include degenerative neurological conditions. Underlying physical causes are treated, and therapy may be necessary to help with psychological causes. Ejaculation may be delayed by altering sexual positions and using the squeeze technique.

## ▶ Age-Related Diseases

In older females and males, pubic hair thins and grays and the external reproductive genitalia acquire a wrinkled and sagging appearance due to a decrease in elasticity. In both older females and males, cancer of the reproductive organs is more common and is frequently related to hormone levels.

Physical changes in the aging female include shrinking of internal reproductive organs, decrease in vaginal secretions and elasticity, and a decrease in breast tissue volume. The pH of vaginal secretions becomes more alkaline, making older women more susceptible to vaginal infections. Increased stimulation and lubrication may be necessary to facilitate sexual intercourse.

Menopause, the cessation of menstrual periods, is not a disease but is a physical change related to aging. Menopause usually takes place between 45 and 55 years of age. As a woman ages, the ovaries produce less estrogen and progesterone, causing cessation of ovulation and menstruation. Removal of the ovaries also causes menopause. Common physical symptoms of menopause include hot flashes, night sweats, and vaginal dryness.

In addition, the hormonal changes brought about by menopause increase a woman's risk of cardiac disease and osteoporosis. Some women also experience psychological symptoms, including depression, sleep disorders, mood swings, and a decreased sex drive. To help protect against cardiac disease and osteoporosis and to relieve menopause symptoms, hormone replacement therapy may be prescribed. Each woman and her physician must weigh the benefits and risks of hormone replacement therapy.

Uterine prolapse is the condition of the uterus dropping or protruding downward into the vagina. This condition results from trauma to the fascia, muscle, and pelvic ligaments during pregnancy and delivery, or atrophy of the pelvic floor muscles with age. The ligaments and muscles become so overstretched they can no longer hold the uterus in place, so the uterus falls or sags downward. Symptoms include feelings of heaviness in the pelvic area, incontinence, and lower back pain. Treatment consists of strengthening the pelvic floor muscles (Kegel exercises), inserting a pessary into the vagina to support the uterus, or a hysterectomy.

Cystocele is a downward displacement of the urinary bladder into the vagina. This condition results from trauma to the fascia, muscle, and pelvic ligaments during pregnancy and delivery, or atrophy of the pelvic floor muscles with age. Symptoms include pelvic pressure, urinary urgency and frequency, and incontinence. Treatment includes Kegel exercises. If cystocele is severe or exercise is ineffective, surgery may be necessary.

A rectocele is the protrusion of the rectum into the posterior aspect of the vagina. This condition results from trauma to the fascia, muscle, and pelvic ligaments during pregnancy and delivery, or atrophy of the pelvic floor muscles with age. Symptoms include discomfort, constipation, and fecal incontinence. Treatment options include surgical repair of the posterior wall of the vagina.

In males, testosterone levels decline gradually and the testes decrease in size. Sperm reduces slightly, and prostate gland secretions are decrease. Increased stimulation may be necessary to achieve erection.

A common problem in older males is enlargement of the prostate gland or benign prostatic hyperplasia. The symptoms result from the enlarged prostate partially blocking the flow of urine from the bladder. If the bladder cannot be fully emptied, residual urine provides a medium for bacterial infection, and cystitis develops. Other symptoms include difficulty starting urination and a weak urine stream.

The blockage of urine outflow places backpressure on the ureters, which causes them to become congested with urine, a condition called hydroureters. This backpressure can extend to the kidneys, which swell with fluid, a condition of hydronephrosis. An imbalance of sex hormones frequently causes prostatic enlargement. The level of testosterone generally decreases with age, but estrogen from the adrenal cortex continues to be secreted, changing the ratio of the two. Treatment for benign prostatic hyperplasia, which is highly symptomatic, is surgical removal.

## ▶ Diagnostic Procedures for Reproductive Diseases

Physical examination of the female reproductive tract begins with a pelvic examination, including examination of the vulva, visual examination of the vagina and cervix through a speculum, Pap smear, and palpation of the internal reproductive organs and breast tissue.

Laparoscopy is used to view the female reproductive organs for abnormalities and to diagnose and treat diseases such as endometriosis, carcinoma of the cervix, carcinoma of the endometrium, choriocarcinoma, and menorrhagia. Under general anesthesia, a small incision is made below or inside the navel, and a gas, such as carbon dioxide or nitrous oxide, is put into the abdomen to expand the abdomen so the reproductive organs can be seen clearly. Into this incision is placed a laparoscope, containing a telescope with a light source. Through another incision is placed an instrument that moves the organs into view. Surgical instruments can be inserted through the scope or through another small incision. After the procedure, the instruments are removed, the gas is released, and the incisions are closed with sutures that dissolve.

Mammography is an x-ray examination of breast tissue. Mammography is used to determine the presence of cysts or tumors. If abnormalities, tumors, or cysts are discovered during diagnostic testing, a biopsy may be performed. Genetic screening is available for malignant neoplasms of the breast.

Ultrasound may be performed on the pelvis to visualize the female reproductive organs' position and size, and to determine the presence of tumors, ectopic pregnancy, and spontaneous abortion.

Female reproductive tract infections are diagnosed by bacterial culture. Menstrual and pregnancy diseases may be diagnosed with hormone and blood tests.

Physical examination of the male reproductive system includes palpation of the testes to determine the presence of tumors. Diagnostic tests for the prostate include the digital rectal examination that allows the physician to feel the prostate for enlargement or tumors, biopsy, and prostate-specific antigen blood test. Urinalysis, urine culture, and serological testing are useful in diagnosing infections of the male reproductive tract.

Diagnosis of gonorrhea or trichomoniasis can be made by examining discharge for the etiological agent. Chlamydia is diagnosed by antibody serologic testing. Syphilis diagnosis includes the VDRL test (Venereal Disease Research Laboratory of the United States Public Health Service). The most sensitive and specific test for syphilis is the TPI test (*Treponema pallidum* immobilization test) that detects specific antibodies against the spirochete. Genital herpes is diagnosed by a positive viral culture on living tissue. Genital warts are diagnosed based on visualization of the warts and biopsy to rule out carcinoma.

Infertility diagnosis in females includes physical examination, charting of the menstrual cycle, urine and blood analysis, STD testing, and visualization of the reproductive tract. Infertility diagnosis in men includes physical examination, including rectal and genital palpi-

tation, semen and blood analysis, and STD testing.

Sexual dysfunction diagnosis includes a physical examination with a medical and sexual history and laboratory tests to rule out physical causes.

## CHAPTER SUMMARY

Disease can affect the reproductive system in many ways. In the female, tumors and cysts develop in the ovary, uterus, and breast. Infections invade the vagina, breasts, fallopian tubes, and endometrium. Menstrual abnormalities result from a diseased organ or from a hormonal imbalance. Pregnancy complications include ectopic pregnancy, spontaneous abortion, toxemia, and placental problems. Aging and childbearing affect the reproductive system. Sexual dysfunction in women may be caused by psychological or physical factors.

Diseases of the male include prostate gland infection, inflammation and enlargement, or tumor formation. Infections of the testes and epididymis can result in sterility. Testicular tumors affect young men and are highly malignant.

HIV/AIDS, a sexually transmitted but also a blood-borne infection, was discussed in Chapter 2 as a failure of the immune system. Gonorrhea and syphilis have far-reaching consequences if untreated. Early detection of these diseases and treatment may prevent numerous complications. Chlamydial infections are the most prevalent STD and cause urethritis, PID, and sterility. There is no cure for genital herpes, which tends to recur periodically. The human papilloma virus that causes genital warts is considered a risk factor for cervical cancer.

## RESOURCES

Centers for Disease Control and Prevention: www.cdc.gov
American Cancer Society: www.cancer.org

# DISEASES AT A GLANCE

## Reproductive System

| DISEASE OR DISORDER | ETIOLOGY | SIGNS AND SYMPTOMS |
|---|---|---|
| Pelvic inflammatory disease | Infection | Lower abdominal pain, fever, chills, leukorrhea |
| Puerperal sepsis | Infection | Fever, chills, profuse bleeding, vaginal discharge, pain in lower abdomen and pelvis |
| Uterine prolapse | Childbirth, aging | Feelings of heaviness in pelvic area, urinary stress, incontinence, lower back pain |
| Cystocele | Childbirth, aging | Pelvic pressure, urinary urgency and frequency, incontinence |
| Rectocele | Childbirth, aging | Discomfort, constipation, fecal incontinence |
| Menopause | Aging | Hot flashes, night sweats, vaginal dryness, depression, sleep disorders, mood swings, decreased sex drive |
| Carcinoma of the endometrium | Aging, no children | Vaginal bleeding |
| Fibroid tumor | Unknown | Abnormal bleeding between periods, excessive heavy menstrual flow, pelvic pain |
| Ovarian neoplasms | Unknown | Pelvic pain, abdominal and digestive disturbances, weight loss, general malaise |
| Hydatidiform mole | Developmental anomaly | Vaginal bleeding, enlarged uterus |
| Choriocarcinaoma | Hydatidiform mole, abortion, normal delivery | Abdominopelvic pain |
| Adenocarcinoma of the vagina | Diethylstilbestrol | Leukorrhea, bloody vaginal discharge |

| DIAGNOSIS | TREATMENT |
|---|---|
| Pelvic examiniation, positive culture | Antibiotics, aspirin, bedrest, fluids |
| Pelvic examination, positive culture | Antibiotics |
| Pelvic examination | Kegel exercises, surgery |
| Pelvic examination | Kegel exercises, surgery |
| Physical examination | Surgery |
| Symptoms, elevated FSH, low estrogen | Hormone replacement therapy |
| Visual examination of the endometrium, biopsy | Radiation, surgery |
| Pelvic examination, ultrasound | Surgery, myolyosis, ultrasound ablation |
| Pelvic examination, laparoscopy | Surgery, hysterectomy, radiation, chemotherapy |
| Elevated HCG without presence of fetus, no fetal heart tones, sonogram | D & C |
| Elevated HCG without presence of fetus, no fetal heart tones, laparoscopy, biopsy | Chemotherapy |
| Pelvic examination, Pap smear, biopsy | Surgery, radiation, chemotherapy |

# DISEASES AT A GLANCE (*continued*)

## Reproductive System

| DISEASE OR DISORDER | ETIOLOGY | SIGNS AND SYMPTOMS |
|---|---|---|
| Malignant neoplasms of the breast | Unknown | Hard, fixed lump in the outer quadrant, swollen lymph node |
| Paget's disease | Unknown | Nipple becomes granular with lesions, nipple discharge, breast skin has pigskin appearance |
| Cystic hyperplasia or fibrocystic disease | Unknown | Fluid-filled cysts in the breast |
| Amenorrhea | Lack of gonadotropic hormone, diseased ovary, hormonal imbalance, extreme depression, worry, stress, eating disorders | No menstrual period |
| Dysmenorrhea | Pelvic infections, endometriosis, other unknown causes | Dull to severe pelvic and lower back pain |
| Menorrhagia | Tumors of uterus, PID, endocrine imbalance, failure to ovulate | Excessive or prolonged bleeding during menstruation |
| Metrorrhagia | Hormonal imbalance | Bleeding between menstrual periods, extreme irregularity of menstrual cycle |
| Toxic shock syndrome | Infection | High fever, rash, skin peeling, decreased blood pressure, gastrointestinal complaints, neuromuscular disturbances |
| Premenstrual syndrome | Unknown | Lower abdominal bloating, breast swelling and soreness, headache, constipation, depression, anxiety, irritability, hostility |
| Endometriosis | Unknown | Pelvic pain, abnormal bleeding, painful menstruation |
| Ectopic pregnancy | Obstruction of the fallopian tube | Intense pain, uterine bleeding |

| DIAGNOSIS | TREATMENT |
|---|---|
| Mammography, biopsy | Surgery, radiation, hormone therapy |
| Biopsy | Surgery |
| Palpation, mammography | Surgery |
| Pelvic examination, hormone level testing | Hormone treatment |
| Pelvic examination, laparoscopy, D & C | Oral contraceptive therapy, anti-inflammatory medications, heat |
| Pelvic examination, laparoscopy, hormone level testing | Surgery, antibiotics, hormone therapy, hysterectomy, endometrial ablation |
| Pelvic examination, hormone level testing | D & C |
| Physical symptoms, elevated liver enzyme levels, history of tampon use | Antibiotics, fluid replacement |
| Daily diary | Dietary changes, exercise, stress management, support groups, antidepressant medication, hormone therapy |
| Laparoscopy | Hormone therapy, surgery |
| Pelvic examination, ultrasound | Surgery |

# DISEASES AT A GLANCE *(continued)*

## Reproductive System

| DISEASE OR DISORDER | ETIOLOGY | SIGNS AND SYMPTOMS |
|---|---|---|
| Spontaneous abortion | Genetic abnormality, hormone imbalances, emotional and psychological factors | Vaginal bleeding with cramping |
| Morning sickness | Unknown but possibly linked to hormonal changes related to pregnancy | Transient nausea or vomiting |
| Hyperemesis gravidarum | Usually unknown, but may be due to increased production of chorionic gonadotropin hormone by the fetus | Excessive vomiting during pregnancy |
| Abruptio placentae | Usually unknown, but may be due to trauma, multiple births, convulsions, chronic hypertension | Severe abdominal pain, vaginal hemorrhage, shock, decreased fetal movement |
| Placenta previa | Unknown | Painless, bright red vaginal bleeding during the third trimester of pregnancy |
| Toxemia of pregnancy | Unknown | Hypertension, albuminuria, edema, weight gain |
| Puerpersal mastitis | Infection | Redness, heat, swelling, pain, bloody discharge from the nipple |
| Female arousal: orgasmic dysfunction | Stress, fatigue, depression, sexual abuse, guilt, anxiety, nerve damage | Lack of sexual desire or response |
| Carcinoma of the cervix | Human papilloma virus | Vaginal discharge and bleeding |
| Gestational diabetes mellitus | Pregnancy | Maternal hypertension, polyhydramnios, excessive weight gain, fetus large for gestational age |

| DIAGNOSIS | TREATMENT |
|---|---|
| Ultrasound | D & C, hormone therapy counseling |
| Symptoms | Usually not necessary |
| Symptoms, weight loss, dehydration | IV fluids, sedatives |
| Ultrasound | Delivery, blood replacement |
| Ultrasound | Delivery, blood replacement |
| Electrolyte levels, elevated blood albumin, increased blood pressure | Dietary changes, diuretics, anticonvulsants |
| Symptoms | Antibiotics, analgesics |
| Physical examination, sexual history | Therapy, arousal devices |
| Pelvic examination, Pap smear, biopsy | Surgery, radiation |
| Glucose tolerance test | Regular blood glucose monitoring, dietary control of blood glucose levels, weight control, insulin injections |

# DISEASES AT A GLANCE (*continued*)

## Reproductive System

| DISEASE OR DISORDER | ETIOLOGY | SIGNS AND SYMPTOMS |
|---|---|---|
| Dyspareunia | Physical, psychological | Painful sexual intercourse |
| Prostatitis | Not always known; may be infection | Pain and burning during urination, tender prostate, pus discharge |
| Benign prostate hyperplasia | Aging | Difficulty starting urination, weak urine stream, inability to completely empty bladder |
| Carcinoma of the prostate | Unknown | Weak urine flow, problems starting/stopping urine flow, need to urinate at night, pain and burning during urination, urinary infections, urinary incontinence |
| Epididymitis | Infection, prostatistis | Severe pain in testes, swelling and tenderness in the scrotum |
| Orchitis | Injury, viral infection | Swelling of the testes, severe pain |
| Cryptorchidism | Developmental error | Undescended testes |
| Testicular tumors | Unknown | Painless lump in testicle |
| Impotence | Emotional disturbances, physiological problems, medications, alcoholism | Inability to achieve and maintain an erection sufficient for sexual intercourse |
| Premature ejaculation | Guilt, anxiety, degenerative neurological conditions | Regular ejaculation during foreplay or immediately after beginning intercourse |
| Gonorrhea | *Neiserria gonorrhoeae* | Pain and burning during urination, pus discharge |
| Syphilis | *Treponema pallidum* | Chancre, rash |
| Genital herpes | Herpes simplex virus type II | Blisters, pain and burning during urination, discharge |

| DIAGNOSIS | TREATMENT |
| --- | --- |
| Symptoms, physical examination | Lubricants, gentle stretching of vaginal opening, treatment of infections, surgery, counseling |
| Urinalysis, urine culture, digital-rectal examination | Antibiotics |
| Aging, hormone imbalance | Surgery |
| Digital-rectal examination, PSA blood test, biopsy | Surgery, hormone therapy |
| Physical examination, urine culture | Antibiotics |
| Physical examination, symptoms, serologic testing | Bedrest |
| Physical examination | Surgery, hormone therapy |
| Physical examination, biopsy | Surgery, chemotherapy, radiation |
| Symptoms, physical examination | Therapy, medication, treatment of physiological cause |
| Physical examination, lab tests | Therapy, treatment of physical cause |
| Physical examination, positive culture | Antibiotics |
| Physical examination, positive culture | Antibiotics |
| Physical examination, serological testing | Suppressive therapy |

# DISEASES AT A GLANCE (continued)

## Reproductive System

| DISEASE OR DISORDER | ETIOLOGY | SIGNS AND SYMPTOMS |
| --- | --- | --- |
| Genital warts | Human papilloma virus | Warts, itching, bleeding |
| Chlamydia | *Chlamydia trachomatis* | Asymptomatic, or genital discharge, burning and itching during urination |
| Trichomoniasis | *Trichomonas vaginalis* | Urethritis, epididymitis, prostatitis in males; itching and burning in genital area, green, frothy vaginal discharge with a fishy odor in females |

| DIAGNOSIS | TREATMENT |
| --- | --- |
| Physical examination, Pap smear, serological testing | Electrocautery, cryosurgery, laser surgery |
| Physical examination, positive culture | Antibiotics |
| Physical examination, positive culture | Antiparasitic medication |

# Interactive Activities

## Cases for Critical Thinking

1. A young woman reports severe pain and cramping in her lower abdomen. Laproscopic examination found ectopic endometrial tissue on the uterine wall and ovaries. Name this disease. What is meant by ectopic endometrial tissue? She was prescribed oral contraceptives. Why would these be useful?

2. A 16-year-old, sexually active woman complains of a green, frothy, fishy-smelling vaginal discharge. What is the possible diagnosis? What test would you perform? What treatment is available?

3. A 63-year-old male says he gets up several times a night to urinate but has difficulty getting urination started. A digital rectal examination reveals a very hard and enlarged prostate gland. What is the possible diagnosis? What tests would you perform? What treatment is available?

## Multiple Choice

1. Which is the most common tumor among females?

   a. ovarian cysts
   b. breast cancer
   c. uterine leiomyomas
   d. cervical cancer

2. Diseases are matched to descriptions. Which match is **INCORRECT?**

   a. recurrent painful sores on genitals: genital herpes
   b. leading cause of PID: chlamydia
   c. transmission to newborns can cause blindness: gonorrhea
   d. caused by *Treponema pallidum:* genital warts

3. Which is **FALSE** about syphilis?

   a. sores of primary syphilis heal after a few weeks
   b. a fetus can be affected and born with major physical and mental abnormalities
   c. mental disorders are a part of tertiary syphilis
   d. secondary syphilis is characterized by lesions that form in several organs

4. Which disease can lead to pelvic inflammatory disease and sterility?

   a. gonorrhea
   b. cystitis
   c. prostatitis
   d. herpes

5. Pelvic inflammatory disease can ascend to the fallopian tubes, this is known as _____.

   a. cervicitis
   b. salpingitis
   c. oophoritis
   d. endometritis

6. Downward displacement of the urinary bladder into the vagina is known as _____.

   a. uterine prolapse
   b. cystocele
   c. rectocele
   d. sepsis

7. Painful or difficult menses is _____.

   a. amenorrhea
   b. dysmenorrhea
   c. menorrhea
   d. metrorrhagia

8. Failure of the testes to descend from the abdominal cavity is _____.

   a. orchitis
   b. prostatitis
   c. cryptorchidism
   d. epididymitis

9. A benign tumor of the placenta is a _____.

   a. choriocarcinoma
   b. teratoma
   c. cyst
   d. hydatidiform mole

10. The sudden separation of the placenta from the uterus prior to or during labor is _____.

    a. placenta previa
    b. abruptio placentae
    c. toxemia
    d. hyperemesis gravidarum

## True or False

_____ 1. Pelvic inflammatory disease can lead to infertility.

_____ 2. The Pap smear detects endometriosis.

_____ 3. Family history is not a risk factor for breast cancer.

_____ 4. Herpes simplex virus causes syphilis.

_____ 5. Benign prostatic hyperplasia is common in men over 50.

_____ 6. Toxic shock syndrome is caused by _Streptococcus pyogenes_.

_____ 7. Frigidity is seldom caused by psychological conditions.

_____ 8. The only certain means of diagnosing endometriosis is to see it.

_____ 9. Vomiting early in pregnancy happens only in the morning.

_____ 10. The cause of PMS is known.

## Fill-Ins

1. Fluid-filled cysts in breast tissue are signs of _____ disease.

2. After mumps, some males experience _____, a painful swelling of the testes.

3. The most prevalent reportable sexually transmitted infection in the United States is

   _____ _____.

4. Human papilloma virus infection is strongly associated with _____.

5. _____ _____ is ejaculation during foreplay or immediately after the start of intercourse.

6. _____ is an STD caused by a protozoan.

7. The herpes type _____ virus causes cold sores; the herpes type _____ virus causes genital herpes.

8. _____ is a white, foul-smelling vaginal discharge.

9. _____ is the cessation of menstrual periods.

10. _____ _____ occurs when bacteria from the nursing baby's mouth or mother's hands enter the breast tissue through the nipple and cause infection.

## MedMedia Wrap-Up

**www.prenhall.com/mulvihill**
Remember to visit this website for extra study practice, including exercises, Internet links, news updates, and an audio glossary.

**Activity CD-ROM**
Check out the CD-ROM in the back of this book. You will find games, exercises, puzzles, and videos to help enhance your understanding of this chapter.

# Diseases of the Endocrine System

**CHAPTER**

# 13

## Learning Objectives

After studying this chapter, you should be able to

- Describe the normal structure and function of the endocrine glands
- Name the hormones secreted from each endocrine gland
- Describe the normal functions of hormones secreted from the endocrine glands
- Identify diseases of the anterior and posterior pituitary glands
- Describe the consequences of hyposecretion and hypersecretion of the anterior pituitary
- Describe the consequences of hyposecretion of the posterior pituitary
- Define the causes and consequences of goiter, hyperthyroid, and hypothyroid
- Identify and describe the diseases of the adrenal cortex and adrenal medulla
- Describe the effect of excessive secretion of parathormone and deficiency of parathormone
- Describe the regulatory function of insulin and glucagon
- Differentiate between type I and type II diabetes
- Identify the warning signs of diabetes
- Describe the complications associated with diabetes
- Distinguish between diabetic coma and insulin shock
- Describe the signs, symptoms, causes, and treatment of gestational diabetes mellitus
- Discuss age-related endocrine system diseases
- Identify and describe the various diagnostic procedures and tests for endocrine function

## Fact or Fiction?

Obesity is caused by a "gland problem," a disorder of endocrine gland function.

*Fiction: Although the thyroid gland controls metabolic rate and thus the rate at which calories are used, obesity is more complicated. An obese person can have a normally functioning thyroid gland. In general, obesity results when more calories are ingested than are expended.*

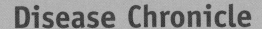

# Disease Chronicle

## Diabetes

Ancient Hindu writings record distinctive signs of diabetes thousands of years ago: large volumes of urine, to which ants and flies were attracted, intense thirst, and a wasting of the body. No treatment or cure existed for this mysterious ailment, which killed children and crippled survivors with its complications. It was not until the late 19th century, when diabetes was observed in dogs that had their pancreas removed experimentally, that the disease could be linked to a specific organ. The key component of the pancreas was eventually isolated and identified as the protein hormone insulin. Today, instead of treating patients with insulin extracted from dog pancreas, human insulin is synthesized using recombinant DNA technology. Early diagnosis, treatment, and effective management have lengthened and greatly improved the lives of diabetics. Still, no cure for diabetes exists.

## MedMedia
www.prenhall.com/mulvihill

## Functions of the Endocrine Glands

The endocrine system consists of a group of organs of internal secretion. These endocrine glands secrete hormones, or chemical messengers, directly into the bloodstream. The major organs of the endocrine system are the hypothalamus, the pituitary gland, the thyroid gland, the parathyroid glands, the pancreatic islets, the adrenal glands, the testes, and the ovaries. The sex glands—the ovaries and testes—are studied with the reproductive system in Chapter 12. Figure 13–1 shows the location of the endocrine glands.

Hormones are released from endocrine glands into the bloodstream, where they affect activity in cells at distant sites. Some hormones affect the whole body, and others act only on target or distant organs. Most hormones are composed of proteins or chains of amino acids; others are steroids or fatty substances derived from cholesterol.

Most glandular activity is controlled by the pituitary, which is sometimes called the master gland. The pituitary itself is controlled by the hypothalamus.

The body is conservative and secretes hormones only as needed. For example, insulin is secreted when the blood sugar level rises. Another hormone, glucagon, works antagonistically to insulin and is released when the blood sugar level falls below normal. Hormones are potent chemicals, so their circulating levels must be carefully controlled. When the level of a hormone is adequate, its further release is stopped. This type of control is called a negative-feedback mechanism. Its importance becomes clearer as specific diseases of the endocrine system are considered.

Overactivity or underactivity of a gland is the malfunction that most commonly causes endocrine diseases. If a gland secretes an excessive amount of its hormone, it is hyperactive. This condition is sometimes caused by a hypertrophied gland or by a glandular tumor.

A gland that fails to secrete its hormone or secretes an inadequate amount is hypoactive. This condition may be caused by disease or tumor, or it may be caused by trauma, surgery, or radiation. A gland that has decreased in size and consequently is secreting inadequately is said to be atrophied. Each endocrine gland is discussed with an emphasis on normal function and importance. The diseases caused by hypoactivity and hyperactivity of each gland are then explained.

## The Structure and Function of the Pituitary Gland

The wonder of the pituitary gland is its tiny size and yet its tremendous functions. It is only the size of a pea suspended from the base of the brain by a small stalk. The pituitary gland fits into a bony depression in one of the skull bones that carefully protects it from injury. The pituitary gland is illustrated in Figure 13–2.

Another name for the pituitary gland is the hypophysis. The hypophysis has two parts to it, each of which acts as a separate gland. Each part is stimulated differently to cause secretion, and each secretes entirely different hormones.

The anterior and larger portion of the hypophysis is the glandular adenohypophysis. It is in direct communication with the hypothalamus of the brain. Portal blood vessels extending through the stalk connect the two. The hypothalamus is an extremely important coordinating center for the brain. It directs which hormones the anterior pituitary gland should secrete at a particular time by sending substances called releasing factors to the anterior pituitary through the connecting blood vessels. The pituitary then secretes the proper hormone.

The posterior pituitary, or neurohypophysis works differently. It receives hormones secreted by the hypothalamus and stores them for subsequent release. These hormones travel over nerve fibers from the hypothalamus to the neurohypophysis. It is because of the neural connection with the hypothalamus that the posterior portion of the pituitary gland is called the neurohypophysis.

What can this little pea-sized structure control that makes it the master gland? The anterior pituitary, the adenohypophysis, secretes six hormones called tropic hormones. Tropic hor-

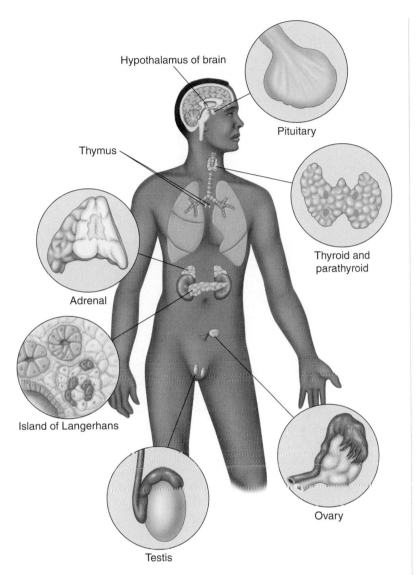

**Figure 13–1**
The endocrine glands.

Hypothalamus of brain

Pituitary

Thymus

Thyroid and
parathyroid

Adrenal

Island of Langerhans

Ovary

Testis

mones travel through the blood from the pituitary and exert their effects on other endocrine glands.

## Hormones of the Anterior Pituitary Gland

Growth hormone (GH; also called somatotropin) affects all parts of the body by promoting growth and development of the tissues. Before puberty, it stimulates the growth of long bones, increasing the child's height. Soft tissues—organs such as the liver, heart, and kidneys—also increase in size and develop under the influence of growth hormone. After adolescence, growth hor-

mone is secreted in lesser amounts but continues to function in promoting tissue replacement and repair.

The thyroid gland regulates metabolism, the rate at which the body produces and uses energy. The anterior pituitary controls secretion of thyroid hormone by the thyroid gland. The pituitary hormone that stimulates the thyroid gland is thyroid-stimulating hormone (TSH; also called thyrotropin). In the absence of TSH, the thyroid gland stops functioning.

The anterior pituitary also regulates the adrenal glands. The adrenal glands have an

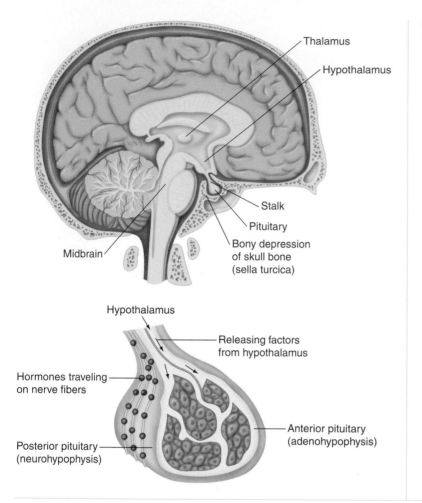

**Figure 13–2**
The pituitary gland and its relation to the brain.

inner part, the adrenal medulla, and an outer portion, the adrenal cortex. It is the cortex that is controlled by the anterior pituitary. The tropic hormone affecting the adrenal cortex is adrenocorticotropic hormone (ACTH).

The anterior pituitary regulates sexual development and function by means of hormones known as the gonadotropins. These are not sex hormones, but they affect the sex organs, the gonads. They are follicle-stimulating hormone (FSH), luteinizing hormone (LH), and prolactin. These gonadotropins regulate the menstrual cycle and secretion of male and female hormones. The relationship between the anterior pituitary and its target organs is seen in Figure 13–3.

## ▶ Diseases of the Anterior Pituitary Gland

### Hyperpituitarism

The most noticeable result of hyperpituitarism is the effect of excessive growth hormone. The condition produces a giant if the hypersecretion of growth hormone occurs before puberty. Normally, at puberty, the ends of the long bones seal with the shafts, and no further height is attained. Excessive growth hormone retards this normal closure of the bones. Sexual development is usually decreased, and mental development may be normal or retarded. Gigantism is

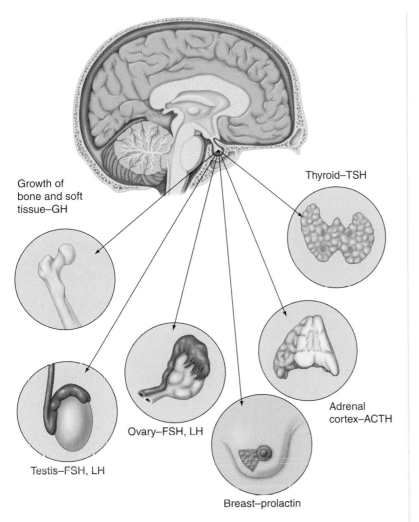

**Figure 13–3**
Anterior pituitary gland and its target organs.

Growth of bone and soft tissue–GH

Thyroid–TSH

Testis–FSH, LH

Ovary–FSH, LH

Breast–prolactin

Adrenal cortex–ACTH

usually the result of a tumor, an adenoma, of the anterior pituitary. Removal of the tumor or radiation treatment to reduce its size decreases the secretion of growth hormone.

If excessive production of growth hormone occurs after puberty, when full stature is attained, the result is the condition of acromegaly. The long bones can no longer grow in length, and bones of the hands, feet, and face enlarge. There is also excessive growth of soft tissues. The features of the face become coarsened; the nose and lips enlarge, and the lower jaw protrudes, producing an overbite that interferes with chewing. The skin and tongue thicken, the latter causing slurred speech. A curvature of the spine

often develops, giving the person a bent appearance. The curvature is caused by an overgrowth of the vertebrae. This hyperactivity of the pituitary gland is generally due to a tumor.

Treatment of acromegaly is complex. Surgery is used to remove or reduce the size of the tumor. Radiation and medication therapy is used to reduce overproduction of growth hormone. These treatments may not return growth hormone levels to normal for several years.

## Hypopituitarism

Hypopituitarism can result from damage to the anterior lobe of the pituitary gland or from an inadequate secretion of hormones. A fracture at the base of the skull, a tumor, or ischemia (lack of bloodflow) can cause pituitary destruction. Lack of bloodflow causes an infarction, and the tissue becomes necrotic. Hypopituitarism can be mild or severe. If the entire anterior lobe of the pituitary is destroyed, the condition is called panhypopituitarism, *pan* meaning all. No pituitary hormones are secreted.

The abnormalities that result from the absence of tropic hormones are numerous. The thyroid gland, for example, is dependent on TSH from the pituitary for its functioning. Without that tropic hormone, the thyroid atrophies, and the functions of the thyroid cease. Mental dullness and lethargy, a condition of drowsiness, develop.

Lack of ACTH causes the adrenal cortex to atrophy. Inadequate cortical hormones result in a salt imbalance and improper metabolism of nutrients. The adrenal cortical hormones are essential to life.

Absence of the gonadotropic hormones depresses sexual functions. The gonads atrophy without stimulation of the tropic hormones. If the lack of hormones exists before puberty, sexual development is impaired. In an adult woman, menstruation ceases; an adult male will lack sex drive or have aspermia, that is, no formation or emission of sperm. Figure 13–4 illustrates the glandular failure caused by severe hypopituitarism.

Hypopituitarism caused by a tumor may show additional symptoms. Pressure of the tumor may cause pain, a headache, or a peculiar form of blindness. Figure 13–5 shows the closeness of the pituitary gland to the optic

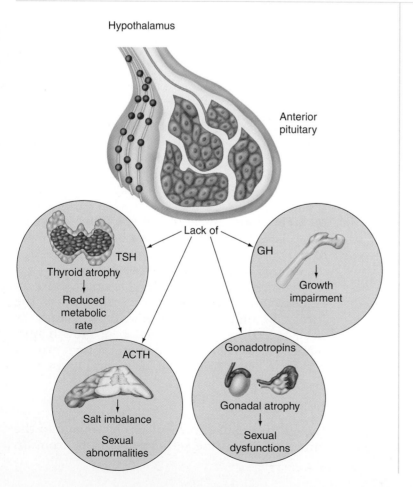

**Figure 13–4**
Effects of pituitary failure.

nerves. As the tumor enlarges, it interferes with these nerves.

The patient suffering from hypopituitarism must be treated with hormonal supplements. Administration of thyroxine, cortisone, growth hormone, and sex hormones can compensate for the dysfunctional glands. It is significant that all these failures result from hypoactivity of the anterior pituitary. For this reason, the anterior pituitary is called the master gland.

A different form of hypopituitarism sometimes occurs in children. Inadequate growth hormone can cause a pituitary dwarf. This patient is mentally bright but small and underdeveloped sexually. All growth processes are retarded; teeth, for example, are late in erupting. Replacement therapy with injections of growth hormone is currently used to treat children with pituitary dwarfism.

### ▶ Function of the Posterior Pituitary Gland

The posterior pituitary, or neurohypophysis, secretes two hormones: oxytocin and vasopressin, also called antidiuretic hormone (ADH). Oxytocin causes contraction of smooth muscle in the uterus and initiates milk secretion. It strengthens contractions during labor and helps prevent hemorrhage after delivery. Antidiuretic hormone prevents excessive water loss through the kidneys and makes the collecting ducts permeable to water. Water is then reabsorbed into the bloodstream by the kidney tubules.

### ▶ Hyposecretion of the Posterior Pituitary Gland

#### Diabetes Insipidus

Diabetes insipidus results from a deficiency of ADH. ADH is produced in the hypothalamus and is stored and released from the posterior pituitary gland. In the absence of ADH, water is not reabsorbed by the kidney and is lost in the urine. Extreme thirst, or polydipsia, and excessive production of dilute urine, or polyuria, results.

A condition of central diabetes insipidus can result from inadequate production of ADH by the hypothalamus or failure of the pituitary gland to release ADH into the bloodstream. Diabetes insipidus can also occur when ADH levels are normal. This condition, nephrogenic diabetes insipidus, involves a defect in the kidney. The kidney fails to concentrate urine in response to the instructions of ADH.

Excessive water loss can lead to dehydration quickly. Whenever possible, the underlying cause of diabetes insipidus must be corrected. Modified forms of ADH may be taken orally, by injection, or by nasal spray to maintain normal urine output. Figure 13–6 shows the normal action of ADH, and Figure 13–7 shows the effects of its absence.

### ▶ Structure and Function of the Thyroid Gland

The activity of the thyroid gland affects the whole body. It regulates the metabolic rate, the rate at which calories are used. The thyroid gland, through its hormone thyroxine, governs

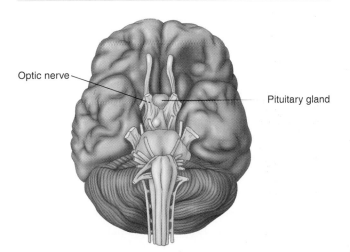

Optic nerve

Pituitary gland

**Figure 13–5** Base of brain showing proximity of pituitary gland to optic nerves.

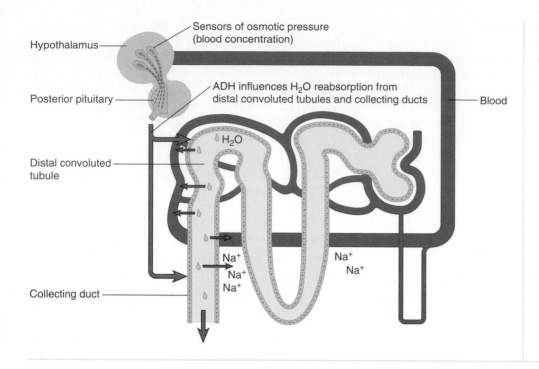

Hypothalamus

Sensors of osmotic pressure
(blood concentration)

Posterior pituitary

ADH influences $H_2O$ reabsorption from
distal convoluted tubules and collecting ducts

Blood

$H_2O$

Distal convoluted
tubule

Na⁺
Na⁺
Na⁺

Na⁺
Na⁺

Collecting duct

**Figure 13–6**
Normal action of
antidiuretic hormone (ADH).

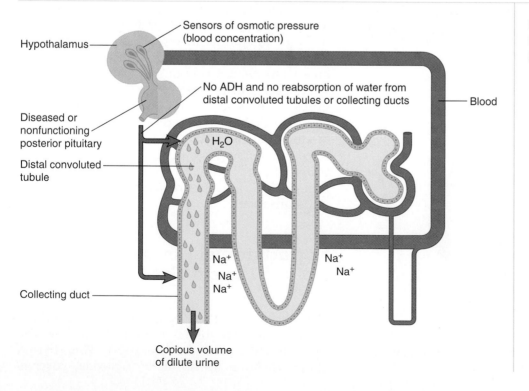

Hypothalamus

Sensors of osmotic pressure
(blood concentration)

Diseased or
nonfunctioning
posterior pituitary

No ADH and no reabsorption of water from
distal convoluted tubules or collecting ducts

Blood

$H_2O$

Distal convoluted
tubule

Na⁺
Na⁺
Na⁺

Na⁺
Na⁺

Collecting duct

Copious volume
of dilute urine

**Figure 13–7**
Effect of antidiuretic
hormone (ADH) deficiency.

cellular oxygen consumption and thus energy and heat production. The more oxygen that is used, the more calories are metabolized ("burned up"). Thyroxine assures that enough body heat is produced to maintain normal temperature even in a cold environment.

A person with a low rate of metabolism requires fewer calories than a person with a higher metabolic rate. Many people blame obesity on an underactive thyroid, a low rate of metabolism. Although there is a relationship between a person's body weight and metabolic rate, diet is still the critical factor in controlling obesity.

## Structure of the Thyroid Gland

The thyroid gland is located in the neck region, one lobe on either side of the trachea. A connecting strip, or isthmus, anterior to the trachea, connects the two lobes. The thyroid gland lies just below the Adam's apple, the protrusion formed by part of the larynx. Figure 13–8 illustrates the thyroid gland. Internally, the thyroid gland consists of follicles, microscopic sacs. Within these protein-containing follicles, the thyroid hormones thyroxine and triiodothyronine are stored. Thin-walled capillaries run between the follicles in a position ideal to receive the thyroid hormones.

## Function of the Thyroid Gland

The thyroid gland synthesizes, stores, and releases thyroid hormones, which contain iodine. In fact, most of the iodide ions of the body are taken into the thyroid gland by a mechanism called the iodide trap. Iodine combines with an amino acid; two of these groups join, and the thyroid hormones are formed.

The hormones are stored until needed and then released into the blood capillaries. In the blood, the thyroid hormones combine with plasma proteins. Tests to determine the activity of the thyroid gland are based on this combination of tri-iodothyronine ($T_3$) and thyroxine ($T_4$) with plasma proteins. In the $T_3$ and $T_4$ tests, a sample of the patient's serum is incubated with radioactive thyroid hormones and resin. The resin absorbs the hormones that are not bound to the blood proteins. Radioactivity counts of the serum and resin are made, and the percentage of thyroid hormones absorbed by the resin is calculated. A low percentage of absorption indicates a poorly functioning thyroid gland. A high percentage of absorption indicates hyperactivity. In the latter case, the patient's own thyroid hormones had saturated the plasma proteins, and the excess radioactive hormones were absorbed by the resin. This is a more accurate

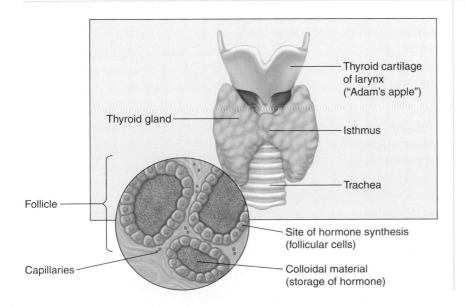

**Figure 13–8**
The thyroid gland.

Thyroid cartilage of larynx ("Adam's apple")

Thyroid gland

Isthmus

Trachea

Follicle

Site of hormone synthesis (follicular cells)

Capillaries

Colloidal material (storage of hormone)

means of measuring thyroid activity than the test used for many years, the BMR, or basal metabolic rate. The term basal metabolic rate, however, is still used, and it refers to a person's oxygen consumption while at rest.

## Effects of Thyroid Hormones

Although there is more than one thyroid hormone, for clarity the thyroid hormones are referred to here as thyroxine, the one that is secreted in the largest quantity. Thyroxine stimulates cellular metabolism by increasing the rate of oxygen use with subsequent energy and heat production.

Keeping in mind that thyroxine stimulates the rate of cellular metabolism, the effect of an increased thyroxine level on heart activity becomes clear. Think of it this way: Faster cellular metabolism increases the cell's demand for oxygen, so more oxygen must be circulated to the cells. Nutrients are converted to energy in the presence of oxygen, and the waste products of metabolism, including carbon dioxide, are formed. These must be carried away from the cells. The circulatory system can meet these needs by increasing bloodflow to the cells. Increased bloodflow is obtained by greater cardiac output, more heart activity.

As cellular metabolism increases, respiration increases. The greater need for oxygen and a corresponding accumulation of carbon dioxide stimulate the respiratory center of the brain. Stimulation of the respiratory center results in a faster rate and greater depth of breathing.

Thyroxin increases body temperature. Heat is produced through cellular metabolism, and thyroxine stimulates this process. In a cold environment, thyroxine secretion increases to assure adequate body heat. If excessive body heat is produced, it is dissipated in two ways. Blood vessels of the skin dilate, increasing bloodflow at the body surface and giving the body a flushed appearance. As the blood flows through the skin's blood vessels, excess heat escapes. The body is also cooled by the perspiration mechanism. Body temperature is controlled by a regulatory center in the brain.

Thyroxine also has a stimulatory effect on the gastrointestinal system. It increases the secretion of digestive juices and the movement of material through the digestive tract. Absorption of carbohydrates from the intestine is also increased under the influence of thyroxine, assuring adequate fuel for cellular metabolism. The effects of thyroxine are illustrated in Figure 13–9.

An understanding of these effects of thyroxine makes the diseases of the thyroid gland meaningful. Many symptoms of thyroid diseases can be related to the effects of inadequate or excessive thyroxine secretion.

## Control of Circulating Thyroxine Level

The anterior pituitary gland stimulates the thyroid by releasing TSH. The thyroid, in turn, releases thyroxine, which circulates in the blood to all cells and tissues. When the level of circulating thyroxine is high, the anterior pituitary is inhibited and stops releasing TSH. This is an example of a negative-feedback mechanism. An adequate level of thyroxine prevents further synthesis of the hormone. When the level of thyroxine falls, the anterior pituitary is released from the inhibition and once again sends out TSH. This feedback mechanism is shown in Figure 13–10.

At times, this control mechanism fails, constituting one basis for a thyroid disease. The

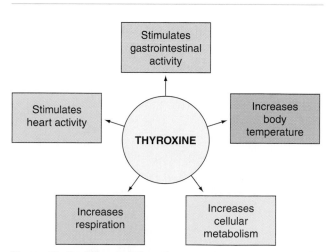

**Figure 13–9** Effects of thyroxine.

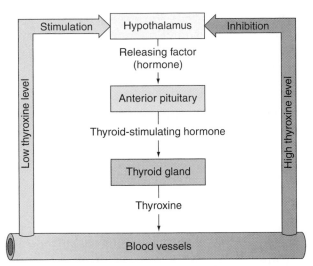

**Figure 13–10** Control of thyroxine secretion through negative feedback.

thyroid gland also functions abnormally if the body's iodine supply is inadequate, if the gland is overstimulated or understimulated by the anterior pituitary, or if the thyroid gland itself becomes diseased. These are some of the conditions that are discussed.

## ▶ Diseases of the Thyroid Gland

### Goiter

Goiter is an enlargement of the thyroid gland. The enlargement may be caused by hypoactivity or hyperactivity of the thyroid or a deficiency in iodine needed to synthesize thyroid hormones.

The most common type of goiter is the diffuse colloidal goiter, or nontoxic goiter. The follicles of the thyroid gland normally contain colloid, a protein material. In this type of goiter, an excessive amount of colloid is secreted into the follicles, increasing the size of the gland. A diffuse colloidal goiter is also called an endemic goiter because it is common in a particular geographic region.

The usual cause of an endemic goiter is insufficient iodine in the diet. Inland areas, such as the Great Lakes region, and mountainous regions, like the Alps, have a very low iodine content in the soil and water. As a result, the inhabitants are unable to synthesize thyroxine adequately.

Normally, when the proper level of thyroxine is circulating, the anterior pituitary stops secreting TSH. In the absence of thyroxine, no

**SIDE by SIDE** ■ Goiter

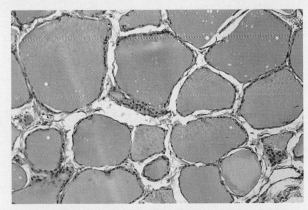

▲ Histology of normal thyroid gland showing follicles containing thyroglobin. (© M. Peres/Custom Medical Stock Photo.)

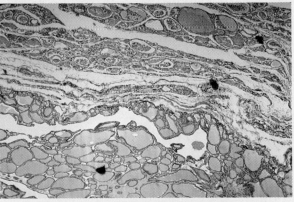

▲ Nodular goiter. Note the distorted follicles. (© O.J. Staats/Custom Medical Stock Photo.)

negative-feedback signal inhibits the anterior pituitary. As a result, the continuous secretion of TSH causes the thyroid gland to enlarge as a compensatory mechanism. The thyroid enlarges in an attempt to meet the demand of TSH.

An enlargement of the neck is generally the only symptom. Usually, enough thyroxine is produced to prevent the symptoms of hypothyroidism. The condition responds well to treatment with iodide, so the use of iodized salt prevents endemic goiter formation. If the goiter is very advanced, surgery may be necessary. A very large goiter puts pressure on the esophagus, causing difficulty in swallowing, or presses on the trachea, causing a cough or choking sensation.

A defect in the thyroxine-synthesizing mechanism also can cause a simple diffuse colloidal goiter. A young girl entering adolescence may develop this type of goiter because of an increased need for thyroxine at this time.

## Hyperthyroidism

Another type of goiter is the adenomatous or nodular goiter. These nodules secrete an excessive amount of thyroxine, a condition of hyperthyroidism.

The effects of thyroxine have been discussed, and an excessive amount of this hormone augments these effects. Hyperthyroidism causes nervousness and tremors, particularly in the hands. Metabolism increases, causing sweating and a rapid pulse. A nodule or adenoma may put pressure on the trachea or esophagus. Surgery is sometimes necessary to remove part of the thyroid gland, but medication is often effective in preventing further enlargement.

Graves' disease is another condition in which goiter develops. In this case, the entire gland hypertrophies, and there are no nodules. The person suffers from severe hyperthyroidism. Graves' disease is far more common in women than in men and usually affects young women.

A person with Graves' disease has a very characteristic appearance. The facial expression is strained and tense, and there is a stare in the eyes. The eyes protrude, a condition called exophthalmos. This is caused by edema in the tissue behind the eyes. The bulging of the eyes

can be so severe that the eyelids do not close, and the swelling sometimes damages the optic nerve. This symptom generally persists even when the hyperthyroidism is corrected.

The person has a tremendous appetite but loses weight to the point of appearing emaciated, as calories are burned up at a rapid rate. Thyroxine speeds the passage of food through the digestive tract. There is no time for the normal reabsorption of water from the large intestine, so diarrhea frequently accompanies the disease.

Tachycardia, rapid pulse rate, and palpitation are also among the symptoms. The person is extremely nervous, excitable, and always tired but has difficulty sleeping because of the hyperactivity of the body. The high metabolic rate causes excessive heat production, which results in profuse perspiration. The skin is always moist, and an insatiable thirst follows the loss of water. The signs and symptoms of Graves' disease are shown in Table 13–1.

Graves' disease is an autoimmune condition in which antibodies to a thyroid antigen stimulate

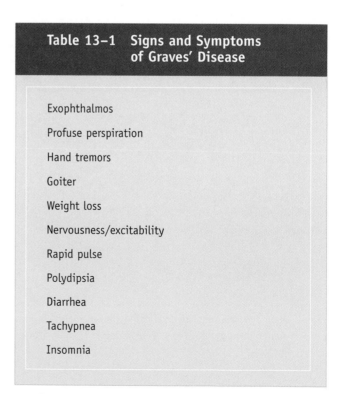

| Table 13–1 Signs and Symptoms of Graves' Disease |
| --- |
| Exophthalmos |
| Profuse perspiration |
| Hand tremors |
| Goiter |
| Weight loss |
| Nervousness/excitability |
| Rapid pulse |
| Polydipsia |
| Diarrhea |
| Tachypnea |
| Insomnia |

hyperactivity of the thyroid gland. This causes the thyroid to produce too much thyroxine.

Graves' disease can sometimes be treated with medication that inhibits the synthesis of thyroxine or by administration of radioactive iodine, which destroys the thyroid gland. Removal of the thyroid gland, however, may be necessary. If the gland is removed, hormonal supplements must be given. Partial removal of the thyroid gland allows the remaining portion to secrete hormones.

## Hypothyroidism

Myxedema is the condition of severe hypothyroidism, an inadequate level of thyroxine. The symptoms are just the opposite of those in Graves' disease. The person's face is bloated, the tongue is thick, and the eyelids are puffy. The skin is dry and scaly, and there is little perspiration. The person has no tolerance of a cold environment.

A person with myxedema experiences muscular weakness and somnolence, sleeping for 14 to 16 hours a day. The mental and physical processes are sluggish, the speech is slurred, and reflexes are slow. Heart rate is decreased, and the slowed circulation causes edema to develop. Left untreated, lack of thyroxine increases the amount of circulating lipids, which leads to the development of atherosclerosis (Chapter 7). The digestive system works sluggishly, so the patient suffers from constipation. Weight gain also accompanies the disease.

Myxedema affects women more than men, and usually affects women of middle age. It can result from radiation damage to the thyroid gland or develop after thyroid surgery if thyroxine is not administered. Myxedema can be a primary disease of the thyroid gland or secondary to pituitary disease. If the pituitary gland does not secrete TSH, the thyroid gland ceases to function. Myxedema is treated by administering thyroxine. A chronic condition requiring long-term medical care, myxedema generally responds well to treatment.

## Cretinism

Cretinism is a congenital thyroid deficiency in which thyroxine is not synthesized. Cretinism can result from an error in fetal development if the thyroid gland fails to form or is nonfunctional. Cretinism sometimes occurs in areas of endemic goiter where the mother suffers from an inadequate iodine supply.

Thyroxine is essential to both physical and mental development. Lack of this hormone in an infant or young child causes mental retardation and an abnormal, dwarfed stature. The cretin has a stocky build with a characteristically protruding abdomen. The sexual organs do not develop, and the face of the cretin is typically misshapen: a broad, sunken nose, small eyes set far apart, puffy eyelids, and a short forehead. A thick tongue protrudes from a wide-open mouth, and the face is expressionless.

The earlier this condition is diagnosed and treated with thyroxine, the more optimistic is the prognosis. Lifelong hormonal therapy will be required.

Even less severe cases of hypothyroidism should be treated in infants. A baby may appear normal at first and only later give indications that the developmental processes are retarded. The baby may be slow in smiling, reaching, sitting, and standing. Newborns are routinely tested for hypothyroidism within two days of birth. Prompt treatment can prevent the effects of hypothyroidism and the development of cretinism.

## ▶ Structure and Function of the Adrenal Glands

The adrenal glands are located on top of each kidney. Each of the glands consists of two distinct parts: an outer part (the adrenal cortex) and an inner section (the adrenal medulla). The cortex and medulla secrete different hormones. The adrenal cortex is stimulated by ACTH, adrenocorticotropic hormone, from the anterior pituitary gland. The adrenal glands are shown in Figure 13–11.

The adrenal cortex secretes many steroid hormones, which can be classified into three groups. One group, the mineralocorticoids, regulates salt balance. The principal hormone of this group is aldosterone. Aldosterone causes sodium

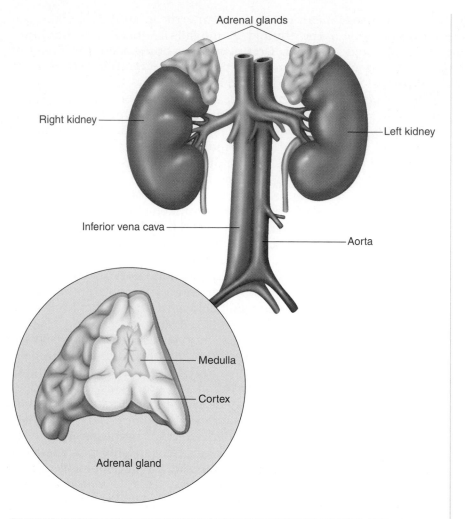

Adrenal glands

Right kidney

Left kidney

Inferior vena cava

Aorta

Medulla

Cortex

Adrenal gland

**Figure 13–11**
The adrenal glands.

retention and potassium secretion by the kidneys. Another group, the glucocorticoids, helps regulate carbohydrate, lipid, and protein metabolism. The principal hormone of this group is cortisol or hydrocortisone. The third group of hormones are sex hormones: androgens, the male hormones, and estrogens, the female hormones.

The adrenal medulla secretes epinephrine and norepinephrine. These hormones are secreted in stress situations when additional energy and strength are needed. Epinephrine causes vasodilatation and increases heart rate, blood pressure, and respiration. Norepinephrine

brings about general vasoconstriction. Together, epinephrine and norepinephrine help shunt blood to vital organs when required.

Hyperactivity of the adrenal cortex is usually caused by hyperplasia (enlargement of the glands), a tumor. Hyperactivity may also result from overstimulation by the anterior pituitary gland.

Hypoactivity of the adrenal cortex sometimes results from a destructive disease, such as tuberculosis. Some steroid hormones can cause the adrenal glands to atrophy by interfering with the normal control mechanism for corticosteroid release.

## ▶ Diseases of the Adrenal Glands

### Hyperadrenalism

Overactivity of the adrenal cortex (hyperadrenalism) can take different forms depending on which group of hormones are secreted in excess. Table 13–2 compares the diagnostic signs and symptoms of different types of hyperadrenalism syndromes. Cushing's syndrome develops from an excess of glucocorticoid hormones, the hormones that raise the blood sugar level. In excess, they cause hyperglycemia. Elevation of blood glucose caused by hypersecretion by the adrenal cortex is called adrenal diabetes. Glucocorticoids mobilize lipids, increasing their level in the blood. A characteristic obesity develops that is confined to the trunk of the body. A fat pad forms behind the shoulders and is referred to as a buffalo hump, but the arms and legs remain normal. The face is round and described as moon-shaped.

The person with Cushing's syndrome retains salt and water, resulting in hypertension, and atherosclerosis develops as a result of excess circulating lipid. Muscular weakness and fatigue accompany the disease, and the person finds it difficult even to climb stairs. The skin is thin and tends to bruise easily. Red striae (stretch marks) develop on the abdomen, buttocks, and breasts as a result of a loss of elastic tissue and fat accumulation. Wounds heal poorly, and the patient is very susceptible to infection. Bones, particularly the vertebrae and ribs, are likely to fracture. These symptoms result from a decrease in protein synthesis. Surgical removal of the enlarged glands or tumor can correct the condition. Hormonal therapy is then required to replace the hormones normally secreted by the adrenal cortex.

Conn's syndrome is another form of hyperadrenalism. In this disease, aldosterone is secreted in excess. This causes retention of sodium and water, and abnormal loss of potassium in the urine. Hypertension develops as a result of the salt imbalance and water retention. Muscles become weak to the point of paralysis. The person has an excessive thirst (polydipsia) caused by the salt retention, and polyuria follows the great intake of water. Conn's syndrome is usually caused by a tumor that can be removed surgically, and the prognosis is usually good.

Adrenogenital syndrome is another form of hyperadrenalism, also called adrenal virilism. In this case, androgens, male hormones, are secreted in excess. If this occurs in children, it stimulates premature sexual development. Sex organs of a male child greatly enlarge. In a girl, the clitoris enlarges, a male distribution of hair develops, and the voice deepens.

This excessive production of androgens is usually caused by a block in the synthesis of cortisol from cholesterol or from other corticosteroids. Cortisone is generally inactive until it is converted to cortisol. Cortisone is prepared synthetically from animal and plant tissue. Inasmuch as steroids cannot be converted to cortisol, because of the blockage in the pathway, they are converted to androgens. Cortisol treatment can prevent this overproduction.

### Table 13–2  Hyperadrenalism Signs and Symptoms

| Disease | Diagnostic Signs and Symptoms |
| --- | --- |
| Cushing's | Excess glucocorticoids; hypertension, hyperglycemia |
| Conn's | Excess aldosterone; hypertension, muscle weakness, polydipsia |
| Adrenal virilism | Excess androgens; premature maturation of sex organs, masculinization in females |
| Pheochromocytoma | Excess epinephrine and norepinephrine; palpitations, tachycardia, hypertension, weight loss |

Excessive androgen secretion in a woman causes masculinization (adrenal virilism). Hair develops on the face, a condition called hirsutism, and the hairline recedes. The breasts diminish in size, the clitoris enlarges, and ovulation and menstruation cease. In an adult, the cause is usually an androgen-secreting tumor of the glands.

Pheochromocytoma is a rare tumor of the adrenal medulla that causes overproduction of epinephrine and norepinephrine. This condition is rare and occurs equally in men and women, most commonly between the ages of 30 and 60. Symptoms of palpitations, increased blood pressure, rapid heart rate, chest pain, and weight loss may appear suddenly and sporadically. The best treatment is to remove the tumor. Medications are also used before surgery to control symptoms caused by excessive epinephrine and norepinephrine.

## Hypoadrenalism

Addison's disease results when the adrenal glands fail to produce corticosteroids—aldosterone and cortisol. The adrenal glands may be destroyed by cancer or infections, or inhibited by chronic use of steroid hormones, such as prednisone. Many cases of Addison's disease are idiopathic.

Aldosterone deficiency renders the patient unable to retain salt and water. The kidneys are unable to concentrate urine and, eventually, dehydration ensues. Severe dehydration can ultimately lead to shock. Cortisol deficiency leads to low blood sugar, impaired protein and carbohydrate metabolism, and generalized weakness.

The pituitary gland produces more corticotropin in response to a deficiency of corticosteroids. Corticotropin normally stimulates the adrenal gland and production of a skin-darkening pigment called melanin. Persons with Addison's disease develop a peculiar yellow-brown discoloration. Normally, pigmented areas such as the areola surrounding the nipples and parts of the genitals become even darker. Areas of the body such as the palms and elbows also darken, and pigment develops in scars.

Addison's disease can be life-threatening and must be treated with corticosteroid replacement. Injectable cortisol treatment is used initially to treat severe cases. Oral cortisol treatment is required for life. Medication to restore normal excretion of salt and water is also administered.

## ▶ Structure and Function of the Parathyroids

### Structure of the Parathyroids

The parathyroids are four tiny glands located on the posterior side of the thyroid gland (Figure 13–12). Before the function of the parathyroid glands was understood, they were sometimes removed with a thyroidectomy. The hormone secreted by the parathyroids is parathormone, also called parathyroid hormone.

### Function of the Parathyroids

The parathyroid glands are extremely important in regulating the level of circulating calcium and phosphate. Ninety-nine percent of the body's calcium is in bone, but the remaining 1% has many important functions. Calcium is essential to the blood-clotting mechanism. It increases the tone of heart muscle and plays a significant role in muscle contraction.

There is a constant exchange of calcium and phosphate between bone and the blood. Two kinds of cells are at work within bone: osteoblasts, which form bone tissue, and osteoclasts, which resorb salts out of bone, dissolving it. These salts are then released into the blood. The balance between these two processes, osteoblastic and osteoclastic, is governed by the parathyroid hormone.

When the blood calcium level falls, parathormone is secreted. The hormone acts at three distinct sites to raise the blood level of calcium to normal. Parathormone increases the amount of calcium that is absorbed out of the digestive tract by interaction with ingested vitamin D. It prevents a loss of calcium through the kidneys and releases calcium from bones by stimulating osteoclastic activity. When the proper level of circulating calcium is restored, parathormone is no longer released. An excess or a deficiency of

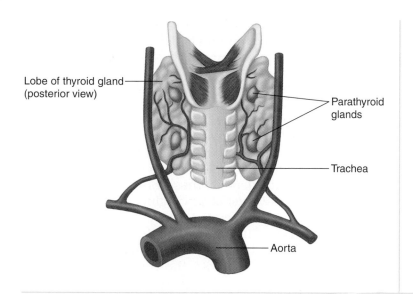

**Figure 13–12**
Parathyroid glands.

Lobe of thyroid gland (posterior view)

Parathyroid glands

Trachea

Aorta

calcium can have disastrous results. These conditions are usually the result of hyperactivity or hypoactivity of the parathyroid glands.

## ▶ Diseases of the Parathyroid Gland

### Hyperparathyroidism

An overactive parathyroid gland secretes too much parathormone (hyperparathyroidism). Excessive parathormone raises the level of circulating calcium above normal, the condition called hypercalcemia. Much of the calcium comes from bone resorption mediated by parathormone. As the calcium level rises, the phosphate level falls.

With the loss of calcium, the bones are weakened. They tend to bend, become deformed, and fracture spontaneously. Giant cell tumors and cysts of the bone sometimes develop. Excessive calcium causes formation of kidney stones because calcium forms insoluble compounds. Calcium deposited within the walls of the blood vessels makes them hard. It may also be found in the stomach and lungs. Effects of hyperparathyroidism are listed in Table 13–3.

Hyperparathyroidism, with its concurrent excess of calcium, causes generalized symptoms. There may be pain in the bones that is sometimes

confused with arthritis. The nervous system is depressed, and muscles lose their tone and weaken. Heart muscle is affected and the pulse slows. Symptoms include gastrointestinal disturbances, abdominal pain, vomiting, and constipation. These symptoms result from deposits of calcium in the mucosa of the gastrointestinal tract. Deposits of calcium sometimes form in the eye, causing irritation and excessive tearing. Hyperparathyroidism usually results from a tumor. If the tumor is removed, parathormone secretion returns to normal, and the level of circulating calcium is again properly controlled.

Hyperparathyroidism can develop from other conditions that reduce the level of circulating calcium. Any decrease in calcium stimulates the parathyroid glands to hypertrophy and to

| Table 13–3 | Complications of Hyperparathyroidism: Hypercalcemia |
|---|---|

Kidney stone formation

Calcification of blood vessels walls

Calcification of organ walls

Spontaneous fractures

increase their rate of secretion. During pregnancy and lactation, the mother's supply of calcium is reduced. This reduction stimulates the parathyroid glands to secrete parathormone.

## Hypoparathyroidism

The principal manifestation of hypoparathyroidism is tetany, a sustained muscular contraction. In hypoparathyroidism, the muscles of the hands and feet contract in a characteristic fashion. The typical tetanic contraction of the hand is seen in Figure 13–13. Laryngeal muscles are very susceptible to these spasms, which can obstruct the respiratory tract, and death may follow.

The low level of calcium in the blood, hypocalcemia, makes the nervous system hyper-excitable. As the nerves discharge spontaneously, the skeletal muscles are overstimulated. Administration of calcium and vitamin D, which assists in the absorption of calcium from the gastrointestinal tract, will correct the condition.

## ▶ Endocrine Function of the Pancreas

The structure of the pancreas and its role as an exocrine gland were described in Chapter 10. The pancreas has another critical function: the control of glucose level in the blood. This is ac-

complished through the secretion of two hormones: insulin and glucagon.

Insulin is secreted by certain cells of the pancreas called beta cells, located in patches of tissue named the islets of Langerhans or pancreatic islets. Glucagon is secreted by the alpha cells of the islets. This arrangement is illustrated in Figure 13–14. These hormones work antagonistically to each other. Insulin lowers the level of blood glucose, and glucagon elevates it. The combined effect of these hormones maintains the normal level of blood glucose.

Insulin is secreted when the blood glucose level rises. Through a complex mechanism, not completely understood, insulin facilitates the entry of glucose into the cells where it is primarily stored as glycogen and metabolized for energy. Glucose enters primarily skeletal muscle cells and fat cells.

As glucose enters cells and is converted to glycogen by the liver, the level of blood glucose falls. The normal level of glucose in the blood is about 90 mg/100 ml (or 90 mg/dl) of blood. This is also expressed as 90 mg percent.

When the level of blood glucose falls below normal, glucagon is released. Glucagon circulates to the liver and stimulates the release of glucose from its stored form, glycogen. This raises the level of blood glucose to normal. The control of glucose is illustrated in Figure 13–15.

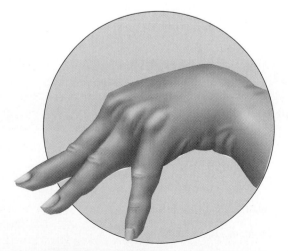

**Figure 13–13**   Tetany of the hand in hypoparathyroidism.

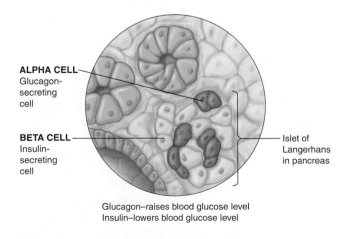

ALPHA CELL
Glucagon-
secreting
cell

BETA CELL
Insulin-
secreting
cell

Islet of
Langerhans
in pancreas

Glucagon–raises blood glucose level
Insulin–lowers blood glucose level

**Figure 13–14**   Islet of Langerhans.

## ▶ Hyposecretion of the Pancreas

### Diabetes Mellitus (Hyperglycemia)

Diabetes mellitus is an endocrine disease in which the beta cells fail to secrete insulin or target cells fail to respond to insulin. In the absence of insulin, glucose cannot enter the cells. The glucose level in the blood increases greatly, resulting in hyperglycemia. A diabetic's sugar level can range from 300 to 1200 mg/dl of blood and even higher. The cells are deprived of their principal nutrient, glucose, for the production of energy.

Insulin-dependent diabetes mellitus (IDDM) or Type I diabetes most commonly occurs before the age of 30. This is the most serious form in which the patient requires multiple injections of insulin daily. Noninsulin dependent diabetes mellitus (NIDDM) or Type II diabetes usually occurs after the age of 45 and becomes more common with advancing age. Type II diabetes frequently accompanies obesity and can often be controlled by weight loss, diet, and exercise.

Development of Type I and Type II diabetes may have a genetic basis. Other less common causes of diabetes are abnormally high levels of corticosteroids, pregnancy or gestational diabetes, and drugs that interfere with production or utilization of insulin. Gestational diabetes is discussed in Chapter 12.

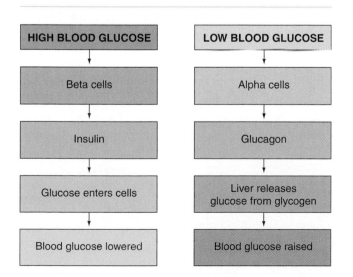

| HIGH BLOOD GLUCOSE | LOW BLOOD GLUCOSE |
|---|---|
| Beta cells | Alpha cells |
| Insulin | Glucagon |
| Glucose enters cells | Liver releases glucose from glycogen |
| Blood glucose lowered | Blood glucose raised |

**Figure 13–15**   Control of blood glucose level.

**Symptoms of Diabetes Mellitus**   One of the principal symptoms of diabetes mellitus is excessive urination, or polyuria (Table 13–4). This is caused by the great amount of glucose that filters into the kidney tubule and the volume of water required to carry it away. The glucose acts as a diuretic. Normally, glucose that enters the kidney tubules is reabsorbed and does not appear in the urine. In diabetes, however, the amount of glucose that the kidney tubules can absorb, the tubular maximum, is surpassed. The excess glucose is excreted in the urine, a condition called glycosuria. Glycosuria is a major sign of diabetes mellitus.

The great loss of water with the glucose could result in dehydration, but the diabetic has an excessive thirst, polydipsia. By drinking large amounts of water, the diabetic compensates for the fluid loss. An unusual thirst is also one of the symptoms of diabetes.

Cells preferentially metabolize glucose, but in its absence, cells metabolize fats first and proteins last. This is known as the protein-sparing effect. Because glucose cannot enter the cells without the action of insulin, the diabetic metabolizes a large amount of fat. Fat metabolism produces a large number of fatty acids and ketone bodies, acetone, and related substances. The presence of ketone bodies in the urine is another sign of diabetes mellitus.

The production of acids lowers the body's pH, and the condition of acidosis results. This is one of the most serious consequences of diabetes. The normal pH range is 7.35 to 7.45. If the pH drops below 6.9 to 7.0, the person goes into a coma and will die if not treated.

Another sign of diabetes mellitus is weight loss, although the diabetic's appetite is good. The patient tires easily and lacks energy. In the absence of glucose to metabolize, the diabetic uses the body's tissue fat and protein, as well as that in the diet, which explains the loss of weight. There is an increased breakdown of tissue protein and a decrease in protein synthesis that results in poor wound healing. Susceptibility to infection also accompanies diabetes.

**Complications of Diabetes Mellitus**   Lipid is mobilized from fat tissue, and the level of blood lipid, particularly cholesterol, increases. Much of this lipid is deposited within the walls of blood ves-

## Prevention ✚ PLUS!

### Obese Children and Type II Diabetes

The number of overweight children is increasing in the United States. Obese children are at increased risk of developing Type II diabetes mellitus as young adults. They also have an increased lifetime risk for heart disease and cancer. These chronic diseases are largely preventable: All children should learn and practice healthful eating and exercise habits.

sels, causing atherosclerosis. This is one of the greatest dangers of untreated long-term diabetes mellitus because blood vessels tend to become occluded. Blockage of a coronary artery causes myocardial infarction, as explained in Chapter 7. Thromboembolic strokes are also frequent complications of untreated diabetes. Occlusion of a leg artery can result in gangrene. Atherosclerosis generally causes poor circulation, which is another reason for poor wound healing.

Another complication of diabetes is diabetic retinopathy, a vascular disorder of the retina that can result in blindness. The minute retinal blood vessels become sclerotic and rupture. The nervous system is affected by poor circulation, as manifested by pain, tingling sensations, loss of feeling, and paralysis. The kidneys are usually affected by long-standing diabetes, and kidney failure is frequently the cause of death in the diabetic. The complications of diabetes are summarized in Figure 13–16.

**Treatment of Diabetes Mellitus** Important factors in treating diabetes are weight loss, diet, and exercise. The insulin dosage prescribed accompanies a carefully regulated diet. The diet cannot be altered without creating an insulin excess or deficiency. A person who exercises actively requires less insulin than one who does not. A diabetic's exercise pattern is a factor in prescribing insulin.

Regulation of the proper insulin dosage takes time. Certain factors—illness or emotional stress—can temporarily alter a patient's needs. There are different types of insulin (fast-, intermediate-, and slow-acting), which are effective

### Table 13–4  Warning Signs of Diabetes

| Type I or Insulin-Dependent Diabetes Mellitus | Type II or Non-Insulin Dependent Diabetes Mellitus |
|---|---|
| Frequent urination | Any of the Type I symptoms |
| Excessive thirst | Frequent infections |
| Extreme hunger | Recurring skin, gum, or bladder infections |
| Weight loss | Blurred vision |
| Fatigue | Cuts and bruises that heal slowly |
| Irritability | Numbness or tingling sensations in the hands or feet |

*From the American Diabetes Association.*

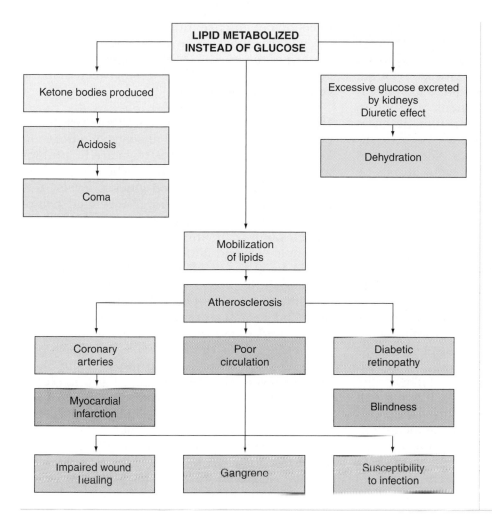

**Figure 13–16**
Complications of diabetes mellitus.

over various time periods. These are often prescribed in combination. Monitoring blood sugar levels is an essential part of diabetes care. Self-monitoring of blood glucose enables the diabetic to determine his or her blood glucose and adjust insulin dosage according to a measured reading. The test involves taking a small sample of blood from a finger prick and checking it with a portable glucose-monitoring device.

Insulin must be given by injection because it is a protein and would be digested in the gastrointestinal tract. There are oral compounds that can be used for some Type II diabetes, but they are not insulin. These are oral hypoglycemic agents, which stimulate secretion of insulin from beta cells that still have some capacity or make

cells more responsive to insulin. There are several choices of injectors and needle sizes that are easy to use. The automatic insulin pump administers a measured dose of insulin into the body via a tube with its tip embedded under the skin.

**Diabetic Coma and Insulin Shock** Diabetic coma develops when a person with severe diabetes fails to take enough insulin or deviates markedly from a prescribed diet. Acidosis and dehydration can follow if proper treatment is not given immediately. One symptom of diabetic coma is deep, labored breathing, which results from the effect of acidosis on the respiratory center of the brain. The person's breath has a fruity, acetone smell. The skin is flushed and dry, and the tongue is dry because of the dehydration. A diabetic coma may have a gradual onset, during which time the person is drowsy and lethargic. If urine and blood samples are taken, a high level of glucose is found.

Treatment of diabetic coma (diabetic ketoacidosis) requires urgent replacement of fluids to correct the dehydration. Insulin, usually given intravenously, is necessary as well. Because diabetic coma adversely affects sodium and potassium, the serum electrolytes must be checked frequently as therapy proceeds.

Insulin shock, also called hypoglycemic shock, results from too much insulin, not enough food, or excessive exercise. The person feels light-headed and faint, trembles, and begins to perspire. Taking sugar in some form—candy or orange juice, for example—may be adequate treatment at this stage. If the glucose level is not raised, the condition becomes more serious. The person's speech becomes thick, and walking becomes unsteady because the low level of glucose affects the brain. Double vision may be experienced; a loss of consciousness may follow.

If the person becomes comatose, it is difficult for the untrained to determine if the cause is a diabetic coma or insulin shock. A significant difference is that the deep, rapid breathing and the acetone breath characteristic of diabetic coma are not present in insulin shock. The person in insulin shock breathes shallowly. Intravenous injections of glucose must be given immediately for insulin shock. The administration of epinephrine raises the blood sugar level. Table 13–5 illustrates the differences between diabetic coma and insulin shock.

**Tests for Diabetes Mellitus** A simple urine test can show the presence or absence of glucose or ketones in the urine. Urine tests are helpful for initial screening and for those who are prone to ketoacidosis. Fasting blood glucose levels, glucose tolerance testing, and glycosylated hemoglobin testing are used to monitor and diagnose diabetes. For the fasting blood glucose level test, a sample of blood is taken after the person has fasted for 8 hours. The glucose tolerance test challenges the body's ability to secrete and use insulin. The test is performed after a 10-hour fast. The patient drinks a standard glucose solution, and blood and urine sample are taken and analyzed for the next three hours. No glucose should appear in the urine, and the blood glucose levels should not exceed 170 mg/dl of blood if insulin is being produced and utilized. Glycosylated hemoglobin determination is a simple blood test that is used to monitor long-term control of diabetes. It generally indicates the average blood glucose levels over the past 90 days. Normal values should be below 6, and levels for diabetics should be less than 7.

## Table 13–5   Differences between Diabetic Coma and Insulin Shock

| Diabetic Coma | Insulin Shock |
| --- | --- |
| Deep, labored breathing due to acidosis | Shallow breathing |
| Skin and tongue dry due to dehydration | Patient perspires |
| Fruity, acetone smell to breath | Odor of breath normal |
| Patient drowsy and lethargic before onset | Patient feels light-headed and faint before onset |
| Comatose | Comatose |
| Requires large dose of insulin | Requires glucose intravenously |
| Fluid and salts needed | |

## Prevention ✚ PLUS!

### Diabetes Control

Nearly three-fourths of adults with diabetes lack basic information that can help control their disease. Studies have shown that better control of diabetes helps prevent serious complications that may develop over time.

## Education of the Diabetic Patient

The American Diabetes Association, physicians, nurses, and dieticians have made a great effort to assist the diabetic patient in leading a normal life. The diabetic who understands the disease knows the importance of weight control, diet, exercise, and either insulin or oral agents for leading a normal life. A safety precaution advised by the American Diabetes Association is that anyone who takes insulin should carry an identification card explaining the emergency treatment required if an insulin reaction occurs.

## Gestational Diabetes Mellitus

Gestational diabetes is diabetes mellitus associated with pregnancy. It occurs in approximately 1% to 2% of all pregnancies, with an incidence that increases with maternal age.

Increased metabolic demands during pregnancy require higher insulin levels, but certain normal maternal physiological changes during pregnancy can result in insufficient insulin levels, which, if uncorrected, result in diabetes. Increased levels of estrogen and progesterone interfere with insulin action, and the placenta inactivates insulin. Moreover, the normal pregnancy-induced elevation of stress hormones such as cortisol, epinephrine, and glucagon raises blood glucose. Insulin requirements continue to rise as pregnancy approaches term. In a normal pregnancy, more insulin is secreted to compensate for these changes, but in some women, insulin levels remain low and blood glucose becomes high. Signs and symptoms of gestational diabetes are similar to insulin-dependent diabetes mellitus, but include maternal hypertension, polyhydroamnios (excessive amniotic fluid), excessive weight gain during the last 6 months of pregnancy, and a fetus large for gestational age.

## ▶ Abnormalities in Secretion of Sex Hormones

The gonads (ovaries and testes) are endocrine glands as well as the source of the ova and sperm (Chapter 12). They secrete the hormones estrogen and testosterone directly into the blood.

### Hypergonadism (Hypersecretion)

Abnormally increased functional activity of the gonads before puberty produces precocious sexual development in both sexes. In a male child, excessive production of testosterone may be caused by a tumor in the testes. This causes rapid growth of musculature and bones but premature uniting of the epiphyses and shaft of long bones. Normal height, therefore, is not attained. Hypersecretion of ovarian hormones in the female is rare because of the negative-feedback mechanism with gonadotropic hormones.

**Hypogonadism in the Male**   Several factors can cause hypogonadism—that is, the decreased functional activity of the gonads. A person may be born without functional testes, the testes may fail to descend and thus atrophy, or the testes may be lost through castration. Testes fail to develop because of lack of gonadotropic hormone.

Loss of the male gonads before puberty causes the condition of eunuchism in which sexual characteristics do not develop. Development of male traits depends on testosterone secreted by the testes. Castration after puberty causes some regression of secondary sexual characteristics, but masculinity is retained. Hormonal therapy, the administration of testosterone, can be effective.

**Hypogonadism in the Female**   Hyposecretion of hormones by the ovaries may be caused by poorly formed or missing ovaries. When ovaries are absent or fail to develop, female eunichism results. Secondary sexual characteristics do not develop. A characteristic of this condition is excessive growth of long bones because the epiphyses do not seal with the shaft of the bone as normally occurs at adolescence.

## ▶ Age-Related Diseases

Some changes in endocrine function occur normally with aging. Of these, none are significant causes of disease alone. However, some changes make the aging person more susceptible to disease.

Growth hormone level decreases with age. This is manifested in men after age 30 as a decrease in lean body mass and decreases in thickness and strength of bone matrix. As the body fat level increases, the growth hormone level decreases further. Increased body fat is correlated with greater risk of diabetes, heart disease, and cancer. Decreased bone density makes bones more susceptible to fracture.

A slight decrease in $T_3$:$T_4$ ratio is seen with age, resulting in decreased metabolic rate. The incidence of autoimmune disease of the thyroid among females increases with age.

Although aldosterone levels remain relatively steady, an age-related decline in the kidney's sensitivity to aldosterone occurs, accompanied by a diminishing capacity of the kidney to secrete renin when needed. The body is less able to deal with the stress of changes in blood pressure, dehydration, and disease in general. There is an increased incidence of abnormalities in blood pressure, sodium and potassium levels, acid-base balances, and osmotic pressure.

The pancreas retains the ability to secrete insulin at normal levels with age, but tissue responsiveness to insulin decreases. Insulin resistance leads to a greater incidence of NIDDM. It is estimated that NIDDM occurs in 10% of those over age 56, 20% of those between 45 and 76, and 40% of people over age 85. Although IDDM is somewhat less common than NIDDM, and its occurrence is unrelated to aging, it remains among the 10 leading causes of death among people over age 65.

Androgen and estrogen levels drop with age. The effects of these changes are discussed in Chapter 12.

## ▶ Diagnostic Procedures for Endocrine Diseases

Indications of pituitary hyperactivity or hypoactivity can be confirmed by serum assays. Growth hormone (GH) levels can detect hyperpituitarism (gigantism and/or acromegaly) and hypopituitarism (dwarfism). Thyroid-stimulating hormone (TSH) assay is useful in confirming primary hypothyroidism or hyperthyroidism. Activity of the posterior pituitary can be evaluated by the water deprivation and vasopressin test. A urine specimen is taken after controlled water deprivation, and a blood sample is drawn. Dilute urine and high osmotic pressure in the blood indicates that water is not being absorbed by the kidney tubules. If vasopressin injection corrects the massive polyuria, diabetes insipidus is confirmed.

Diseases of the thyroid gland are diagnosed on the basis of the $T_3$ and $T_4$ tests previously described and by the serum level of TSH. An elevated TSH indicates low $T_4$ function. A low TSH indicates an excess of $T_4$ caused by a functioning adenoma or carcinoma. A thyroid scan provides visualization of the thyroid gland after administration of radioactive iodine. It is usually recommended after discovery of a mass, an enlarged gland, or an asymmetric goiter. Thyroid ultrasonography evaluates characteristics of thyroid nodules and distinguishes between solid or cystic masses in the gland.

Diagnostic tests for parathyroid gland activity measure parathyroid hormone and calcium levels in the blood and can detect hyperparathyroidism.

Adrenal gland activity can be evaluated by the level of plasma cortisol from the adrenal cortex. Abnormal levels indicate hypersecretion (Cushing's syndrome) or hyposecretion (Addison's disease). Urine tests measure steroid level and detect hyperactivity of the gland.

A fasting blood glucose test helps detect diabetes mellitus and evaluate the clinical status of diabetic patients. An oral glucose tolerance test challenges the ability of the pancreas to secrete insulin in response to large doses of glucose.

## CHAPTER SUMMARY

The endocrine system provides a means of chemical communication between body parts. The tiny anterior pituitary gland controls activities of the thyroid, adrenals, and sex glands. It also stimulates growth, development, and tissue repair. The pituitary is called the "master gland" for these reasons. Pituitary activity is governed by the hypothalamus of the brain.

Hyperpituitarism causes an excess of growth hormone. This condition, if present before puberty, results in gigantism. In an adult, excessive production of growth hormone leads to abnormal enlargement of facial bones, bones of hands and feet, and soft tissue. This growth in an adult is called acromegaly.

Severe hypopituitarism impedes growth and development in a child, causing the child to be dwarfed in stature. Glands dependent on stimulation by the anterior pituitary, the thyroid, adrenals, and sex glands cease functioning in hypopituitarism at any age. The posterior pituitary gland secretes vasopressin, also called antidiuretic hormone, and oxytocin. Hypoactivity of this gland causes diabetes insipidus.

The rate of metabolism is controlled by the thyroid gland. An enlargement of this gland is a goiter. Hyperthyroidism, an excess of thyroxine, accelerates heart and respiratory activity, increases metabolic rate, and raises body temperature. Graves' disease is an example of severe hyperthyroidism. A congenital lack of thyroxine results in cretinism, a condition of mental and physical retardation. Myxedema is a disease of severe hypothyroidism in an adult.

Hormones of the adrenal cortex are essential to life. Aldosterone regulates salt balance, and cortisol affects the metabolism of nutrients. The sex hormones estrogen and androgen are also produced by this gland. Hypoactivity of the adrenal cortex is called Addison's disease.

Hyperactivity of the adrenal cortex causes different diseases, depending on which hormones are in excess. Cushing's syndrome results from an excess of cortisol, and Conn's syndrome results from excessive aldosterone. Precocious puberty and adrenal virilism develop from too much androgen secretion.

The parathyroid hormone, parathormone, regulates the level of circulating calcium and phosphate. Hyperactivity of the parathyroids causes hypercalcemia. The high level of calcium is primarily from bone resorption that weakens the bones. Hypoparathyroidism reduces the level of calcium in the blood. This causes the nervous system to become hyperexcitable, skeletal muscles are overstimulated, and tetany results. Hormones of the pancreas, insulin and glucagon, control blood sugar level. Lack of insulin causes an increase in blood glucose, the condition of diabetes mellitus.

Hypoglycemia, abnormally low blood glucose, results from insulin excess. This condition can develop in the diabetic from an overdosage of insulin. A tumor of the insulin-producing cells of the pancreas can also cause hypoglycemia. The absence of glucocorticoids in an Addison's disease patient results in low blood glucose.

## RESOURCES

*The Merck Manual of Diagnosis and Therapy,* 17th ed., John Wiley & Sons, 1999.

*Professional Guide to Diseases,* 6th ed., Springhouse, 1998.

# DISEASES AT A GLANCE

## Endocrine System

| DISEASE | ETIOLOGY | SIGNS AND SYMPTOMS |
|---|---|---|
| Gigantism | GH hypersecretion beginning in childhood due to adenoma of anterior pituitary | Bone length increases rapidly, delayed sexual development |
| Acromegaly | GH hypersecretion beginning in adulthood due to adenoma of anterior pituitary | Enlargement of feet, hands, face as bones grow in diameter; soft tissue growth, nose, lips, lower jaw protrude, tongue and skin thicken |
| Pituitary dwarfism | GH hyposecretion beginning in childhood due to pituitary damage or ischemia | Normal mental development, slow growth, sexual development lacking |
| Panhypopituitarism | No pituitary hormones secreted due to anterior pituitary damage | General lack of endocrine activity; mental slowness, lethargy, salt imbalance, abnormal nutrient metabolism, lack of sexual function |
| Diabetes insipidus | Central: hyposecretion of ADH by hypothalamic nuclei due to vascular lesion, neoplasm, trauma to base of skull, or inherited abnormality on chromosome 20<br>Nephrogenic: kidney insensitive to ADH due to X-linked gene or due to polycystic disease or pyelonephritis | Polyuria, polydipsia |
| Hyperparathyroidism | Neoplasm | Weak bones deform and fracture easily, kidney stones, pain in bones, depressed nervous system, weak muscles, slow heart rate, abdominal pain, vomiting, constipation |
| Hypoparathyroidism | Complication of thyroidectomy; also rare X-linked syndrome | Overexcited muscular and nervous system, characteristic tetany in hands, laryngeal spasm |
| Endemic and similar goiters | Insufficient iodine in diet | Enlargement of neck, difficulty swallowing, cough, choking sensation, reduced thyroxine |

| DIAGNOSIS | TREATMENT |
| --- | --- |
| Serum assay for GH | None |
| Serum assay for GH | None |
| Serum assay for GH | Hormone replacement therapy |
| Serum assay for GH, TSH, thyroxine, cortisol | Thyroxine, cortisol, GH, sex hormones |
| Urinalysis in water deprivation vasopressin test | Administer ADH |
| High serum calcium, patient history, kidney stones | Surgical removal of tumor, medication to lower calcium |
| Low serum calcium, patient history | Administer vitamin D and calcium |
| Ultrasound, thyroid scan, serum assay for thyroxine | Add iodine to diet |

# DISEASES AT A GLANCE (*continued*)

## Endocrine System

| DISEASE | ETIOLOGY | SIGNS AND SYMPTOMS |
|---|---|---|
| Adenomatous and similar goiters | Adenoma of thyroid | Exophthalmos, increased nervous activity, tremor, high metabolic rate, sweating and thirst, rapid pulse, increased appetite and weight loss, diarrhea, difficulty sleeping |
| Myxedema | Autoimmune disease or complication of thyroid surgery or radiation treatment of thyroid | Edema, weight gain, dry skin, little sweat, low body temperature, muscular weakness, somnolence, slow heart rate, atherosclerosis, constipation |
| Cretinism | Congenital absence of thryoid gland or autoimmune disease in childhood | Mental retardation, retarded growth, weak muscles, protruding abdomen, no sexual development, characteristic facial features—protruding tongue, broad nose, short forehead, small wide-set eyes, expressionless |
| Cushing's syndrome | Hypersecretion of ACTH by pituitary or a tumor; may be induced by high therapeutic levels of cortisol | Hyperglycemia, adrenal diabetes, obesity of trunk, buffalo hump, moon face, hypertension, atherosclerosis, muscle weakness and fatigue, thin skin, easily bruised, stretch marks, increases susceptibility to infections, poor wound healing, weak bones |
| Conn's syndrome | Adenoma of adrenal cortex | Weak muscles, polydipsia, polyuria, hypertension water retention |
| Adrenogenital syndrome | Adenoma of adrenal gland | Virilization, male secondary sexual characteristics in females |
| Addison's disease | Most idiopathic; probably autoimmune; linked to stress, chronic infection, inflammation, tumors | Dehydration, salt loss, low blood pressure, muscle weakness, weight loss, fatigue, gastrointestinal disturbances, dark skin pigmentation |
| IDDM (insulin-dependent diabetes mellitus) | Hyposecretion of insulin due to autoimmune disease; genetic | Polyuria, polydipsia, increased appetite, with weight loss, glycosuria, hyperglycemia, ketone bodies in urine, acidosis, poor wound healing, increased susceptibility to infections |

| DIAGNOSIS | TREATMENT |
|---|---|
| Ultrasound, thyroid scan, serum assay for thyroxine | Radioactive iodine, medication, surgery |
| Ultrasound, serum assay for thyroxine | Administer thyroid hormone |
| Serum assay for thyroxine | Administer thyroid hormone |
| Serum cortisol, urinalysis, physical exam | Surgery and hormone replacement |
| Serum aldosterone, urinalysis | Surgical removal of adenoma |
| Physical exam, serum androgen | Surgical removal of tumor |
| Serum cortisol and aldosterone | Administer cortisol and aldosterone |
| Urinalysis, fasting blood glucose, oral glucose tolerance test, physical exam, history | Diet, insulin, exercise |

# DISEASES AT A GLANCE (*continued*)

## Endocrine System

| DISEASE | ETIOLOGY | SIGNS AND SYMPTOMS |
| --- | --- | --- |
| NIDDM (non-insulin dependent diabetes mellitus) | Hyposecretion of insulin or insulin resistance in tissues; genetic, obesity | May or may not have polyuria, polydipsia, increased appetite, weight loss, often obese, gradual onset, nonspecific symptoms including itching, recurrent infections, visual changes, abnormal sensations |
| Diabetic coma | Insufficient insulin and low blood sugar | Ketosis, acidosis, dehydration, deep labored breathing, fruity acetone odor of breath, skin flushed, tongue dry, gradual onset, drowsiness, lethargy |
| Insulin shock | High insulin levels | Light-headedness, faintness, trembling, perspiration, double vision, speech thick, unsteady walk, loss of consciousness, shallow breathing, breath odor normal |
| Hypergonadism | Hypersecretion of sex hormones caused by tumors | Precocious sexual development |
| Hypogonadism | Hyposecretion of sex hormones caused by undeveloped gonads | Lack of sexual development, eunuchism |

| DIAGNOSIS | TREATMENT |
|---|---|
| Urinalysis, fasting blood glucose, oral glucose tolerance test, physical exam, history | Diet, oral hypoglycemic medications, exercise |
| High blood and urine glucose | Insulin, fluids, sodium chloride, sodium bicarbonate, electrolytes |
| Low blood sugar | Sugar (candy, orange juice), IV glucose if unconscious, epinephrine |
| Serum sex hormones | Administration of sex hormones |
| Serum sex hormones | Administration of sex hormones |

# Interactive Activities

## Cases for Critical Thinking

1. A mother brings her 5-year-old son to the pediatrician with complaints that her son has been "wetting the bed" consistently. The child has a good appetite, drinks a lot of water, and has a "high metabolism" according to the mother. On examination, the doctor notes that the child has lost 10 pounds since his last physical 6 months ago. What diseases should be ruled out?

2. A 59-year-old woman reports to the doctor's office with a chief complaint of "terrible headaches" especially between her eyes. Her blood pressure, blood sugar, and cholesterol level are high. The doctor also notes a terrible bruise on her leg that was there since her last examination 2 months ago. What diseases should be ruled out?

3. A 45-year-old man reports to the emergency room with terrible dehydration. He has a yellowish appearance and can hardly stand without assistance. His blood level of potassium is extremely high and his legs feel "tingly." His heartbeat is very rapid, and his breathing is shallow. What diseases does this man possibly have?

## Multiple Choice

1. Acromegaly results from hyperactivity of the _____.

   a. thyroid
   b. parathyroid
   c. anterior pituitary
   d. posterior pituitary

2. This hormone increases the blood calcium level.

   a. glucagon
   b. parathormone
   c. androgen
   d. insulin

3. Hypoglycemia is a sign in _____.

   a. Cushing's disease
   b. Addison's disease
   c. diabetes
   d. Graves' disease

4. The trunk is obese in _____.

   a. Graves' disease
   b. Cushing's disease
   c. Addison's disease
   d. Conn's disease

5. A deficiency of ADH is the cause of _____.

   a. IDDM
   b. NIDDM
   c. diabetes insipidus
   d. ketoacidosis

6. Which of these is associated with hypersecretion of thyroxine?

   a. Graves' disease
   b. gigantism
   c. cretinism
   d. myxedema

7. Which gland secretes epinephrine and norepinephrine?

   a. pancreas
   b. parathyroid
   c. testes
   d. adrenal

8. A deficiency in corticosteroids is associated with _____.

   a. Addison's disease
   b. Conn's disease
   c. diabetes insipidus
   d. pheochromocytoma

9. A person in insulin shock should receive _____ immediately.

   a. sodium
   b. insulin
   c. water
   d. glucose

10. Iodine is required for the body to make _____.

   a. bone
   b. insulin
   c. thryoxine
   d. glucose

## True or False

_____ 1. Kidney stones are likely to form in hypoparathyroidism.

_____ 2. Hypercalcemia causes tetany.

_____ 3. Glucagon prevents hyperglycemia.

_____ 4. Steroids that suppress the inflammatory response, as in arthritis, are produced by the thyroid.

_____ 5. Hypertension accompanies Addison's disease.

_____ 6. Cretinism results from a congenital thyroid deficiency.

_____ 7. A person with Graves' disease is very sensitive to cold.

_____ 8. Dehydration can develop in diabetes mellitus.

_____ 9. Cushing's syndrome results from an excess of glucocorticoids.

_____ 10. Glucagon elevates blood glucose level.

## Fill-Ins

1. Overproduction of growth hormone before puberty is called _____.

2. An overproduction of growth hormone after puberty is called _____.

3. The posterior pituitary secretes _____ and _____.

4. Chronic hypoadrenalism, accompanied by weight loss and muscle weakness, is known as _____ _____.

5. A tumor of the adrenal medulla, or _____, causes overproduction of epinephrine and norepinephrine.

6. Insulin is secreted by cells of the pancreas called _____ _____.

7. A blood pH of 6.9 is a condition called _____.

8. Tropic hormones are secreted by the _____ _____.

9. Dwarfism is associated with hyposecretion of _____ _____.

10. Sexual characteristics do not develop in the rare condition called _____ _____.

# MedMedia Wrap-Up

**www.prenhall.com/mulvihill**
Remember to visit this website for extra study practice, including exercises, Internet links, news updates, and an audio glossary.

**Activity CD-ROM**
Check out the CD-ROM in the back of this book. You will find games, exercises, puzzles, and videos to help enhance your understanding of this chapter.

CHAPTER

14

# Diseases of the Nervous System and Special Senses

## Learning Objectives

After studying this chapter, you should be able to

■ Recognize the basic structure and functions of the nervous system

■ Name the causes and primary treatments for the common headache, cluster headache, and migraine

■ Describe infectious diseases of the nervous system, eye, and ear, and list their specific causes, symptoms, and treatment

■ List and describe degenerative diseases of the nervous system, including multiple sclerosis, Parkinson's disease, and amyotrophic lateral sclerosis

■ Describe inherited and congenital diseases of the nervous system

■ Describe the causes, signs, and treatment of seizures

■ List and describe the effects of trauma in the nervous system

■ Identify the causes, effects, and treatment of CVA (stroke)

## Fact or Fiction?

Benign brain tumors are not very serious and therefore are not cause for concern.

*Fiction:* Benign tumors tend to grow and crowd out precious cranial space and, thus, apply pressure or restrict blood flow to particular brain regions. If these benign growths are inoperable or uncontrolled, they will kill the victim. Malignant brain tumors may be lethal, but they may also be surgically removed or reduced with medication or radiation. All brain tumors require attention and may be lethal if left untreated. Treatment with surgery, medication, or radiation is most successful for slow-growing, encapsulated tumors.

# Disease Chronicle

## Phineas Gage and Neuroscience

The brain is a very complex and integrated organ. At approximately three pounds, this organ governs much of the body and how it responds to its environment. Occasionally, even small disruptions in this organ of millions of neurons can cause the body and mind to fail or die. In 1847, Phineas Gage, a hard working Irishman, was busy rock blasting on a mountainous construction project. One fateful day an explosion sent an iron bar completely and cleanly through the front part of his head. Incredibly, he survived being impaled; still more amazing, though, is that he retained his intelligence and memory. However, his personality changed drastically. Phineas became fitful, irreverent, and very profane.

This accidental injury taught medical scientists the importance of the frontal lobes in personality and behavior, and it inspired the practice of frontal lobotomies, a type of psychosurgery in which a defined portion of the brain is removed for therapeutic purposes. By 1955 over 40,000 such psychosurgeries had been performed, many by questionably trained personnel, which no doubt resulted in many premature patient deaths. Today, drugs and psychosocial therapy, including counseling, have replaced surgery as the treatments of choice for abnormal behavior.

## MedMedia
www.prenhall.com/mulvihill

Use the web address to the left to access the free, interactive Companion Website created for this textbook. It features chapter-specific exercises, Internet links, news links, and an audio glossary. Additionally, explore the CD-ROM that accompanies this book to discover Disease Focus videos and a rich array of activities that accompany this chapter.

## ▶ Structural Organization of the Nervous System

The nervous system monitors the external and internal environment and, along with the endocrine system, controls the body's functions.

The basic organization of the nervous system includes two major divisions: the central nervous system (CNS) and the peripheral nervous system (PNS). The CNS is composed of the brain and spinal cord. It integrates information and controls the peripheral nervous system. The PNS comprises all those nerves outside the CNS, beginning with the 12 pairs of cranial nerves and 31 pairs of spinal nerves. The nerves carry information to and from the CNS. Nerves consist of motor nerves, which carry information to muscles and glands, and sensory nerves, which carry sensory information from sense receptors to the CNS. Certain organs are highly specialized for gathering sensory input; these are called organs of the special senses and include the eyes, ears, and nose. We consider diseases of the eye and ear in this chapter; diseases involving the nose were described in Chapter 9.

The basic unit of the nervous system is the neuron, or nerve cell. The neuron consists of a cell body to which are attached filamentous extensions called dendrites that carry information toward the cell body and a filamentous axon that carries information away from the cell body. A neuron is shown in Figure 14–1. Some neurons are sensory nerve cells, capable of detecting environmental changes and transmitting messages to the brain or spinal cord. Other neurons, the motor neurons, convey messages from the central nervous system to muscles, causing contraction, or to glands, triggering secretion. The fibers of sensory and motor neurons are insulated by a lipoprotein covering called the myelin sheath, which facilitates the rate of transmission of an impulse. Deterioration of this sheath is characteristic of multiple sclerosis, a disease to be described.

### The Brain

Three coverings, the meninges, protect the delicate nerve tissue of both the brain and spinal cord. The innermost covering is the pia mater, the middle layer is the arachnoid, and the toughest, outermost covering is the dura mater. Meningitis is an inflammation of these coverings.

The brain has three major anatomical areas: the cerebrum, cerebellum, and brain stem. The largest portion of the brain is the cerebrum, comprised of two cerebral hemispheres. The cerebral surface is highly convoluted with many elevations (gyrus) and depressions (sulci). The outer surface of the brain, the cortex, consists of gray matter, where nerve cell bodies are concentrated. The inner area consists of white matter, the nerve fiber tracts. Deep within the white matter are concentrations of nerve cell bodies known as basal ganglia, also called basal nuclei, which help control position and subconscious movements. It is the basal ganglia (also gray matter) that are affected in Parkinson's disease.

Within the brain are four spaces called ventricles where cerebrospinal fluid (CSF) is formed and

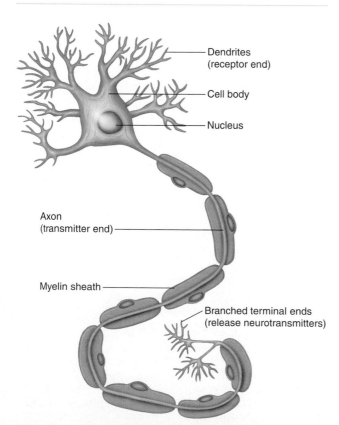

**Figure 14–1** Typical neuron.

Dendrites
(receptor end)

Cell body

Nucleus

Axon
(transmitter end)

Myelin sheath

Branched terminal ends
(release neurotransmitters)

which are continuous with the central canal of the spinal cord. CSF is derived from plasma and flows out of the ventricles through small openings to circulate over the brain and spinal cord, forming a watery, protective cushion. CSF is reabsorbed into the venous sinuses of the dura mater, and new fluid is formed. Obstruction of cerebrospinal fluid circulation results in hydrocephalus, which is described in this chapter.

The cerebellum controls voluntary movements, such as riding a bicycle. The brain stem is called the "vital center" because it regulates heart and breathing rates.

## The Spinal Cord

The spinal cord is housed within the vertebral column and is continuous with the brain stem (Figure 14–2). Numerous tracts of nerve fibers within the cord ascend to and descend from the brain, carrying messages to and from muscles, organs, and glands.

## The Autonomic Nervous System

A division of the PNS is the autonomic nervous system. This system controls internal functioning of the body. The autonomic nervous system contains the sympathetic and the parasympathetic nervous systems, which often work antagonistically to each other. The hypothalamus, located within the brain, controls certain activities of the autonomic nervous system, and is known as the center for homeostasis.

The autonomic nervous system controls arterial blood pressure, heart rate, gastrointestinal functions, sweating, temperature regulation, and many other involuntary actions. Whereas some peripheral nerves affect skeletal or voluntary muscle, the autonomic nervous system acts on smooth or involuntary muscle and cardiac muscle. Diseases of the digestive system such as stress ulcers, regional enteritis, and ulcerative colitis (Chapter 10) are influenced by the autonomic nervous system.

## The Sensory Nervous System

Sensations detected by sensory neurons in specialized organs such as the eye and ear, as well as in skin, muscles, tendons, and internal organs, are transmitted to the central nervous system. The spinal cord receives simple sensations and directs simple reflex responses, as when one touches a hot stove and quickly withdraws the hand. Complex sensory information must travel to specialized parts of the brain. Impulses reaching the brain stem and cerebellum bring about many unconscious automatic actions, but sensory information involving thought processes must reach the highest area of the brain, the cerebral cortex.

The cerebral cortex has specialized areas to receive sensory information from all parts of the body, such as the feet, the hands, and the abdomen. Visual impulses are transmitted to the posterior part of the brain, whereas olfactory and auditory impulses are received in the lateral parts. Association areas of the brain interpret deeper meaning of the sensations, and all the sensory messages are integrated and stored as memory. Creative thought becomes possible through use of sensory input.

## The Motor Nervous System

Just as the cerebral cortex has areas specialized for the reception of sensory information, it has areas that govern motor activity. The primary motor cortex controls discrete movements of skeletal muscles. Because the nerve fibers cross over in the medulla and/or spinal cord, stimulation on one side of the cerebral cortex affects particular muscles on the opposite side of the body.

Anterior to the primary motor cortex is the premotor cortex, which controls coordinated movements of muscles. This process is accomplished by stimulating groups of muscles that work together. The speech area is located here and is usually on the left side, especially in right-handed people. Specialized areas of the brain are shown in Figure 14–3.

## ▶ Diseases of the Nervous System

## Common Headache

Moderate to severe head pain characterizes the common headache. Nausea, vomiting, and sensitivity to noise and light may accompany more severe cases. Tension or inflammation of muscles

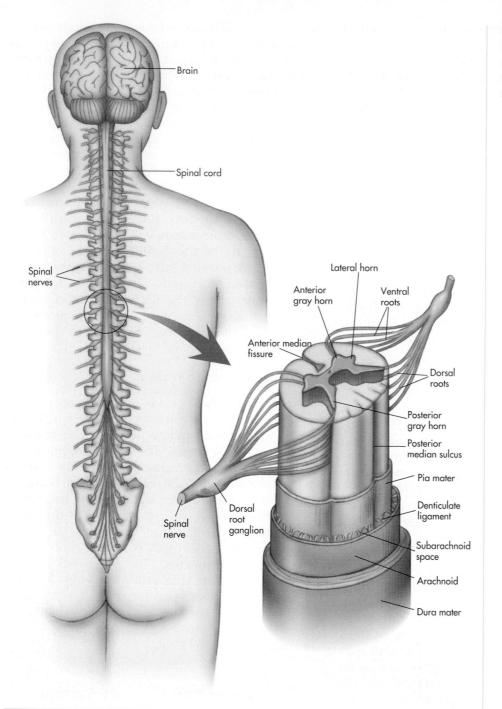

**Figure 14–2**
The brain, spinal cord, and spinal nerves. An expanded view of the spinal cord is shown.

in the head, eyes, neck, and shoulders may cause the common headache. Other causes include dilation of cerebral blood vessels, allergies, chemical fumes, extreme temperatures, and constipation.

Common household treatments are NSAIDs (nonsteroid anti-inflammatory drugs) such as aspirin, ibuprofen (Advil), and acetaminophen (Tylenol); rest in a dark room; and application of a cold compress.

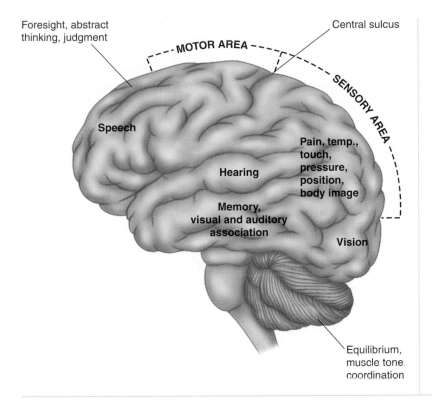

Foresight, abstract thinking, judgment

Central sulcus

MOTOR AREA

SENSORY AREA

Speech

Pain, temp., touch, pressure, position, body image

Hearing

Memory, visual and auditory association

Vision

Equilibrium, muscle tone, coordination

**Figure 14–3**
Specialized areas of the brain.

Two of the more intense and episodic forms of headache are the cluster headache and the migraine.

## Cluster Headache

Cluster headache affects 1 to 4 per 1000, and men are five times more likely to be affected than women. The cluster headache occurs suddenly, producing very severe, sharp, and stabbing pain particularly near one eye or temporal area. The headaches may occur two to three times per day for weeks, or may occur over 1 to 3 months, subside, and recur months or years later. The pain may develop any time, but usually occurs at night and tends to last from 30 minutes to several hours. The pain is so severe that many individuals cannot lie down and may instead pace about. In contrast with migraine, however, light intensity, sounds, or strange odors do not elicit nausea or vomiting.

Alcohol and nicotine may trigger these painful headaches. This condition tends to run in families, although the genetics have not been clarified. Treatment requires medications like those

for migraines described below, plus biofeedback, reduction of stress, and oxygen therapy.

## Migraine Headache

Migraine headaches are more common in women and usually begin in the teen years or early 20s. The symptoms are throbbing (moderate) pain on one or both sides of the head plus sensitivity to light and/or noise or certain odors. Because migraines tend to cause nausea and vomiting, they are referred to as a "sick headache." Sometimes, an aura or premonition precedes the migraine onset. Additional symptoms include numbness, dizziness, or visual blurring. The headaches last from a few hours to a few days and may recur once a month or once every few years. A history of the symptoms helps diagnose migraine.

Specific causes have not been identified. Some women find relief when they discontinue their birth control pills or when they attain menopause. Bedrest in a dark, quiet room is beneficial. Drug treatment is aimed at prevention and relief of symptoms. NSAIDs may not provide adequate relief, but prescription drugs like opioids, codeine, and mependine are often effective.

## ▶ Infectious Diseases of the Nervous System

Certain pathogenic microorganisms are neurotropic in that the virus or bacterium has an affinity for nervous system tissue. Pathogens obtain access to the nervous system by many routes, including by way of wounds, trauma, and systemic infections.

### Meningitis

Meningitis is an acute inflammation of the first two meninges that cover the brain and spinal cord: the pia mater and the arachnoid. A contagious disease, it usually affects children and young adults and may have serious complications if not diagnosed and treated early. The symptoms of meningitis are high fever, chills, and a severe headache caused by increased intracranial pressure. A key symptom is a stiff neck that holds the head rigidly. Movement of neck muscles stretches the meninges and increases head pain. Nausea, vomiting, and a rash may also be symptomatic. The high fever often causes delirium and convulsions in children, and they may lapse into a coma.

There are many forms of meningitis, and some more contagious than others. The most common cause is the bacterium *Neisseria meningitidis,* also called the meningococcus, but other bacteria, as well as viruses, cause meningitis. The infecting organisms can reach the meninges from the middle ear, upper respiratory tract, or frontal sinuses; or they can be carried in the blood from the lungs or other infected sites. Healthy children may be carriers of the bacteria and spread the organisms by sneezing or coughing. Viral meningitis may be caused by mumps, polio viruses, and occasionally by herpes simplex.

Diagnosis of meningitis is made by performing a lumbar puncture (Figure 14–4) or spinal tap, in which a hollow needle is inserted into the spinal canal between vertebrae in the lumbar region. This procedure is possible because the spinal cord terminates at or near the first lumbar vertebra although a sac containing cerebrospinal fluid extends down to the sacrum. The spinal tap will reveal cerebrospinal fluid at increased pressure. The infected fluid contains an elevated protein level, numerous polymorphs (WBCs), and infecting organisms. The level of glucose in the cerebrospinal fluid is below normal because the bacteria use the sugar for their own growth.

The prognosis depends on the cause of meningitis and prompt treatment. Treatment with antibiotics is very effective if the meningitis is bacterial. If not treated, permanent brain damage usually results, manifesting itself by sight or hearing loss, paralysis, mental retardation, or death. Another complication is blockage of the fourth ventricle by a pyogenic infection, which results in the accumulation of cerebrospinal fluid in the brain, a form of hydrocephalus.

### Encephalitis

Encephalitis, an inflammation of the brain and meninges, is caused by several types of viruses. Some of these viruses may be harbored by wild birds and transmitted to humans by mosquitoes.

Symptoms of encephalitis range from mild to severe and include headache, fever, cerebral dysfunction, disordered thought patterns, and seizures. In serious cases involving extensive brain damage, convalescence is slow and requires prolonged physical rehabilitation. Nerve damage may cause paralysis. Personality changes may occur as well as emotional disturbances that require therapy.

There are many forms of the disease, and they may occur in epidemics. Lethargic encephalitis, or "sleeping sickness," is one type of encephalitis with persistent drowsiness and delirium that sometimes results in coma. Secondary encephalitis may develop from viral childhood diseases such as chicken pox, measles, and mumps.

Diagnosis of encephalitis is made by lumbar puncture. Treatment is essentially aimed at the symptoms, control of the high fever, maintenance of fluid and electrolyte balance, and careful monitoring of respiratory and kidney function.

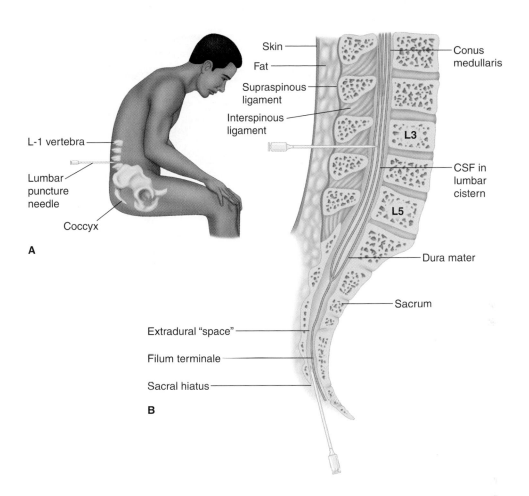

**Figure 14–4** (A) Lumbar puncture, also known as spinal tap. (B) Section of the vertebral column showing the spinal cord and membranes. A lumbar puncture needle is shown at L3-4 and in the sacral hiatus.

## Poliomyelitis

Poliomyelitis is an infectious disease of the brain and spinal cord caused by a virus. Motor neurons of the medulla oblongata and of the spinal cord are primarily affected.

As a result, muscle tissue is not stimulated; it weakens and finally atrophies. If the respiratory muscles are affected, artificial means of respiration are required.

Symptoms of poliomyelitis are stiff neck, fever, headache, sore throat, and gastrointestinal disturbances. When diagnosed and treated early, severe damage to the nervous system and paralysis can be prevented. Those who survive paralytic polio may be left with a limp or need a walking aid such as crutches or a wheelchair.

Excessive fatigue, muscular weakness, pain, and other difficulty may occur 20 to 30 years after the onset of the disease. This condition is known as post-polio syndrome (PPS), and its exact cause remains unknown. Additional rest seems to offer some relief for PPS.

Once a highly prevalent disease that killed or crippled primarily children, polio has been nearly eradicated through the development of the Salk and Sabin vaccines. Dr. Jonas Salk's vaccine consisted of inactivated poliovirus injected intramuscularly, which stimulated production of antibodies against poliovirus. With the institution of immunization programs, cases of polio dropped immediately. Dr. Albert Sabin developed an oral vaccine more convenient to administer, particularly to large groups, and it is extremely ef-

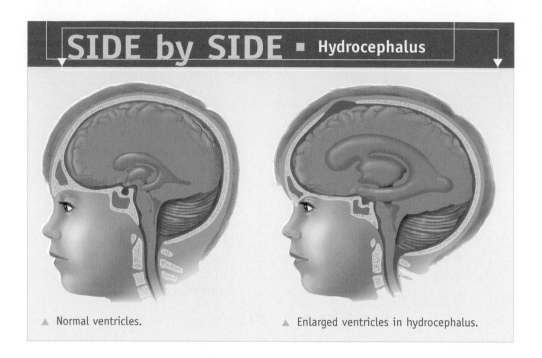

## SIDE by SIDE ■ Hydrocephalus

▲ Normal ventricles.　　　　▲ Enlarged ventricles in hydrocephalus.

fective. The Sabin vaccine is taken orally and stimulates the production of antibodies within the digestive system, where the viruses reside. Unlike the Salk vaccine, the Sabin destroys the viruses in the digestive system, thus preventing transmission and eliminating carriers. Many researchers believe, however, that the Salk vaccine is the better choice because it employs killed virus and ensures that the vaccine itself will not transmit polio. The Centers for Disease Control and Prevention has recommended a combination of Sabin and Salk vaccines.

The World Health Organization projects that by 2006 polio will be eradicated as smallpox has been. Between 1988 and 1998, polio declined 85% worldwide, and today, polio has been eliminated in the United States and from much of the world. A tragic exception is Africa, especially Nigeria, where under-vaccination has enabled many epidemics to break out. Clearly, it remains important to continue immunization, both locally and globally, in order to control this disease.

## Rabies

Rabies is an infectious disease of the brain and spinal cord caused by a virus that is transmitted by secretions (saliva, urine) of an infected animal. Rabies is primarily a disease of warm-blooded animals such as dogs, cats, raccoons, skunks, wolves, foxes, and bats, but it can be transmitted to humans through bites or scratches from a rabid animal.

The virus passes from the wound along nerves to the spinal cord and brain, where it causes acute encephalomyelitis. The incubation period is long, 30 to 60 days or more, depending on the distance of the wound from the brain. Bites on the face, neck, and hands are the most serious. The mode of tetanus and rabies transmission to the central nervous system is illustrated in Figure 14–5.

Symptoms of rabies include fever, pain, mental derangement, rage, convulsions, and paralysis. Rabies affects the areas of the brain that control the muscles of the throat for swallowing and also for breathing. As a result, spasms occur within the throat and voice box, causing a painful paralysis. Because of the inability to swallow or clear the throat, the infected animal or human produces profuse, sticky saliva, and thus tends to "foam" at the mouth. Hydrophobia is an aversion to water related to rabies. The disease is fatal in humans once it reaches the central nervous system and the symptoms described have developed.

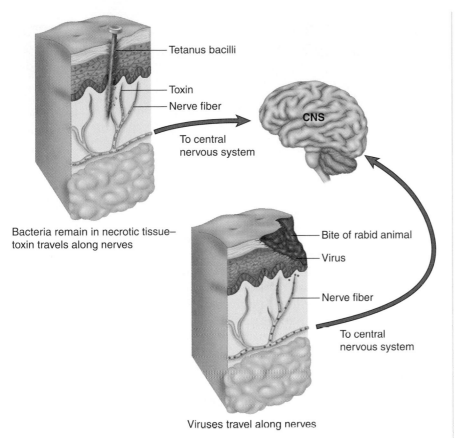

**Figure 14–5**
Nerve involvement in tetanus and rabies.

Tetanus bacilli

Toxin

Nerve fiber

CNS

To central nervous system

Bacteria remain in necrotic tissue– toxin travels along nerves

Bite of rabid animal

Virus

Nerve fiber

To central nervous system

Viruses travel along nerves

**Figure 14–5**
Nerve involvement in tetanus and rabies.

In the case of an animal bite, it is extremely important to know if the animal is rabid, and investigation of the animal must be made whenever possible. If rabies is suspected, immunization and globulin injections are started on the infected person. The person receives repeated injections of an altered virus to stimulate antibody production and an immune serum to provide passive immunity.

The severity of rabies explains the critical need for the vaccination of dogs and cats against the disease. Certain signs indicate that an animal is rabid. The animal goes through several stages, the first of which is an anxiety stage manifested by a change of temperament. For example, a wild animal may act friendly. A furious stage follows in which the animal bites at everything. When paralysis of the throat occurs, the animal cannot swallow, and it foams at the mouth. The last stage of rabies is called the dumb stage. The animal appears to have something caught in the throat but makes no attempt to remove it, and death follows.

Prevention of rabies is achieved by taking a series of three vaccinations over 28 days. The vaccine is required for field workers and medical associates who work with animals and tissues that may carry the rabies virus.

## Shingles (Herpes Zoster)

**Shingles** is an acute inflammation of nerve cells caused by the chicken pox virus, herpes zoster. It is manifested by pain and a rash characterized by small water blisters surrounded by a red area. The lesions follow a sensory nerve, forming a streak toward the midline of the torso. The rash is generally confined to one side of the body and does not cross the midline. The lesions dry and become encrusted. They cause severe itching, pain, and scarring. The optic nerve can be affected, causing severe conjunctivitis. If

## Prevention ✚ PLUS!

### Spelunking

The rabies vaccine and goggles are essential if you are the adventurous type who enjoys exploring caves—spelunking—because you might find yourself crawling through a cave inhabited by bats, with a mist of urine in the air and a floor covered with fecal droppings. Although you may escape bat bites, any exposed open wounds or moist mucous membranes also serve as potential routes of infection.

not properly treated, ulcerations can form on the cornea and cause scarring.

Shingles can develop from exposure to a person with shingles in the infectious stage. It may also develop from exposure to chicken pox and has an incubation period of about 2 weeks. It sometimes accompanies other diseases, such as pneumonia or tuberculosis. Shingles may also result from trauma or reaction to certain drug injections.

Treatment of shingles is directed toward relieving the pain and itchiness. Dry ice pads and lotions such as calamine may provide relief. Glucocorticoids may also be prescribed to suppress the inflammatory reaction.

## Reye's Syndrome

Reye's syndrome is a potentially devastating neurological illness that sometimes develops in children after a viral infection. Viruses associated with Reye's syndrome include Epstein-Barr, influenza B, and varicella, which causes chicken pox. Use of aspirin during these infections is associated with Reye's syndrome. The actual cause of the disease is unknown.

Manifestations of Reye's syndrome include persistent vomiting, often a rash, and lethargy about 1 week after a viral infection. Neurologic dysfunction can progress from confusion to seizures to coma. The encephalopathy includes cerebral swelling with elevated intracranial pressure.

Management is geared toward lowering intracranial pressure and monitoring of vital signs, blood gases, and blood pH. The outcome is very satisfactory when diagnosed and treated early, with a recovery rate of 85% to 90%.

## Tetanus

Tetanus, commonly called "lockjaw," is characterized by rigid, contracted muscles that are unable to relax. Tetanus is caused by the tetanus toxin, which is produced by a rodlike tetanus bacillus that lives in the intestines of animals and human beings. The organisms are excreted in the fecal material and persist as spores indefinitely in the soil. The bacilli are prevalent in rural areas and in garden soil fertilizer containing manure, especially from horse farms or racetracks.

A laceration, puncture, or animal bite introduces the bacterium deep into the tissues, where it flourishes in the absence of oxygen. Thus, deep wounds with ragged, lacerated tissue contaminated with fecal material (manure or contaminated soils) are the most dangerous type.

Tetanus has an incubation period ranging from 1 week to a few weeks. The toxin travels slowly, so the distance from the wound to the spinal cord is significant. The tetanus toxin (Figure 14–5) anchors to motor nerve cells and stimulates them, which in turn stimulate muscles. Muscles become rigid, and painful spasms and convulsions develop. The jaw muscles are often the first to be affected, hence the name lockjaw. Because these muscles cannot relax, the mouth holds tightly closed. The neck is stiff, and swallowing becomes difficult. If the muscles of respiration are affected, asphyxiation occurs. Death can result from even a minor wound if the condition is not treated.

Treatment includes a thorough cleansing of the wound, removal of dead tissue and any foreign substance. Immediate immunization to inactivate the toxin before it reaches the spinal cord is crucial. The type of immunization administered depends on the patient's history. If the patient has had no previous immunization, tetanus antitoxin is given. If 5 years have elapsed since the previous tetanus injection, the person receives a booster injection of tetanus toxoid to increase the antitoxin level.

Additional treatment includes the administration of antibiotics to prevent secondary infections and the use of sedatives to decrease the frequency of convulsions. Oxygen under high pressure is also used because the bacillus is anaerobic; that is, it thrives in the absence of oxygen.

Tetanus may be prevented by adequate immunization. Tetanus toxoid, which stimulates antibody formation, should be given to infants and small children at prescribed times. This inoculation may be done in combination with diphtheria toxoid and pertussis vaccine, which prevents whooping cough.

## Abscess of the Brain

Pyogenic organisms such as streptococci, staphylococci, ameobae, and *E. coli* can travel to the brain from other infected areas and cause a brain abscess. Infections of the middle ear, skull

bones, or sinuses, as well as pneumonia and endocarditis, are potential sources for brain abscess. Figure 14–6 shows abscesses of the brain.

The symptoms of brain abscess may be misleading. Symptoms may include fever and headache, which can suggest a tumor. Analysis of cerebrospinal fluid shows increased pressure and the presence of neutrophils and lymphocytes, indicating infection.

Once the diagnosis of a brain abscess has been made, the abscess must be opened surgically and drained, and the patient must be treated with antibiotics. Brain abscesses are not as common today in the developed world because most infections are held in check by antibiotics.

## ▶ Diseases of Special Senses: Eye and Ear

Two special sensory organs assist daily life immensely by allowing one to see and to hear. Here we consider the diseases of the eye and ear. Diseases related to the nose were considered in Chapter 9.

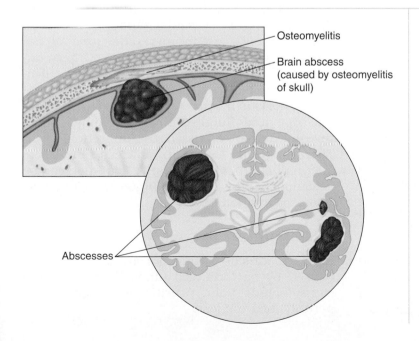

Osteomyelitis

Brain abscess
(caused by osteomyelitis
of skull)

Abscesses

**Figure 14–6**
Abscesses of the brain.

## Conjunctivitis

Conjunctivitis is an inflammation of the superficial covering of the visible sclera (white of the eye) and the inner linings of the eyelids. Red, swollen eyes with some discomfort are the usual symptoms.

Various fumes, such as from peeled onions or bathroom cleansers, may initiate the inflammatory response. However, viruses and normal bacterial flora such as *Staphylococcus aureus* also cause conjunctivitis. Bacterial infections are quite contagious, and therefore patients, usually children, are instructed to stay home from school or social occasions. Re-infections may occur due to lack of hygiene and to rubbing or touching the eye unnecessarily. Topical antibiotics control the "pink eye."

Chronic conjunctivitis, or trachoma, results when the infecting agent invades the conjunctiva. These cases are often highly contagious and when severe may disrupt the corneal surface and impair vision. The infective agent in this case is *Chlamydia trachomatis*, the same organism responsible for the STD (Chapter 12). Infected mothers pass on this infection to the newborn. When this situation develops an erythromycin ointment is usually administered.

## Glaucoma

Glaucoma is an insidious disease that typically results from a pressure building up in the anterior chamber of the eye in front of the lens.

The aqueous humor made by the ciliary body apparatus is made at a fairly constant rate and normally drains away. But, in glaucoma, fluid accumulates and increases pressure within the eye. Pressure exceeding twice the normal intraocular pressure causes the retina to start losing its ability to distinguish images clearly. This slow progression of events continues until a partial to total and rather painless blindness occurs. Peripheral vision is reduced, then lost, as "tunnel vision" continues to deteriorate the eyesight.

A glaucoma gene, GLCA1 on chromosome 1, may account for 10% of the 80,000 to 100,000 new cases per year. The incidence of glaucoma among black Americans is four times that of white Americans. This disease affects nearly 2% of the population over age 35, which is about 3 million persons in the United States.

Drugs like timolol reduce fluid production, and pilocarpine promotes aqueous humor flow. Surgery involves piercing the anterior chamber with a laser, which promotes draining and improves vision.

## Cataracts

Cataracts are clouding of the lens. The cause of cataracts is not known, but they have been attributed to a congenital defect, eye trauma, the effects of toxins, and aging. The main symptom is fading and distortion of vision. Usually in the eighth decade, cataracts become evident. With outpatient lens replacement, normal vision is restored in 95% of patients.

## Macular Degeneration

Macular degeneration is the reduction or loss of acute vision. Macular degeneration develops in 10% of the elderly, and affects both eyes, affecting only central vision and leaving peripheral vision intact. There are two forms of macular degeneration: the atrophic (dry) version, comprising 70% of the cases, and the exudative (wet, hemorrhagic) type.

Causes for this degeneration are not well understood, but it is known that obstructed blood-flow, followed by revascularization, as occurs in atherosclerosis, compromises the area of the retina responsible for acute vision. Other contributing factors are injury, inflammation, infection, and heredity.

Diagnosis is by direct eye exam with ophthalmascope and fluorescein angiography, which reveal leaking vessels in the subretinal area. There is no cure for the atrophic case, but 5% to 10% reduction in the exudative condition can be accomplished by using an argon laser to cause photocoagulation.

## External Otitis

External otitis or "swimmer's ear" is an infection caused by bacteria and fungi. Symptoms and signs include pain, pruritis, fever, and (temporarily) hearing loss.

The pathogens of external otitis are found in contaminated swimming pools or beaches. Drying the external ear opening after bathing or swimming, and cleaning earphones, earplugs, and earmuffs can prevent it. Treatment with antibiotics is effective for bacterial infections, but some fungus infections may be more stubborn to control.

Acute otitis media is a middle ear infection that affects primarily infants and children. Symptoms include pain and edema, with pus, and left unchecked may cause perforation of the tympanic membrane (ear drum). In recurrent cases, scarring of the eardrum, auditory ossicles, and inner ear components occurs. There is potential for invasion of the nearby mastoid process, a honeycombed sinus area, and this results in mastoiditis. With mastoiditis comes the possibility of brain infection and abscess formation. In undeveloped countries with inadequate access to health care and antibiotics, chronic otitis media and its complications are very common among both adults and children.

Otitis media often follows pneumonia or an upper respiratory infection (URI), such as sinusitis. Most often, bacteria are the cause. Children are more susceptible than adults to middle ear infections because their nearly horizontal auditory tubes prevent adequate drainage.

Pain can be controlled with analgesics, and swelling is reduced by use of decongestants.

## ► Degenerative Neural Diseases

Some diseases of the nervous system involve the degeneration of nerves and brain tissue. Abnormalities in muscle and sensory function often result from degeneration of nervous tissue. Note that Alzheimer's disease is discussed in Chapter 15, although it, too, can be considered a type of neurodegenerative disease.

### Multiple Sclerosis

Multiple sclerosis (MS) is a chronic, progressive, degenerative disorder of the central nervous system that usually affects young adults between the ages of 20 and 40.

At first, the disease manifests itself by muscle impairment, beginning with a loss of balance and coordination. Tingling and numbness ensue and are accompanied by a shaking tremor and muscular weakness. Clear speech becomes difficult, and urinary bladder dysfunction frequently develops.

Vision may suddenly become impaired, and double vision frequently occurs. Lesions on the optic nerve can lead to blindness. The person may have nystagmus, an involuntary, rapid movement of the eyeball. Emotional changes may also accompany the disease. Signs and symptoms of MS typically enter periods of remission and exacerbation, with greatly different rates of progression.

The disease is difficult to diagnose in the early stages, as many disorders of the nervous system have similar symptoms. Diagnosis is based on the specific tissue changes that accompany MS.

The degeneration of nervous tissue in MS involves the breaking up of the neuronal myelin sheath due to chronic inflammation. Therefore, patchy areas of demyelination appear and become sclerotic. Because the myelin sheath protects the neuron and acts as an insulator to promote the velocity of the nerve impulse transmission, the degeneration of myelin impairs nerve conduction. MRI (magnetic resonance imaging) demonstrates plaques of demyelinated nerve fibers.

The cause of MS has variously been attributed to viruses or immunologic reactions to a virus, bacteria, trauma, autoimmunity, and heredity, but the findings of this research have remained inconclusive.

To date, there is no effective specific treatment for MS. Physical therapy enables the person to use the muscles that are operable. Muscle relaxants help reduce spasticity, and steroids are often helpful. Psychological counseling is advantageous in dealing with the emotional changes brought about by the disease.

### Amyotrophic Lateral Sclerosis (ALS)

Amyotrophic lateral sclerosis, also known as Lou Gehrig's disease, is a chronic, terminal neurological disease with a progressive loss of motor neurons. ALS occurs late in life, most commonly in the 50s and 60s, and is slightly more common in men than in women.

ALS is characterized by disturbances in motility and atrophy of muscles of the hands, forearms, and legs because of degeneration of neurons in the ventral horn of the spinal cord. Also affected are certain cranial nerves, particularly the hypoglossal, trigeminal, and facial nerves, which impair muscles of the mouth and throat. Swallowing and tongue movements are affected, and speech becomes difficult or impossible.

Cause of the disease is not known. ALS is diagnosed by an electromyogram (EMG), which shows a reduction in the number of motor units active with muscle contraction. Also observed are *fasciculations*, the spontaneous, uncontrolled discharges of motor neurons seen as irregular twitchings.

ALS requires early education of the patient and the patient's family so that a proper management system may be provided to anticipate and prevent certain hazards. Specifically, the prevention of upper airway obstruction and pathologic aspiration—drawing of vomitus or mucus into the respiratory tract—is the main focus. Aspiration can occur from weakened respiratory musculature and ineffective cough. Death usually occurs within 3 to 5 years after onset of symptoms and generally results from pulmonary failure. However, as the renowned British scientist Stephen Hawking attests, survivorship of ALS does vary.

## Parkinson's Disease

Parkinson's disease (PD) is a degenerative disease that affects muscle control and coordination. PD normally strikes at midlife, about age 45. Approximately 1.5 million people are affected in the United States.

Symptoms are progressive and include tremor, rigid muscles, and loss of normal reflexes. A masklike facial expression is noticed along with faltering gait and mental depression.

In the earlier stages, physical therapy and exercise help maintain flexibility, motility, and mental well-being. Relaxation is particularly important for PD patients because stressful situations worsen the condition. Figure 14–7 summarizes possible effects of PD.

The degeneration of nerve cells occurs in the basal ganglia, the nerve tissue that normally produces a neurotransmitter, dopamine, which regulates certain involuntary muscle movements.

Treatment includes the administration of L-dopa, the form of dopamine that passes the blood–brain barrier. The drug does not stop the degeneration, but it restores dopamine levels in the brain and reduces symptom severity. In later stages, physical therapy, including heat and massage, helps reduce muscle cramps and relieve tension headaches caused by the rigidity of neck muscles. Psychological support is needed while learning to cope with the disability. In terminal stages, an increased risk for suicide has been noted.

A new method of deep brain stimulation with electrodes implanted into the thalamus is showing promise. The person may turn on/off an implanted pulse generator, a small pacemaker-like device implanted under the collarbone, by passing a magnet over it. Normally, a constant trickle of charge is sent to the thalamus in order to interrupt tremor-causing signals, similar to surgical techniques that destroy part of the thalamus to limit involuntary movements.

Another treatment suggested is a sort of "brain transplant," in which dopamine-producing neural tissue from a mouse or pig is implanted in the brain to replenish the missing dopamine.

The cause of Parkinson's disease in unknown, but environmental factors, particularly undetected viruses, are suspected.

## Essential Tremor

About 2 million people in the United States have essential tremor. This disorder is often confused with Parkinson's disease even though it usually becomes symptomatic in adolescence. Like PD, essential tremor progresses with the passage of time. Moving or shaking of the head and hands, and a halting or quivering voice are characteristic of this condition. There is a familial pattern, but the genetics are not clear. Drugs help approximately 40% of the patients, and a noticeable improvement occurs in about 60% of the patients receiving brain implant devices. Still,

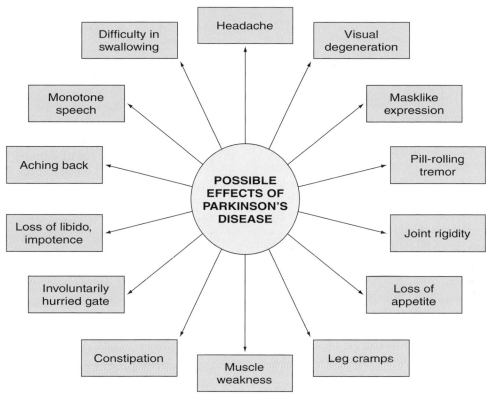

**Figure 14–7** Summary of Parkinson's disease effects.

some of those afflicted choose to leave the disease untreated until it interferes with basic routines of living.

## Huntington's Disease (Huntington's Chorea)

Huntington's chorea is a progressive degenerative disease of the brain that results in the loss of muscle control. Chorea refers to involuntary, ceaseless, rapid, jerky movements. The disease affects both the mind and body. Personality changes include carelessness, poor judgment, and impaired memory, ultimately deteriorating to total mental incompetence, dementia. The physical disabilities include speech loss and a difficulty in swallowing coupled with involuntary jerking, twisting, and muscle spasms.

Huntington's disease is an inherited disease, but symptoms may not appear until middle age. If either parent has the disease, the children have a 50% chance of inheriting it, because it is a dominant trait (see Chapter 5 for genetic

transmission). The responsible gene has been identified on chromosome 4. Some abnormality of neurotransmitters underlies the abnormal muscle activity and dementia.

There is no cure for Huntington's chorea. Carriers can be identified with gene testing.

## ▶ Convulsions

A convulsion is a sudden, intense series of involuntary muscular contraction and relaxation. Causes of convulsions include accumulation of waste products in the blood, such as occurs in uremia, toxemia of pregnancy, drug poisoning, or withdrawal from alcohol. Infectious diseases of the brain, such as meningitis and encephalitis, and high fevers, especially in young children, are frequently accompanied by convulsions.

The basis for convulsions is abnormal electrical discharges in the brain, which abnormally stimulates muscles to contract.

## Epilepsy

Epilepsy is a group of uncontrolled cerebral discharges that recurs at random intervals. The seizures associated with epilepsy are a form of convulsion. Brain impulses are temporarily disturbed, with resultant involuntary convulsive movements. Epilepsy can be acquired as a result of injury to the brain, including birth trauma, a penetrating wound, or depressed skull fracture. A tumor can irritate the brain, causing abnormal electrical discharges to be released. Alcoholism can also lead to the development of epilepsy. Most cases of epilepsy are idiopathic, but a predisposition to epilepsy may be inherited.

Epilepsy may manifest itself mildly, particularly in children. Loss of consciousness may last only a few seconds, during which time the child appears absent-minded. Some muscular twitching may be noticed around the eyes and mouth, and the child's head may sway rhythmically, but the child may not fall to the floor. This form of epilepsy is known as petit mal and usually disappears by the late teens or early 20s.

Major seizures of epilepsy involve a loss of consciousness during which the person falls to the floor. Generalized convulsions are mild to severe, with violent shaking and thrashing movements. Hyper-salivation causes a foaming at the mouth. The individual tends to lose control of the urinary bladder and sometimes bowels. These features are characteristic of grand mal epilepsy.

Individuals sometimes have a warning of an approaching seizure that gives them time to lie down or reach for support. This warning, known as an aura, may come as a ringing sound in the ears, a tingling sensation in the fingers, spots before the eyes, or various odors. The signs described are characteristic of grand mal epilepsy. After a seizure, the person is groggy and unaware of what happened. Seizures last for varying lengths of time and appear with varying frequencies.

Epileptic seizures may take different forms. The classification system adopted by the World Health Organization is called the International Classification of Epileptic Seizures. It classifies seizures into four categories:

1. Partial seizures begin locally and may or may not involve a larger area of brain tissue.
2. Generalized seizures are bilaterally symmetrical and without local onset.
3. Unilateral seizures generally involve only one side of the brain.
4. Unclassified epileptic seizures.

Diagnosis of epilepsy can be made on the results of an electroencephalogram (EEG), a recording of brain waves. X-ray films are also used to identify any brain lesions. Family histories of epilepsy are very important in diagnosing the condition. The diagnosis of epilepsy and the seizure type has become more accurate with new techniques for imaging the brain. Computerized tomography (CT), using x-rays, and MRI, using magnetic fields, visualize brain anatomy.

Medication is very effective in controlling epilepsy, particularly the anticonvulsant drugs, such as Dilantin. Alcohol must be avoided with these types of medication. Molecular neurobiology research is providing new information on how nerve cells control electrical activity, thus making development of more effective anti-epileptic drugs possible. It is now known which drugs are best for treating the various kinds of seizures. Assistance or treatment during a seizure is directed toward preventing self-injury to the individual. Finally, epilepsy does not appear to interfere with mental prowess or creative talents for those afflicted.

## ▶ Developmental Errors

### Spina Bifida

Spina bifida is a condition in which one or more vertebrae fail to fuse, leaving an opening in the vertebral canal. The consequences of spina bifida depend on the extent of the opening and the involvement of the spinal cord. One form of spina bifida, spina bifida occulta (hidden), may not be apparent at birth. Most lesions are located in the lower part of the vertebral column. The opening can be seen on x-ray films. Other malformations, such as hydrocephalus, cleft palate, cleft lip, club-foot, and strabismus (crossed eyes), that tend to accompany this developmental error may point to this disorder. Muscular abnormalities, such as incorrect posture, inability to walk, or lack of bladder and bowel control, appear later. A slight dimpling of the skin and tuft of hair over the vertebral defect indicates the site of the lesion.

One form of spina bifida noticeable at birth is a meningocele. In this condition, meninges protrude through the opening in the vertebra as a sac filled with cerebrospinal fluid. The spinal cord is not involved in this defect.

Meningomyelocele is a serious anomaly in which the nerve elements protrude into the sac and are trapped, thus preventing proper placement and development. The child with this defect may be mentally retarded, fail to develop, lack sensation, or be paralyzed. The consequences of the defect depend on the part of the spinal cord affected. Surgical corrections of various forms of spina bifida have been very effective. Some procedures are intrauterine, to repair the defect of the fetus, and these new operations look promising.

The most severe form of spina bifida is myelocele, in which the neural tube itself fails to close and the nerve tissue is totally disorganized. This condition is usually fatal. The various forms of spina bifida are shown in Figure 14–8.

## Hydrocephalus

Hydrocephalus is a condition of excess CSF on the brain. The formation, circulation, and absorption of CSF were described earlier in this chapter. In hydrocephalus, this fluid accumulates abnormally, causing the ventricles to enlarge and push the brain against the skull.

An obstruction in the normal flow of CSF is the usual cause of hydrocephalus. A congenital defect like stenosis of an opening from the ventricles or an acquired lesion can block the CSF flow. Meningitis, a tumor, or birth trauma may result in acquired hydrocephalus. The error may also be a failure to absorb the fluid into the circulatory system.

There are two types of hydrocephalus: *communicating* and *noncommunicating*. In the communicating type, the increased CSF enters the subarachnoid space. In the noncommunicating hydrocephalus, the increased pressure of the CSF is confined within the ventricles and is not evident in a lumbar puncture.

The head of a child born with hydrocephalus may appear normal at birth, but it will enlarge rapidly in the early months of life as the fluid

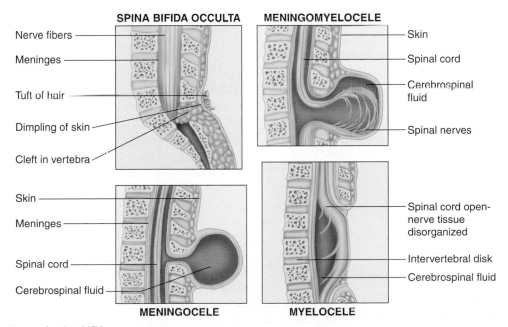

**Figure 14–8**  Forms of spina bifida.

accumulates. The brain is compressed, the cranial bones are thin, and the sutures of the skull separate under the pressure. The appearance of a hydrocephalic infant is typical: The forehead is prominent and the eyes bulge, giving a frightened expression. The scalp is stretched, and the veins of the head are prominent. The weight of the excessive fluid in the head makes it impossible for the baby to lift its head. The infant fails to grow normally and is mentally retarded.

There have been cases of self-arrested hydrocephalus in which expansion of the head stops. A balance is reached between production and absorption of the fluid. The cranial sutures fill in and the skull bones thicken. The extent of brain damage before the arrest determines the degree of retardation.

Success in relieving the excessive CSF has been achieved by placing a shunt between the blocked cranial ventricle and the veins (Figure 14–9), to the heart, or peritoneal cavity. This connection allows the fluid to enter the general circulation.

## ▶ Brain Injury

### Cerebral Palsy

Cerebral palsy is a motor function disease of the brain manifested by motor impairment and perhaps varying degrees of mental retardation that become apparent before age 3. The brain damage may be due to injury at or near the time of birth, a maternal infection such as rubella (German measles), or infection of the brain even after birth. Lack of oxygen or incompatible blood cause brain injury. An Rh⁻ mother may produce antibodies against the blood of an Rh⁺ fetus. The

result is excessive destruction of fetal blood cells that causes hyperbilirubinemia, which is toxic to the brain. Often, cerebral palsy is idiopathic.

There are three forms of cerebral palsy: spastic, athetoid, and atactic. The largest percentage of cerebral palsy victims have the spastic type of condition; muscles are tense, and reflexes are exaggerated. In the athetoid form, there are constant, purposeless movements that are uncontrollable. A continuous tremor or shaking of the hands and feet is present. Cerebral palsy sufferers with the atactic form have poor balance and are prone to fall. Poor muscular coordination and a staggering gait is characteristic of this disease.

Depending on the area of the brain affected, there may be seizures along with visual or auditory impairment. If the muscles controlling the tongue are affected, speech defects result. Intelligence may be normal, but often there is mental retardation. Treatment depends on the nature of the brain injury. Muscle relaxants can relieve spasms; anticonvulsant drugs reduce seizures; casts or braces may aid walking; and traction or surgery is helpful in some cases. Muscle training is the most important therapy, and the earlier it is started, the more effective it is.

## ▶ Stroke or Cerebrovascular Accident (CVA)

The main cause of cerebral hemorrhage is hypertension. Prolonged hypertension tends to result from atherosclerosis, which leads to arteriosclerosis, explained in Chapter 7. The combination of high blood pressure and hard, brittle blood vessels is a predisposing condition for cerebral hemorrhage. Aneurysms, weakened areas in vascular

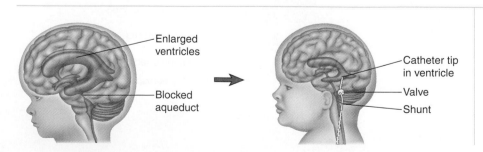

**Figure 14–9**
Hydrocephalus.

Enlarged ventricles

Blocked aqueduct

Catheter tip in ventricle

Valve

Shunt

walls, are also susceptible to rupture (Figure 14–10). Surrounding the pituitary gland is the circle of Willis, a major crossroads of cerebral vascularity, vulnerable to weakness. As the collection of blood within the cranial cavity mounts, the intracranial pressure dangerously increases. When this pressure increase is controlled or alleviated early, countless victims are spared brain damage and death. The pressure relief may come in the form of medication or emergency surgical procedure. Any subsequent hemorrhage into the brain tissue damages the neurons, causing a sudden loss of consciousness. Death can follow, or, if the bleeding stops, varying degrees of brain damage can result. When detected, swift surgical repairs of aneurysms save lives.

## Thrombosis and Embolism

Blood clots that block the cerebral arteries cause infarction of brain tissue. Thromboses develop on walls of atherosclerotic vessels, particularly in the carotid arteries. The clots take time to form, and some warning may precede the occlusion of the vessel. The person may experience blindness in one eye, difficulty in speaking, or a generalized state of confusion. When the cerebral blood vessel is completely blocked, the individual may lose consciousness.

Because an embolism is a traveling clot, it may suddenly occlude a blood vessel and cause ischemia. The embolism is most frequently a clot from the heart, aorta, or carotid artery, but it can travel from another part of the body. Consciousness is generally lost suddenly.

Tissue plasminogen activator (TPA), called a "clot buster," may be used to dissolve clots and restore blood flow. However, if TPA is given in hemorrhagic cases of cerebrovascular accidents (CVAs), intracranial bleeding may continue, and the individual could die. Crucial decisions must be made in acute cases, and because most cerebrovascular accidents are of the ischemic form, TPA is a ready agent for the physician.

The site and extent of the brain damage, regardless of its cause, determines the outcome for the patient. Consciousness is usually regained, but immediately after the stroke, speech is often impaired. Loss of speech, aphasia, requires therapy, but the ability to speak is often restored.

Damage to the motor nerves at the point passing down the spinal cord causes weakness, paresis, or paralysis on the side of the body opposite the brain lesion due to the crossover of nerve fibers in the brain stem. Paralysis on one side of the body is referred to as hemiplegia.

Various procedures make it possible to determine the site of blockage in a cerebral blood vessel. Angiography, a process in which radiopaque material is injected into cerebral arteries, allows x-rays to locate the lesion.

A blockage in a carotid artery can be treated surgically. Endarterectomy, the more common procedure, removes the thickened area of the inner vascular lining. Carotid bypass surgery

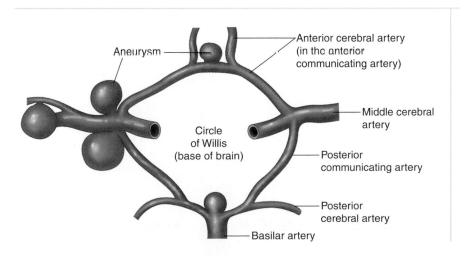

Figure 14–10
Aneurysms.

Aneurysm

Anterior cerebral artery (in the anterior communicating artery)

Circle of Willis (base of brain)

Middle cerebral artery

Posterior communicating artery

Posterior cerebral artery

Basilar artery

removes the blocked vascular segment, and a graft is inserted to allow bloodflow to the brain.

## Transient Ischemic Attack (TIA)

Transient ischemic attacks are caused by brief but critical periods of reduced bloodflow in a cerebral artery. The reduced flow may be due to an atherosclerotic narrowing of the blood vessel or to small emboli that temporarily lodge in the vessel. The attacks may last for a minute or two or up to several hours, with the average attack lasting 15 minutes. Manifestation is often abrupt and can include visual disturbances, transient hemiparesis (muscular weakness on one side), or sensory loss on one side. Lips and tongue may become numb, causing slurred speech. TIAs often precede a complete stroke and often serve as warning of a cerebral vascular disturbance. Further diagnostic testing such as a cerebral angiogram or CT scan may be indicated.

## ▶ Traumatic Disorders

### Concussion of the Brain

A concussion is a transient disorder of the nervous system resulting from a violent blow on the head, or a fall. The person typically loses consciousness and cannot remember the events of the accident. Although the brain may not actually be damaged, the whole body is affected; the pulse rate is weak, and when consciousness is regained, the person may experience nausea and dizziness. A severe headache may follow, and the person should be watched closely, since a coma may ensue.

A person suffering from a concussion should be kept quiet, and drugs that stimulate or depress the nervous system, such as painkillers, are contraindicated. The condition usually corrects itself with rest.

### Contusion

In a contusion, there is an injury, a bruise, to brain tissue without a breaking of the skin at the site of the trauma. The brain injury may be on the side of the impact or on the opposite side, where the brain is forced against the skull. Blood from broken blood vessels may accumulate in the brain, causing swelling and pain. The blood clots and necrotic tissue form and block the flow of CFS, causing a form of hydrocephalus.

### Skull Fractures

The most serious complication of a skull fracture is damage to the brain. A fracture at the base of the skull is likely to affect vital centers in the brain stem. The pressure that increases due to accumulation of CSF must be reduced by medications. Another danger of skull fractures is that bacteria may be able to access the brain.

### Hemorrhages

Hemorrhages can occur in the meninges, causing blood to accumulate between the brain and the skull. A severe injury to the temple can cause an artery just inside the skull to rupture. The blood then flows between the dura mater and the skull: This is called an extradural or epidural hemorrhage (Figure 14–11). The increased pressure of the blood causes the patient to lose consciousness. Surgery is required immediately to tie off the bleeding vessel and remove the blood. No blood is found in a lumbar puncture because the blood accumulation is outside the dura mater.

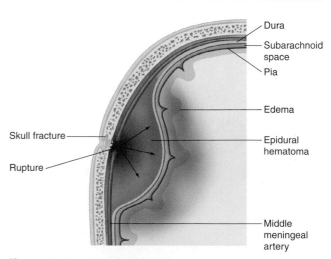

**Figure 14–11** Extradural hematoma.

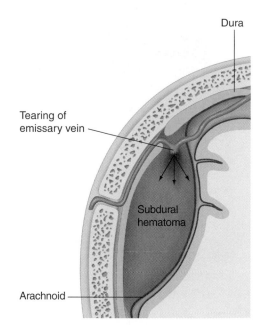

**Figure 14–12**  Subdural hematoma.

A hemorrhage under the dura mater, a subdural hemorrhage (Figure 14–12), is from the large venous sinuses of the brain rather than an artery. This may occur from a severe blow to the front or back of the head. The blood clots, and CSF accumulates into a cystlike formation. Intracranial pressure increases, but the cerebral symptoms may not develop for a time. Subdural hemorrhages are sometimes chronic in alcoholics and abused children.

The surface membrane of the brain may be torn by a skull fracture, causing a subarachnoid hemorrhage. Blood flows into the subarachnoid space where CSF circulates. Blood is found in the CSF with a lumbar puncture. Rupture of an aneurysm can also cause a subarachnoid hemorrhage.

## ▶ Brain Tumors

Tumors of the brain may be malignant or benign. Because benign tumors may grow and compress vital nerve centers, they are consid-

ered serious growths. Benign tumors are usually encapsulated, and they can be completely removed surgically. Malignant tumors have extensive roots and are extremely difficult or impossible to remove in their entirety. Most malignant tumors of the brain are metastatic from other organs. Primary malignant tumors of the brain are called gliomas, tumors of the glial cells that support nerve tissue rather than of the neurons themselves.

Brain tumors manifest themselves in different ways depending on the site and growth rate of the tumor. Astrocytomas are basically benign, slow-growing tumors. Glioblastomas are highly malignant, rapid-growing tumors. Brain function is affected by the increased intracranial pressure. Blood supply to an area of the brain may be reduced by an infiltrating tumor or by edema, causing the tissue to become necrotic.

Symptoms of brain tumors may include a severe headache because of the increased pressure of the tumor. Personality changes, loss of memory, or development of poor judgment may signal a brain tumor. Visual disturbances, double vision, or partial blindness often occur, and the ability to speak may be impaired. The person may be unsteady while standing and develop seizures. A drowsy condition can progress to a coma.

## ▶ Cranial Nerve Disease

### Trigeminal Neuralgia

Individual cranial nerves may be affected by degeneration or unknown causes and thus involved with various ailments. The fifth (V) cranial nerve, or trigeminal nerve, may become inflamed, causing severe intermittent pain usually on one side of the face. This condition, known as trigeminal neuralgia or *tic doulourex*, affects one individual per 25,000 (Figure 14–13). Victims, usually age 40 or older, complain of severe pain, especially around the oral cavity, the tongue, lips, and gums. This recurring pain may or may not respond readily to pain medication. Sometimes drugs or agents

**Sensory distribution**

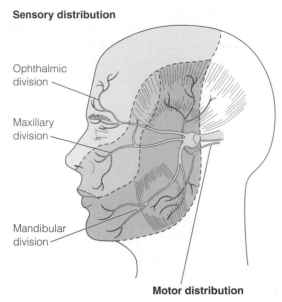

Ophthalmic
division

Maxillary
division

Mandibular
division

**Motor distribution**

**Figure 14–13** Sensory and motor distribution of the trigeminal nerve. There are three sensory divisions: opthalmic, maxillary, and mandibular.

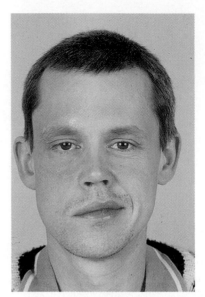

**Figure 14–14** Bell's palsy, showing typical drooping of one side of the face.

like alcohol or phenol are injected directly into the nerve as it exits the skull to reduce the pain, or surgery may be required to cut sensory elements to give relief.

## Bell's Palsy

Bell's palsy involves the inflammation of the seventh (VII) cranial nerve, or facial nerve. The cause is usually unknown, but viruses, autoimmunity, and vascular ischemia are probable culprits. This nerve may also be traumatized, compressed, or invaded by pathogens. Because the seventh cranial nerve innervates facial muscles and salivary glands, the attacks cause sagging of the facial muscles on one side of the face and a watery eye, and the person may drool and have slurred speech (Figure 14–14). In these cases, massage or heat treatment may help. Time seems to work best, and recovery may take weeks. Some corticoid medications or antiviral agents assist as well. Therefore, relief of symptoms may not always be quick or simple. Bell's palsy is rare in children; it usually strikes between ages 25 and 50 years of age. If the situa-

tion fails to be resolved, a facial contracture develops; however, the prognosis is generally good.

## ▶ Age-Related Diseases

Neurological disease affects individuals at all stages of life. Glaucoma and cataracts are age-related visual problems, as is presbyopia, a lens condition that occurs usually in the mid-40s. In presbyopia, the lens becomes less resilient and remains relatively flat, leaving distance vision intact but impairing near vision. Corrective lenses are very common after age 43 to 45. Alzheimer's disease (Chapter 15) is a prominent concern for seniors. The incidence of dementia and of Parkinson's disease rises with age.

Finally, with age, the 3-pound brain reduces in weight and size with loss of neurons and synapses. Thus, it is understandable that functional losses in hearing, sight, and coordination would be experienced in the elderly. Reaction times are reduced, and so is agility, increasing risks for falls and injury.

## ▶ Diagnostic Procedures for the Nervous System

Neurologic laboratory tests include CSF examination obtained by a lumbar (puncture) spinal tap as previously described. Angiography allows visualization of the cerebral circulation through the injection of radiopaque material. Computed tomographic (CT) scans are particularly valuable for diagnosing pathologic conditions such as tumors, hemorrhages, hematomas, and hydrocephalus. Electromyelography (EMG) is a radiographic process by which the spinal cord and spinal subarachnoid space are viewed and photographed after injection of contrast medium into the lumbar subarachnoid space. Myelography is used to identify spinal lesions caused by trauma or disease, such as amyotrophic lateral sclerosis (ALS). Electroencephalography (EEG) records the electrical activity of the brain (brain waves). It is used to diagnose lesions or tumors, and seizures, in impaired consciousness. Magnetic resonance imaging (MRI) uses magnetic fields in conjunction with a computer to view and record tissue characteristics at different planes. MRI is excellent for visualizing brain soft tissue, spinal cord, white matter diseases, tumors, and hemorrhages. Some diagnoses depend on the relief of symptoms as may be found in Parkinson's disease.

## CHAPTER SUMMARY

The nervous system enables the human body to respond to changes in the external and internal environment, and is affected by many diseases in various ways, including aging. Microorganisms that enter the nervous system by various routes cause infectious diseases, such as meningitis, encephalitis, polio, tetanus, rabies, Reye's syndrome, and shingles. Infections enter the eye and ear, causing acute and sometimes permanent damage.

A degeneration of nerves and brain tissue results in multiple sclerosis, amyotrophic lateral sclerosis, Parkinson's disease, and Huntington's chorea. A manifestation of these progressively degenerative diseases is a correspondingly abnormal functioning of the muscles.

Convulsions often result from some chemical imbalance that causes irritation to nerve cells. The seizures of epilepsy are a form of convulsions resulting from abnormal electrical discharges in the brain.

Hydrocephalus and the various forms of spina bifida are caused by developmental errors, obstruction to the flow of cerebrospinal fluid, and failure of the vertebral column to close. Damage to the brain during fetal life or at birth can result in cerebral palsy, which is manifested by various forms of muscular abnormalities. Cerebrovascular accidents (CVA), cerebral hemorrhages, and blood clots damage brain tissue. The results of the damage depend on the site and extent of the brain lesion.

A severe head injury that causes hemorrhaging within the brain or in the meninges has serious effects on the nerve tissue and may even be fatal. Tumors of the brain, both malignant and benign, strangle nerve fibers and obstruct bloodflow.

## RESOURCES

Beers, M. H. and Berkow, R. *The Merck Manual,* 17th ed. John Wiley & Sons, 1999.

Martini, F.H., Timmons, M.J., Tallitsch R.B. *Human Anatomy,* 5th ed. Prentice Hall, 2003.

Kemper, D.W., Wiss, C.A. (Ed.). *Healthwise Handbook.* Healthwise Publishers, 1999.

Tamparo, C. & Lewis, M.A. *Diseases of the Human Body,* 3rd ed. F. A. Davis, 2001.

# DISEASES AT A GLANCE

## Nervous System

| DISEASE | ETIOLOGY | SIGNS AND SYMPTOMS |
|---|---|---|
| Glioma, glioblastoma | Idiopathic | Severe headache, personality changes, loss of speech, unsteady movement, seizures, coma |
| Meningitis | Bacterial, viral | High fever, chills, severe headache, stiff neck, nausea, vomiting, rash, delirium, convulsions, coma |
| Encephalitis | Viral | Mild to severe headache, fever, cerebral dysfunction, disordered thought, seizures, persistent drowsiness, delirium, coma |
| Poliomyelitis | Viral | Stiff neck, fever, headache, sore throat, GI disturbances, paralysis may develop |
| Tetanus | Clostridium tetani | Rigidity of muscles, painful spasms and convulsions, stiff neck, difficulty swallowing, clenched jaws |
| Rabies | Viral | Fever, pain, mental derangement, rage, convulsions, paralysis, profuse sticky saliva, throat muscle spasm produces hydrophobia |
| Shingles | Varicella, herpes zoster | Painful rash of small water blisters with red rim, lesions follow a sensory nerve, confined to one side of body, severe itching, scarring |
| Reye's syndrome | Idiopathic or viral; Epstein-Barr, influenza B, varicella | Persistent vomiting, rash, lethargy about 1 week after a viral infection, may progress to coma; linked with use of aspirin |
| Abscess | Pyogenic bacteria | Fever, headache |
| Multiple sclerosis (MS) | Idiopathic, suspect viral or autoimmune | Muscle impairment, double vision, nystagmus, loss of balance, poor coordination, tingling and numbing sensation, shaking tremor, muscular weakness, emotional changes, remission and exacerbation |

| DIAGNOSIS | TREATMENT |
|---|---|
| CT scan, MRI | Surgery, chemotherapy, radiation |
| Lumbar puncture (spinal tap) | Antibiotics if bacterial infection |
| Lumbar puncture (spinal tap) | Control fever, control fluid and electrolyte balance, monitor respiratory and kidney function |
| Physical exam | Supportive; preventive vaccination |
| Physical exam, patient history | Antitoxin, symptom relief, preventive vaccination |
| Physical exam, history of animal bite | Vaccination before disease develops; fatal once CNS involved |
| Physical exam | Alleviation of symptoms and pain relief, steroids |
| Patient history, liver enlargement, hypoglycemia, ammonia in blood | Supportive; close monitoring necessary |
| Lumbar puncture (spinal tap) | Surgical draining of abscess, antibiotics |
| Physical exam, patient history, MRI | None effective; physical therapy and muscle relaxants, steroids, counseling |

# DISEASES AT A GLANCE *(continued)*

## Nervous System

| DISEASE | ETIOLOGY | SIGNS AND SYMPTOMS |
|---|---|---|
| Amyotrophic lateral sclerosis (ALS), or Lou Gehrig's disease | Idiopathic | Disturbed motility; fasciculations; atrophy of muscles in hands, forearms, and legs; impaired speech and swallowing; death from pulmonary failure in 3 to 4 years |
| Huntington's disease (Huntington's chorea) | Genetic | Involuntary, rapid, jerky movements; speech loss; difficulty swallowing; personality changes; carelessness; poor judgment; impaired memory; mental incompetence |
| Convulsion: epilepsy | Trauma, chemical, idiopathic | Involuntary contractions or series of contractions; a seizure is a sign of illness, not a disease. Petit mal: brief loss of consciousness, "absence seizure" Grand mal: often preceded by aura (various sensations), total loss of consciousness, generalized convulsions, hypersalivation; incontinence may occur |
| Spina bifida | Congential, lack folate | Opening in vertebral canal spina bifida occulta: hidden Meningocele: meninges protrude Meningomyelocele: nerve elements protrude Myelocele: nerve tissue disorganized |
| Hydrocephalus | Congenital, idiopathic | Enlarged head develops |
| Cerebral palsy | Birth trauma, rubella infection | Seizures, visual or auditory impairment, speech defects Spastic: muscles tense, reflexes exaggerated Athetoid: uncontrollable, persistent movements, tremor Atactic: poor balance, poor muscular coordination, staggering gait |
| Transient ischemic attacks (TIA), "mini strokes" | Ischemia, aneurysm, hypertension | Visual disturbances, transient muscle weakness on one side, sensory loss on one side, slurred speech; attacks last minutes to hours, average 15 minutes |
| Cerebrovascular accident (CVA) stroke, brain attack | Trauma | Severe, sudden headache; muscular weakness or paralysis; disturbance of speech; loss of consciousness |

| DIAGNOSIS | TREATMENT |
|---|---|
| Electromyelography (EMG) | Supportive |
| Patient history (inherited disease) and physical exam | No cure; genetic counseling for family |
| Observation of seizure, electroencephalogram (EEG), x-ray, family history, CT scan, MRI | Removal of cause once detected; anticonvulsive drugs |
| Physical exam, CT scan, MRI, EEG | Surgical, physical therapy |
| Physical exam, CT scan, MRI, spinal tap | Implant shunt to drain CSF |
| Physical exam | Muscle relaxants, anticonvulsive drugs, casts, braces, traction, surgery, physical therapy |
| Cerebral angiogram, CT scan | Depends on cause; surgical treatment of blocked vessels |
| Angiography, CT scan, MRI | Clot-dissolving drugs, surgery, endarterectomy |

# Interactive Activities

## Cases for Critical Thinking

1. J.A. has had a severe headache for the last 12 hours, a fever of 102, plus a stiff neck. Following a lumbar puncture, *Streptococcus pneumoniae* was found in culture along with low sugar levels and higher protein values. What disease best explains these findings? What is the prognosis and treatment?

2. At age 78, K.B. started rubbing her eyes and constantly cleaning her (old) glasses for a better view. The right eye particularly was not very good, and she hoped the problem, which she first noticed months ago, would finally go away. The vision in the right eye was foggy, dim, and not focused. There was essentially no pain. What do the symptoms suggest? What are the prognosis and treatments for this elderly woman?

3. T.C. complained of an earache, and after a recent bout with a bad cold, he was rather irritable. The ear was "beet red" and felt warm. He could hardly hear on that side, but he knew there was nothing intentionally or accidentally poked into the ear. What disease best explains these symptoms? Give some recommendations on treatment.

## Multiple Choice

1. Rabies is caused by a _____.
   a. bacterium
   b. virus
   c. fungus
   d. tick

2. Epilepsy can be caused by _____.
   a. a birth trauma
   b. injury to the brain
   c. a penetrating wound
   d. all of these

3. The brain stem controls _____.
   a. sensory function
   b. muscle action
   c. memory
   d. heart rate and breathing

4. An acute inflammation of the first two meninges of the brain and spinal cord, the pia mater and the arachnoid, is known as _____.
   a. thrombophlebitis
   b. meningitis
   c. prostatitis
   d. encephalitis

5. Which of the following is true of polio?
   a. is caused by a virus
   b. affects sensory neurons
   c. is found in most people by age 80
   d. was wiped out in 1976

6. Which of the following applies to MS?
   a. only in males
   b. primarily in east European cultures
   c. damaged myelin sheath
   d. strikes adults age 20 or beyond

7. Within 3 to 4 hours, what clot-buster may be used to treat the most common form of CVA?
   a. aspirin
   b. TPA
   c. ATP
   d. hemolase

8. Petit mal is a mild form of _____.
   a. polio
   b. MS
   c. epilepsy
   d. encephalitis

9. What is the lesion in Parkinson's disease?
   a. no dopamine
   b. no myelin
   c. autoimmunity
   d. cerebral blood clot

10. Pauly, a first grader, woke one fall morning to discover a blood-shot right eye and a yellowish mass near the medial corner of his eye. What is the problem?
    a. common cold
    b. trachoma
    c. conjunctivitis
    d. osteitis

## True or False

_____ 1. Rabies is a viral infection.

_____ 2. The Sabin vaccine works in the digestive tract.

_____ 3. Oxygen under high pressure is effective in treating rabies.

_____ 4. Blood is not normally found in cerebrospinal fluid.

_____ 5. Dopamine deficiency causes epilepsy.

_____ 6. Transient ischemic attacks are characterized by loss of consciousness.

_____ 7. An aura is a flashback of previous contusion events.

_____ 8. Viral meningitis requires quarantine isolation procedures.

_____ 9. Excess Dilantin may cause Parkinson's disease.

_____ 10. Conjunctivitis is usually a viral attack in adults.

## Fill-Ins

1. _____, commonly called lockjaw, is an infection of nerve tissue caused by the tetanus bacillus that lives in the intestines of animals and human beings.

2. Amyotrophic lateral sclerosis is diagnosed by _____.

3. _____ _____ is a chronic, progressive disease of the central nervous system with myelin destruction.

4. _____ _____, also known as shaking palsy, is a disease of brain degeneration that appears gradually and progresses slowly.

5. The common drug given to victims of Parkinson's disease is _____.

6. _____ headaches are severe, unilateral, involve the periorbital and orbital area, and typically occur in men.

7. Tic douloureau, or _____ _____, causes severe pain elicited from cranial nerve V.

8. _____ _____ is a unilateral dysfunction of muscles in the face that leaves the person with slurred speech and a watery eye.

9. _____ is called Lou Gerhig's disease.

10. _____ is the worst form of spina bifida.

# MedMedia
# Wrap-Up

**www.prenhall.com/mulvihill**

Remember to visit this website for extra study practice, including exercises, Internet links, news updates, and an audio glossary.

**Activity CD-ROM**

Check out the CD-ROM in the back of this book. You will find games, exercises, puzzles, and videos to help enhance your understanding of this chapter.

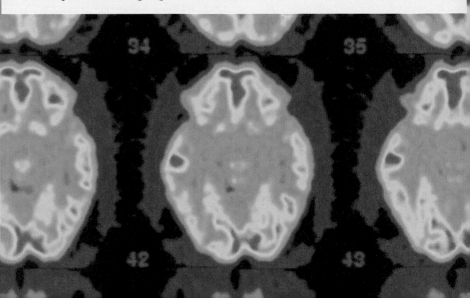

# Mental Illness

**CHAPTER**

# 15

## Learning Objectives

After studying this chapter, you should be able to

- Describe the warning signs of mental illness
- Identify signs, symptoms, etiology, and treatment of the following:

    Developmental disorders

    Disruptive behavior disorders

    Mood disorders

    Substance use disorder

    Schizophrenia

    Anxiety disorders

    Eating disorders

    Personality disorders

- Recognize environmental, genetic, and biological factors associated with mental illness
- Describe diagnostic approaches for mental illness
- Identify the warning signs of suicide

## Fact or Fiction?

Mental illness is a weakness of character.

*Fiction:* Mental illness has physical and/or biological causes, just as do the diseases of the other systems discussed in this text. For every 100 people born, one ends up with schizophrenia, one develops bipolar disorder, and 20 experience some form of depression. Heredity may account for as much as 80% of the risk for these illnesses.

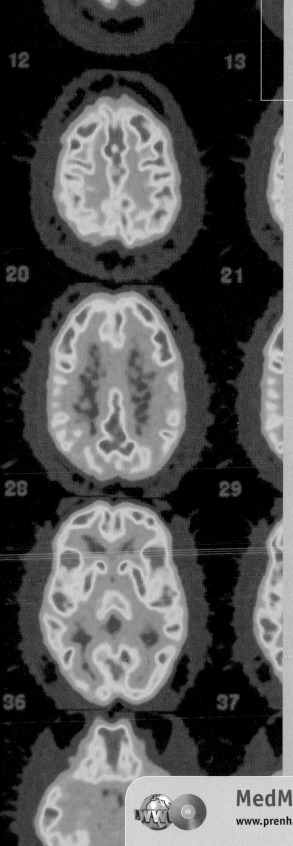

# Disease Chronicle

## Sybil

Sybil Dorsett was a woman with sixteen different personalities. Her behavior shifted from one personality to another without any prior recollection of the previous personality. For instance, one personality named Victoria Antoinette Scharleau was a self-assured, sophisticated, attractive blond, while another was a male carpenter named Mike Dorsett. Unable to cope with childhood torture and sexual abuse, Sybil had a complete break of consciousness. Through years of empathy and psychotherapy, Sybil was able to confront the memories and integrate her separate personalities into one. Sybil was fortunate to receive empathetic treatment. Prior to the 20th century, mental illnesses were primarily attributed to human fault and hostility, magic, or divine forces. The mentally ill were treated by confinement in prisons and asylums. Reforms in the treatment of the mentally ill started after the French Revolution with Franz Mesmer, an Austrian physician, who established rapport with patients. Emil Kraepelin began the modern classification of psychiatry in the 19th century. Modern psychiatry, founded in the 20th century by Sigmund Freud, is credited with a comprehensive approach to understanding psychic development, emotion, behavior, and psychiatric illness. Several schools of psychology, medical treatments, and scientific advancements continue to evolve, guiding further understanding into the biological, chemical, environmental, social, and behavioral mechanisms of mental illness.

# ▶ Mental Illness

Mental Illness refers to a group of psychiatric disorders characterized by severe disturbances in thought, mood, and behavior. Psychiatry is the medical specialty that diagnoses and prescribes medical treatment for mental illness, whereas psychology is the discipline that studies normal and abnormal behavior, and applies counseling methods to treat mental illness.

Mental illness affects one of every four Americans and is associated with social stigma, disability, and death. Many people suffering from mental illness may not look as though they are ill, while others may appear detached and withdrawn from society. Warning signs of mental illness are listed in Table 15–1.

Over 200 psychiatric diagnoses for adults and children are categorized in the Diagnostic and Statistical Manual of Mental Disorders, or DSM. The DSM-IV is the most recent edition, and is used internationally to classify, assess, and guide treatment for mental illness. Because it is difficult to provide a single definition that accounts for all mental illness, disorders are categorized in the DSM-IV according to groups of symptoms or diagnostic criteria. Psychiatric diagnoses are assigned five axes that address developmental, medical, psychosocial, and overall adaptive issues that contribute to the primary psychiatric diagnosis (Table 15–2). All DSM-IV diagnoses require evidence that the symptoms impair academic achievement, occupational performance, and social relationships.

# ▶ Causes of Mental Illness

## Biological Basis for Mental Illness

Current biological theories of mental illness describe anatomical differences, genes, and chemical messengers or neurotransmitters that are implicated in mental illness. Anatomical differences such as brain size and altered neural connections develop from physical insults to the brain, degenerative processes, and genes. Genes within the brain's DNA are inherited from both parents and contain all the necessary information to build the structures that mediate the specialized function of neurotransmitters.

| Table 15–1 Warning Signs of Mental Illness |
|---|
| • Aggression |
| • Changes in eating or sleeping habits |
| • Confusion |
| • Decline in school or work performance |
| • Depression |
| • Euphoria alternating with depression |
| • Excessive fear |
| • Frequent complaints of physical illnesses |
| • Hearing voices |
| • Substance abuse |
| • Thoughts of suicide |
| • Withdrawal from family and friends |

| Table 15–2 Five Axes of Psychiatric Diagnoses |
|---|
| **Axis I:** Primary diagnosis (clinical disorders and other conditions that may be a focus of clinical attention) |
| **Axis II:** Primary diagnosis (personality disorders, mental retardation, learning disabilities) |
| **Axis III:** General medical conditions |
| **Axis IV:** Psychosocial and environmental problems |
| **Axis V:** Global assessment of functioning |
| Primary Psychiatric Diagnosis is indicated on Axis I or II. |

Neurotransmitters are produced, stored, and released from neurons, or nerves cells, within the central and peripheral nervous system. Voluntary and involuntary physical and psychological processes, such as heart rate and blood pressure, behavior, emotions, mood, sleep, and sex drive, are regulated by intricate neurotransmitter activity. Inadequate regulation of neurotransmitters as well as excess neurotransmitter activity in distinct areas of the brain are associated with mental illness. The regulatory action of neurotransmitters and their associated mental illnesses are listed in Table 15–3.

## Environment and Mental Illness

Environmental causes of mental illness shaped the fundamental basis for the diagnosis and treatment of mental illness for many years. Family interactions, age, gender, race, culture, and socioeconomic status alter biological and psychological vulnerability for mental illness

and define learned behaviors, attitudes, and perception of health and illness.

Persons of different age groups and gender are at risk for different mental health problems and illnesses. Mood disorders such as depression, anxiety disorders, and eating disorders occur more frequently in women, whereas disorders with externalizing behaviors such as antisocial personality disorder and associated substance abuse are more common in males. Attention deficit hyperactivity disorder (ADHD) is a development behavioral disorder that appears more commonly in males prior to the age of 7 years. Disorders involving memory and irritability, such as Alzheimer's disease and Huntington's chorea, are more evident with an aging population.

Access to medical care and acceptance of psychiatric illness is influenced by race, cultural beliefs, and socioeconomic status. Mental illness affects all cultures, races, and socioeconomic classes. The highest rates of mental illness are found among the lowest social classes where adverse living circumstances increase

**Table 15–3   Neurotransmitters, Regulatory Actions, and Psychiatric Disorders Associated with Changes in Neurotransmitter**

| Neurotransmitter | Regulatory Action | Mental Illness |
|---|---|---|
| Dopamine | Mood, behavior, thought process, muscle movement, physical activity, heart rate, blood pressure, feeding, appetite, satiety | Schizophrenia, depression, ADHD, bipolar disorder, eating disorder, autism, Tourette's syndrome |
| Norephinephrine | Mood, anxiety, vigilance, arousal, heart rate, blood pressure | Depression, anxiety disorders, ADHD, bipolar disorder |
| Serotonin | Perception of pain, feeding, sleep–awake cycle, motor activity, sexual behavior, temperature regulation | Depression, aggression, suicidality, bipolar disorder, eating disorders |
| Acetylcholine | Learning, memory, muscle tone | Alzheimer's disease, Parkinson's disease, Huntington's chorea, Tourette's syndrome |
| Gamma aminobutyric acid (GABA) | Interacts with a wide range of neurotransmitters to enhance inhibition | Anxiety disorders, alcoholism, Tourettes syndrome, sleep disorders |

social stress and contribute to poor mental hygiene.

## Mental Illness in Children and Adolescents

Mental illness in childhood can have far-reaching academic, social, developmental, and physical consequences. Common complications of childhood-onset mental illness include learning delays with school failure, low self-esteem, impaired relationships with family and friends, and social rejection and withdrawal.

Though many psychiatric disorders begin in childhood, many are not diagnosed until adulthood. In the United States, about 1 in 10 children and adolescents have a mental disorder. However, only about 20% of these children receive needed treatment.

Some disorders have slightly adapted criteria for children. Unlike adults, children often do not verbalize their feelings and as such present with behavioral problems such as boredom, irritability, and conduct problems. The outcome of childhood mental illness depends on the ability of the family to cope and seek treatment, the severity of the illness, and the ability of the child to compensate for and adapt to mental health deficits.

## ▶ Disorders Usually First Diagnosed in Infancy, Childhood, or Adolescents

### Disruptive Behavior Disorders

Disruptive behavior disorders, including conduct disorder and oppositional defiant disorder, are characterized by willful disobedience. Conduct disorders affect males more often than females, and commonly overlap with other psychiatric disorders. Many of these children come from broken homes and are exposed to domestic violence, poverty, and shifting parental figures. Harsh parental discipline with physical punishment appears to lead to aggressive behavior; however, genetic heritability of antisocial and aggressive behaviors has been identified.

Defiance of authority, fighting, school failure, and destruction of property are common indicators of conduct disorder. During adolescence, fire setting, theft, sexual promiscuity, and criminal behaviors may develop. The risk for disruptive behavior disorders increases with inconsistent parenting and punitive disciplinary techniques, parental alcohol and drug abuse, and parental antisocial personality disorder.

### Attention Deficit Hyperactivity Disorder

Attention deficit hyperactivity disorder (ADHD) is a neurobiological condition characterized by prominent symptoms of inattention and/or hyperactivity and impulsivity. ADHD affects males more often than females and persists into adolescence and adulthood. Family and twin studies provide evidence of genetic susceptibility, and molecular DNA studies implicate the role of genes in ADHD. Imaging techniques show anatomic and metabolic differences in ADHD subjects compared to non-ADHD subjects.

The DSM-IV defines three subtypes of ADHD: predominantly inattentive, predominantly hyperactive-impulsive, and combined inattentive, hyperactive and impulsive. Children with the inattentive subtype tend to be described as "spacey" and socially withdrawn, and they have fewer conduct and behavioral problems than the hyperactive-impulsive subtype. Hyperactive ADHD children tend to run around excessively, fidget, and have difficulty playing or engaging in quiet activities. Impulsivity in ADHD is characterized by the inability to wait turns, blurting out answers, and interrupting others.

Contrary to common belief, ADHD is not limited to childhood. ADHD has a chronic lifelong course and, if untreated, results in school and work failure, substance use disorders, legal difficulties, car accidents and fatalities, and sexual indiscretions. ADHD commonly occurs with depressive disorders, anxiety disorders, conduct disorder, oppositional defiant disorder, and learning disorders. The majority of children with ADHD are effectively treated with stimulant medications. Stimulant medications are the oldest and most established pharmacological agents in children with ADHD. Behavior therapy can improve academic achievement and reduce targeted conduct problems, especially in children with a co-occurring conduct disorder.

## ▶ Developmental Disorders

### Mental Retardation

The diagnosis of mental retardation requires the presence of low intelligence accompanied by deficits in social and language skills and adaptive functioning. Mental retardation is the result of psychosocial factors, biological factors, or a combination of the two. Often, the exact cause cannot be identified. Parental intelligence, psychosocial involvement, material resources, and availability of social support services influence the course of mental retardation.

### Autistic Disorder

Autistic disorders include deficits in reciprocal language and social interactions, with associated behavioral peculiarities such as repetitive stereotyped behaviors. Autism may be apparent in infancy; however, in some patients, the full disorder does not appear until after 3 years of age. Suggested causes of autism include illnesses that result in central nervous system dysfunction such as rubella, seizures, encephalitis, and toxins. The concordance rate of occurrence of autism among identical twins is about 90%, and the rate of autism is higher in families with a history of language-related disorders.

The most notable deficits in autism are severe deficits in reciprocal social interactions. Eye contact with caregivers and peers is minimal, language development is delayed, and disinterest in social interactions with peers is usually observed during the toddler years. When speech does develop, it usually is illogical and echolike, as words that are heard are repeated. Repetitive and stereotypic behaviors include odd posturing, hand flapping, self-injurious behavior, abnormal patterns of eating and drinking, and unpredictable mood changes.

Patients fortunate enough to have early access to multimodal treatment, including medication, behavioral modification, occupational therapy, and speech therapy, show significant improvement. Similar to other childhood illness, parental guidance and assurance is critical for obtaining appropriate medical and psychosocial support. Informed parents contribute to the child's learning of self-care and adaptive skills, and to long-term outcomes.

### Tic Disorders

A tic is a sudden, rapid, involuntary stereotyped movement or vocalization that may be temporarily suppressed by conscious efforts. All forms of tics are exacerbated by stress, anxiety, boredom, or fatigue, and typically decrease in severity when the child is concentrating on an enjoyable task. Tics occur more commonly in boys than girls, and are presumed to result from a neurotransmitter imbalance.

Complications of tic disorders include shame and impaired self-esteem that results from being teased and rejected by peers and adults. Severe symptoms may interfere with forming intimate friendships. The unemployment rate in adults with tics has been reported as high as 50%.

Transient tics usually do not require treatment. Complicated tic disorders require carefully titrated medication therapy. Medication therapy is usually complicated by high rates of side effects, and difficulty in finding effective combinations of medications due to the disorder's natural waxing and waning course.

### Dementia

Dementia is a degenerative syndrome characterized by deficits in memory, language, and mood. The most common form of dementia is Alzheimer's disease, which develops gradually and occurs most commonly after the age of 60 years. Vascular dementia has a more abrupt onset and is caused by physical insults from high blood pressure, diabetes, and strokes. Poor nutrition, head injuries, with chronic alcohol intake may result in alcohol-related dementia. Parkinson's disease is a degenerative neurological movement disorder characterized by dementia in late stages of the disease.

The earliest manifestation of Alzheimer's disease is loss of short-term memory. Psychosis, aggression, and profound personality changes are associated with advanced disease. With severe disease, judgment is lost, personal care is neglected, and physical illnesses ultimately may lead to death.

Physical findings in Alzheimer's disease include degeneration of neurons and plaque formation on and around neurons. Plaques or deposits of proteins build up around neurons and interrupt communication between neurons by neurotransmitters. Abnormal collections of proteins form neurofibrillatory tangles that are detected by brain scans. Acetylcholine is the neurotransmitter that is most affected by Alzheimer's disease. Decreases in acetylcholine are correlated with memory loss. Alterations in norepinephrine, GABA, and serotonin have been documented and may play a role in mood, behavior, and aggression.

The two most significant risk factors for Alzheimer's disease are advanced age and family history. The prevalence of Alzheimer's disease is 25% to 30% in the 85- to 90-year-old population. Mutations in chromosomes and inheritance of two high-risk genes are associated with a greater risk for developing Alzheimer's disease.

**Treatment of Alzheimer's Disease**  Medications are used to slow the progression of Alzheimer's disease and to treat symptoms of depression, aggression, and anxiety. Medications that replace acetylcholine improve memory. Antidepressants and antianxiety medications are prescribed to manage depression and anxiety. Social support is needed to improve the quality of life and maximize personal care. Vitamin E may prevent the progression of Alzheimer's disease by decreasing oxygen-free radicals that accelerate cell death.

## ▶ Substance Use Disorders

Substance use disorders include drug and alcohol abuse and addiction. Drug abuse is a social problem with extensive emotional and economic consequences. Individuals who abuse drugs and alcohol often make bad choices, harm their health and personal relationships, place themselves or other people in danger, and frequently end up in prison.

Substance abuse is a conscious choice to use drugs or alcohol. Informative and punitive measures such as Drug Abuse Resistance Education (DARE) in schools and legal charges for driving under the influence are useful in reducing drug abuse. Despite interventions, the pleasurable effects of drugs and alcohol produce changes in the brain that ultimately lead to addiction, which is a chronic, compulsive, relapsing illness. Addicts cannot quit by themselves, and treatment is necessary to break the craving, social manipulation, and risky tactics the addict uses to obtain drugs or alcohol.

Core symptoms of drug and alcohol dependence include compulsive use, physical and psychological cravings, tolerance, and withdrawal. The addict is unable to function without the use of drugs and/or alcohol, and his or her daily life is preoccupied with activities centered on obtaining the substance. Initial pleasurable effects of the abused substance are replaced by strong physical and psychological cravings for which greater amounts are needed to reproduce the same effect.

Warning signs of substance use disorders include use that is physically damaging and persistent use regardless of medical, social, economic, and legal consequences. The addict will continue to drink alcohol or abuse drugs regardless of health problems and medical recommendations. Family and friends may feel manipulated or deceived as the addict denies the severity of the addiction and makes excuses to continue to use drugs or alcohol. A legal charge for driving under the influence often imposes professional evaluation and treatment for substance abuse.

Stressful events, medical uses of an addictive substance, untreated or undertreated mental disorders, neurochemical changes, and genetics influence the development of substance use disorders. Addicts frequently come from broken homes or from disturbed families with inconsistent parenting, abuse, and hostility. For adolescents and adults, drugs and alcohol relieve feelings of isolation, loneliness, anger, and depression. Untreated or undertreated ADHD or bipolar disorder is associated with significant risk for substance use disorders. Alterations in dopamine in reward centers of the brain and the subsequent use of alcohol or drugs simulates pleasure and reward in susceptible individuals. Family and twin studies have led to identification of genes that are implicated in addiction.

In addition to physical and psychological dependence, abuse of drugs and alcohol leads to devastating health consequences, including death. As tolerance and financial troubles develop, the addict will go to great lengths to obtain drugs. Young men and women may sell sex in exchange for drugs or money for alcohol at the risk of contracting HIV and other diseases. Sharing needles is a common source of hepatitis and HIV infection. Damage to the lungs, liver, brain, heart, and kidney from nutritional deficiencies, and physical insults from drugs or alcohol, are common causes of death. Addiction, with its health consequences, may be viewed as a death wish, although nonchemical means, such as gunshots, are more commonly used methods to commit suicide.

**Treatment of Substance Abuse** Medical, psychological, and social interventions are needed to restore health and provide alternatives for drug and alcohol use. Understanding that addiction is a common relapsing illness is necessary for a commitment for lifelong treatment. Twelve-step programs provide a safe place for the addict to gain support and socialization away from situations that lead them to drug and alcohol abuse. Families benefit from 12-step programs that provide insight on how family interactions enable the addict to continue to use drugs or alcohol.

## ▶ Schizophrenia

Schizophrenic disorders are complex illnesses characterized by psychosis or a loss of contact with reality accompanied by severe disturbances in social functioning, bizarre thoughts, changes in affect or emotional state, withdrawal from social relations, and unpredictable behavior. The onset of schizophrenia is mostly noted in late teenage years or early adulthood when family and friends observe that the patient has no regard for daily life activities such as work, education, socialization, and self-care.

The characteristic presentation of schizophrenia is a gradual withdrawal from people, activities, and social contacts, with increasing concern for abstract and sometimes eccentric ideas. Some patients experience only a single episode and remain symptom-free for most of their lives. The course of the illness can fluctuate over many years and can get worse if episodes reoccur. Depression, anxiety, suspiciousness, difficulty in concentrating, and restlessness are among the early symptoms of schizophrenia, and they intensify or diminish as the illness progresses Table 15–4.

Disturbances in perception, or hallucinations, and false beliefs, or delusions, are reflected in behavior and thoughts that are vague and detached from reality. Schizophrenics may experience auditory or visual hallucinations in which they may hear or see things that are not present. Delusions are commonly persecutory (belief that they are being watched, followed, or plotted against), grandiose (belief that they have special powers, influence, or wealth), or somatic (physi-

### Table 15–4  Schizophrenia

- Trouble concentrating or organizing thoughts

- Inappropriate emotional reactions—crying at a joke, for example

- Inability to keep a job or build healthy relationships

- False beliefs or delusions

- Hearing, seeing, or smelling things that are not there (auditory and/or visual hallucinations)

- Disordered thought and speech—for example, shifting from one thought to another

- Behavioral problems, including making odd, repetitive movements such as constantly shaking the head, wearing inappropriate clothing for the season, and ignoring personal hygiene

- Rejection of friends and family, avoidance of eye contact

cal belief that something is rotting inside their bodies).

Affect, or "feeling tone," refers to the outward expression of emotion. The schizophrenic affect may be extremely unstable with rapid shifts from sadness to happiness for no obvious reason, or it may be flattened, with no signs of emotion in tone of voice or facial expression. Patients may state that they no longer respond to life with normal intensity or that they are "losing their feelings."

Motor disturbances in schizophrenia may be catatonic or rigid, or disorganized or agitated. Catatonic features may range from a total reduction in movement, or "zombie-like state," to a wild, aggressive, and agitated state. Disorganized conduct is usually blunted or dull, bearing no relationship to social signals.

Genetics, neurobiology, family influences, and social and environmental attributes provide details about the development of schizophrenia. There may be a common event in a predisposed individual that is reported to have either triggered the development of or worsening of schizophrenia. In other patients, a precipitating event is not reported, because psychological stresses may be difficult to describe as the individual retreats from a painful reality.

Abnormalities in the brains of individuals with schizophrenia include faulty brain development, atypical brain anatomy, and alterations in chemical regulation of the neurotransmitter dopamine.

**Treatment of Schizophrenia**  Schizophrenia has remained the most serious psychiatric illness known for the past 200 years. The suicide rate among schizophrenics is 10%, and the average life expectancy is lower than that of the general population. Comprehensive medical and psychosocial treatment has improved the quality of life of patients and their families. Medications that control dopamine effectively normalize overt behavior and thought processes, and allow the patient to communicate coherently. Compliance with psychosocial therapy in combination with medication helps patients establish a life that is free from symptoms and enriched by personal, social, and occupational achievements.

# ▶ Mood Disorders

Mood disorders are characterized by marked periods of sadness and euphoria. While it is normal for people to experience ups and downs during their lives, those who have major depression, or bipolar disorder experience debilitating symptoms that result in vocational failure, social withdrawal, and dysfunctional relationships.

## Major Depression

Complaints of sadness, hopelessness, and despair vary widely in depressed individuals. Major depression occurs at any age and, if untreated, may result in suicide. Women are diagnosed with major depression about twice as often as men. Depression in the elderly is often masked by concurrent physical illness and is attributed to normal aging processes. School failures, irritability, loss of appetite, social withdrawal, and pretending to be sick are signs of depression in children.

A major depressive disorder consists of at least one episode of serious mood depression accompanied by a number of changes in behavior. Complaints frequently include a loss of interest and pleasure, and withdrawal from activities. Feelings of guilt, worthlessness, anxiety, and shame are reported because individuals with major depression view their illness as a moral deficiency. Physical symptoms that suggest emotional distress include unexplained weight loss or weight gain, disturbed sleep, decreased energy, poor eye contact, monosyllabic speech, and indifference to pleasure or joy.

Subcategories of depression include seasonal affective disorder, postpartum depression, dysthymia, and premenstrual dysmorphic disorder. Seasonal affective disorder is believed to be due to decreased sunlight exposure during the winter months. Postpartum depression usually occurs 2 weeks to 6 months following the birth of a child. Persistent care of the newborn, sleep deprivation, social stresses, and hormonal changes all play a role in the development of postpartum depression. Chronic depression or dysthymia is diagnosed when symptoms persist for more than 2 years. Cyclic depressive symptoms prior to menstruation may occur regularly for some women.

Heredity is currently the most important predisposing factor for major depression. The risk for major depression is higher in families with a history of mood disorders. Depression in a parent contributes to depression in genetically vulnerable children, via modeling, emotional unavailability, and decreased capacity for caregiving activities. While stressful life events trigger sadness, despair, and grief, stressful factors alone do not cause major depression (Table 15–5).

The most prominent theory for depression focuses on regulatory disturbances in neurotransmitters. The neurotransmitters serotonin, norepinephrine, and dopamine are widely distributed in the central nervous system and are implicated in regulation of mood, arousal, movement, and sleep. Medications that increase serotonin, norepinephrine, and dopamine effectively reduce symptoms of depression.

Major depression may occur with a number of physical and psychological disorders. Physical disorders such as thyroid disease or Cushing's disease induce depression by altering hormone levels. Chronic heart disease or cancer produce depressive symptoms from associated disability, fatigue, and physical pain. Direct physical causes of depression include HIV infections and seizure disorders that damage the brain and central nervous system. Psychological disorders such as anxiety disorders, eating disorders, and developmental disorders are often referred to as co-morbid disorders because they commonly occur with major depression.

Various prescription medications and substance abuse induce depression by altering brain function and regulation of hormones and neurotransmitters. Heart medications, for example, alter neuronal responses to norepinephrine, leading to fatigue and depressive symptoms. Corticosteroid medications induce behavioral changes, psychosis, and major depression especially in susceptible individuals. Alcoholic beverages as well as many commonly abused substances depress the central nervous system.

**Treatment of Depression**  A trial of antidepressant medication that restores regulation of norepinephrine, dopamine, and/or serotonin is indicated for most cases of major depression. Optimal reduction of symptoms is usually noticed 14 to 21 days after starting medication. Psychosocial treatment is often required to improve social functioning and to change depressive thought processes.

### Bipolar Disorder

Bipolar disorder, or manic-depressive illness, is a mood disorder that causes unusual shifts from depression to mania, or an overly elevated, energetic, irritable mood. Periods of highs and lows are called *episodes* of mania and depression. Bipolar disorder affects more than 2 million American adults. Bipolar disorder typically

---

**Table 15–5  Symptoms of Major Depression**

- Prolonged sadness or unexplained crying spells

- Significant changes in appetite and sleep patterns

- Irritability, anger, worry, agitation, anxiety

- Pessimism, indifference

- Loss of energy, persistent lethargy

- Unexplained aches and pains

- Feelings of guilt, worthlessness, and/or hopelessness

- Inability to concentrate

- Indecisiveness

- Inability to take pleasure in former interests

- Social withdrawal

- Excessive consumption of alcohol or use of chemical substances

- Recurring thoughts of death or suicide

develops in late adolescence or early adulthood. However, some people have their first symptoms during childhood, and some develop them late in life. It is often not recognized as an illness, and people may suffer for years without a diagnosis or proper treatment (Table 15–6).

Mania can vary from extreme elation, hyperactivity, and irritability to extreme aggression, with little need for sleep, and risky behaviors that are later regretted. An overly enthusiastic mood at times may attract others; however, mood shifts with delusions may lead to alienation of friends and family, and to irresponsible behaviors such as spending ones life savings or sexual indiscretions.

A distinct period of an abnormally elevated mood that is not induced by the physiologic effects of a drug substance followed by a distinct period of depression is central to diagnosis of a bipolar disorder. Different categories of bipolar disorder are determined by patterns of symptoms or severity of highs and lows. Bipolar I disorder is associated with periods of intense mania and depression that last for several weeks. Bipolar II disorder is associated with less severe episodes of mania, but depression may continue for several weeks. A chronic fluctuating mood, with mild symptoms of both depression and mania, or cyclothymic disorder, often is undiagnosed and may eventually result in a more severe form of bipolar disorder.

The causes of bipolar disorder are unclear, though genetic, biochemical, and environmental causes have been identified. Like other mental illnesses, several genes acting together may ultimately identify patients who will develop bipolar disorder. Bipolar disorder runs in families, and stressful experiences may trigger some symptoms. Changes in neurotransmitter regulation that lead to bipolar disorder may be affected by the presence of another illness, stress, substance abuse, changes in diet and exercise, and hormonal changes.

**Treatment of Bipolar Disorder**   Medical treatment of bipolar disorder is complex. Patients often require prolonged treatment with medications called mood stabilizers, such as lithium or certain antiepileptic medications, antidepressants, sedative medications or "sleep aids," and major tranquilizers or antipsychotic medications. Family and individual patient counseling improves social functioning by providing psychological support and treatment that stabilizes extreme characteristics of mania or depression (Figure 15–1).

## ▶ Anxiety Disorders

Anxiety disorders include a number of disorders in which the primary feature is abnormal or inappropriate anxiety that interferes with daily school, work, recreational, and family activities. Anxiety is a normal phenomenon in which our mind and body reacts to flee from danger, also known as "fight or flight." Heart rate, respiratory rate, blood pressure, and muscle tension increases at the onset of a stressful event.

| Table 15–6   Symptoms of Mania |
| --- |

- Increased physical and mental activity and energy

- Heightened mood, exaggerated optimism and self-confidence

- Excessive irritability, aggressive behavior

- Decreased need for sleep without experiencing fatigue

- Grandiose delusions, inflated sense of self-importance

- Racing speech, racing thoughts, flight of ideas

- Impulsiveness, poor judgment, distractibility

- Reckless behavior such as spending sprees, rash business decisions, erratic driving, and sexual indiscretions

- In the most severe cases, delusions and hallucinations

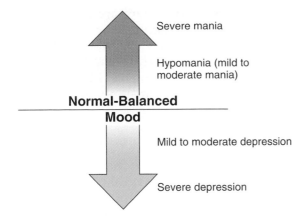

Severe mania

Hypomania (mild to moderate mania)

**Normal-Balanced Mood**

Mild to moderate depression

Severe depression

**Figure 15–1** The spectrum of mood disorder in bipolar disorder.

Symptoms of anxiety become a problem when they occur without any recognizable cause or when the cause does not require an intense response.

Anxiety disorders affect adults and children, and may persist for many years without proper treatment. As with many other mental illnesses, family and friends often label those that suffer anxiety disorders as weak and unable to "snap out of their condition." Some people's lives become so restricted that they avoid normal, everyday activities such as grocery shopping or driving. In some cases, they become housebound.

## Types of Anxiety Disorders

Physical symptoms and behaviors vary slightly with each subtype of anxiety disorder. Panic disorder, generalized anxiety disorder, phobic disorders, social phobia, obsessive compulsive disorder, and posttraumatic stress disorder share the common theme of excessive, irrational fear.

**Panic Disorder** A panic attack involves a sudden onset of fear and terror accompanied by physical symptoms in vital organs such as the heart and lungs. Shortness of breath, chest pains, and palpitations peak within 10 minutes and usually resolve within 30 to 60 minutes. Because of the unpredictability of a panic attack, people who

have them develop anticipatory anxiety, or a persistent pattern of worry regarding when and where the attack will take place. Physical complaints often lead patients to seek emergency medical care.

**Generalized Anxiety Disorder** Severe persistent worries that are out of proportion to the circumstance describe a typical day for sufferers of generalized anxiety disorders. Common worries related to work, money, health, and safety are difficult to control. Additional complaints of restlessness, fatigue, muscle tension, impaired concentration, and disturbed sleep may often be misdiagnosed as depression.

**Phobic Disorders** An irrational fear of something, or specific phobia, that poses little or no danger is the most common type of anxiety disorder. Some phobias, such as a fear of the dark, of strangers, or of large animals, begin in childhood and disappear with age. Hyperventilation, or rapid breathing, may accompany a fear of heights, flying, closed spaces, insects, and rodents. Although adults with phobias realize that these fears are irrational, they often find facing the feared object or situation brings on a panic or severe anxiety attack.

**Social Phobia** Social phobia involves excessive worry and self-consciousness in everyday social situations. Intense fears of being humiliated in social situations interfere with ordinary activities. Physical symptoms that accompany social anxiety include blushing, profuse sweating, nausea, and difficulty talking.

**Obsessive-Compulsive Disorder** Anxious, irrational thoughts and images, also known as obsessions, lead to the need to perform rituals to prevent or get rid of the obsessive stimulus. Rituals are patterns of irrational behaviors, or compulsions, that provide temporary relief from the anxiety. Obsessions centered on cleanliness and fear of germs, for example, may lead to compulsive hand washing. Other rituals may include the need to repeat certain words and phrases to ward off danger, or repetitive counting of objects. Patients with obsessive-compulsive disorder (OCD) are aware that their compulsion and corresponding ritual is irrational, but cannot stop it. OCD affects both men and women, and symptoms may ease over time with appropriate treatment.

**Posttraumatic Stress Disorder**  Exposure to an overwhelming traumatic incident such as the events of September 11, 2001, or encounters of trauma such as rape, violence, child abuse, or war, may lead to symptoms and diagnosis of posttraumatic stress disorder, or PTSD. Victims of trauma develop persistent frightening thoughts and memories months or years after the event. The traumatic event is repeatedly experienced as nightmares and flashbacks or numbing recollections of the event throughout the day. The person avoids reminders of the event, startles or feels frightened easily, and may feel detached and numb. PTSD sufferers may lose interest in things they used to enjoy, avoid affection, and become irritable or aggressive. People with PTSD often feel guilty about surviving the event or about behaving destructively, as in case of veterans of war.

Imaging techniques in persons with anxiety disorders have focused on the role of brain structures that mediate communication and process information to memory. The amygdala is an almond-shaped structure located deep within the brain, and it may play a role in fear and phobias. The hippocampus is a structure of the brain that processes and stores information to memory. The size of the hippocampus appears smaller in persons with posttraumatic stress disorder, which may explain the memory deficits and flashbacks in individuals with PTSD.

The genetic basis for anxiety disorders originates from family studies. Anxiety disorders are common among relatives of affected individuals. The risk for phobias is greater in relatives of individuals with both depression and panic disorder. In cases of PTSD, genetic factors may explain why only certain individuals exposed to trauma develop PTSD.

Head injuries, overactive thyroid gland, cardiovascular disease, respiratory disease, altered regulation of neurotransmitters, and certain medications may cause anxiety disorders. Individuals with anxiety disorders are more sensitive to medications that increase heart rate, blood pressure, and fear behaviors. Abnormal neurotransmission of the neurotransmitter serotonin as a cause of OCD is recognized by a reduction of symptoms with medications that increase serotonin.

## Treatment of Anxiety Disorders

Anxiety, as a learned response to a stimulus and corresponding biochemical changes in brain chemistry, responds to treatment with medications and psychotherapy. Medications that increase serotonin are effective in the treatment of OCD, though psychotherapy is often required to gain understanding of underlying emotional conflict. Antianxiety medications that increase the effect of the neurotransmitter gamma-aminobutyric acid (GABA) have a calming effect and work quickly. The use of antianxiety medications is limited, however, by their potential for addiction.

## ▶ Eating Disorders

Eating disorders involve serious disturbances in eating behavior. Fashion trends, ad campaigns, social attitudes, and athletics promote leaner body weight and a preoccupation with body shape and weight. Extreme attitudes surrounding weight and food, combined with psychological and medical complications, define the disabilities that meet the criteria for eating disorders.

## Symptoms of Eating Disorders

Anorexia nervosa and bulimia nervosa occur primarily in young women who develop a paralyzing fear of becoming fat. In anorexia nervosa, fear of obesity causes excessive restriction of food, resulting in emaciation. Bulimia involves massive binge eating followed by purging or excessive dieting and exercise to prevent weight gain.

**Anorexia Nervosa**  Anorexia means lack of appetite. Ironically, individuals with anorexia nervosa are hungry and yet are preoccupied with dieting and limiting food intake to the point of starvation. There is an intense fear of gaining weight or becoming fat even though anorectics become dangerously thin. The process of eating becomes an obsession, with rituals centered on meal plans, calorie counts, compulsive exercise, and self-induced vomiting despite little food intake.

The typical anorectic is an adolescent female who has lost 15% of her body weight, fears obesity, stops menstruating, and otherwise looks healthy. Other notable signs include low blood pressure, decreased heart rate, and edema or swelling of tissues. Metabolic changes, including dehydration and depletion of electrolytes (sodium, potassium, and chloride), can result in abnormal heart rhythm, heart failure, sudden cardiac arrest, and death.

Usually described as the honor-roll student or state champion, the individual denies that anything is wrong and typically does not seek medical care until prompted into treatment by friends and family. Depression is common as anorectics withdraw from social affairs involving food and festivities.

**Bulimia Nervosa** Similar to anorexia nervosa, bulimics are excessively concerned with body weight and physical shape. Unlike anorectics, bulimics binge by eating an excessive amount of food within a restricted period of time, followed by compensatory purging behavior such as self-induced vomiting or misuse of laxatives or diuretics. Rigorous dieting and exercise may also follow binges to prevent weight gain. There is a feeling of loss of control during the binging episode, followed by intense distress and guilt. Body weight may be normal, which makes it easy for bulimics to hide their illness.

The medical consequences of bulimia nervosa can be devastating. Stomach acid and digestive enzymes from vomiting erode tooth enamel and cause injury and inflammation to the esophagus and salivary glands. Severe dental caries and gum disease eventually require removal of teeth. Vomiting and laxative and diuretic abuse lowers blood potassium levels, causing muscle cramping and abnormal heart rhythms. In cases of severe potassium loss, death may result from cardiac arrest. Prolonged and excessive laxative abuse may severely damage the bowel. If the bowel ceases its function, surgery

is required to form a colostomy, an opening from the bowel to the abdominal wall to allow removal of the feces into a bag attached to the outer abdominal wall.

Bulimics are aware of their behavior and feel intense guilt and shame. Bulimics are generally outgoing, impulsive, and prone to depression and alcohol or drug abuse. Unlike anorectics, bulimics are more likely to talk about their illness and desperately seek help from physicians and friends.

Patterns of psychological and interpersonal issues most consistently provide insight into the causes of eating disorders. Low self-esteem and persistent feelings of inadequacy shape attitudes of perfectionism for the anorectic and severe self-criticism for the bulimic. Troubled family relationships, difficulty expressing feelings and emotions, and a history of physical or sexual abuse are reported more often in bulimics than anorectics. Social attitudes that value thinness and limit beauty to specific body weight and shape influence body image and contribute to extreme dieting and exercise for both anorectics and bulimics.

The biological basis for eating behavior involves a complex network of brain structures and neurotransmitters. The hypothalamus regulates hunger, monitors fullness of the stomach, and determines how much food is eaten. The limbic system influences emotions and selection of foods to appease the appetite. The prefrontal region of the brain controls decisions about when, where, and how to eat. Future studies on the biology of appetite control and behavior may lead to development of new medications to treat eating disorders.

### Treatment of Eating Disorders

Successful treatment of and recovery from eating disorders requires the realization that starvation, binging, and purging is destructive. Medical treatment to restore nutrition and replace fluids and electrolytes is crucial to prevent death from organ failure. Medication to relieve depression and anxiety may improve mood and thought processes. Group, family, individual, and nutritional counseling provide support to break down delusions that shape eating behavior and distortions in body image.

# ▶ Personality Disorders

Persistent, inflexible patterns of behavior that affect interpersonal relationships describe pers-onality disorders. Personality disorders appear in adolescence or early adulthood and remain sta-ble throughout an individual's lifetime. The DSM-IV describes three major categories of per-sonality disorders based on "clusters" of symp-toms.

Personality disorders occur along with med-ical and psychiatric illnesses. Relations with family, friends, and caregivers are often strained by inflexible and maladaptive personality char-acteristics. People with severe personality disor-ders are more vulnerable to psychiatric break-downs and are at risk for alcoholism, substance abuse, reckless sexual behavior, eating disor-ders, and violence.

## Symptoms of Personality Disorders

### Cluster A: Paranoid and Schizoid

**Paranoid Personality**   The paranoid personality type is indifferent, suspicious, and hostile. His or her relationships are shallow because of a ten-dency to respond to positive acts or kindness with distrust. The paranoid personality type interprets positive statement such as "You look like a million bucks" to mean "My friend is after my money."

**Schizoid Personality**   People with schizoid per-sonality appear cold and isolated. Often called introverted, schizoid personality types appear self-absorbed and withdrawn. They often deal with their fears through superstitions, magical thinking, and unusual beliefs.

### Cluster B: Antisocial, Borderline, Histrionic, and Narcissistic

**Antisocial Personality**   Callous disregard for others and manipulation of people for personal gratification characterize antisocial personality types. Antisocial personality may start as a con-duct problem in childhood, manifested as disre-spect for authority and for personal and public property. Adolescents and adults with antisocial personalities are at risk for alcoholism, drug abuse, sexual improprieties, and violence.

**Borderline Personality**   Borderline personality disorders often occur in women who were de-prived of adequate care during childhood. Their moods are unstable and characterized by crisis and anger alternating with depression. Threats of real or imagined abandonment elicit impulsive behaviors such as promiscuity and substance abuse. The individual with a borderline person-ality disorder is vulnerable to brief psychotic episodes, substance abuse, and eating disorders.

**Histrionic Personality**   Persons with histrionic personality are theatrical and exaggerate their emotions. Friendships are initially formed be-cause others are attracted to the histrionic per-sonality's energetic and entertaining behavior. Hysteria and flamboyant behaviors often result in negative responses and feelings of rejection.

**Narcissistic Personality**   The narcissistic per-sonality type has an exaggerated self-image and a tendency to think little of others. Narcissists expect others to admire their grandiosity and feel they are entitled to have their needs at-tended to. When rejected by others through crit-icism or defeat, the narcissist becomes enraged or severely depressed.

### Cluster C: Avoidant, Dependent, and Obsessive-Compulsive

**Avoidant Personality**   Avoidant personality types appear shy and timid, as if they have a so-cial phobia. They fear relationships, although they have a strong desire to feel accepted. They are hypersensitive to criticism and rejection and are susceptible to depression, anxiety, and anger for failing to develop social relationships.

**Dependent Personality**   Dependent personality types have an extremely poor self-image. They appoint others to make significant decisions out of fear of expressing themselves or offending others. Extended illness may bring out a depen-dent personality in adults.

**Obsessive-Compulsive Personality**   The obses-sive-compulsive personality types are depend-able, meticulous, orderly, and intolerant of mis-takes. They are often high achievers, attending to details while failing to complete the task at hand. Individuals with an obsessive-compulsive personality avoid new situations and relationships because these new elements cannot be methodically controlled.

## Treatment of Personality Disorders

Most people with personality disorders do not see a need for treatment. Often, secondary medical and psychiatric illnesses force persons with personality disorders to seek treatment. Rigid thoughts and behavior often complicate compliance with treatment and are frustrating for the health-care providers. Individual, family, and group therapy is required to point out consequences of behavior. Medication is often helpful to relieve anxiety, depression, and psychosis.

## ▶ Suicide

Suicide is almost always associated with mental illness. Suicide attempts are irrational and impulsive self-directed acts of aggression. People consider suicide when they are hopeless and unable to see alternative solutions to confusion, mental and physical anguish, and chaos in their life. Risks for suicide include substance abuse, previous suicide attempts, a family history of suicide, a history of sexual abuse, and impulsive or aggressive character. More than four times as many men as women die by suicide; however, women attempt suicide more often during their lives than do men. Suicidal behavior occurs most often when people experience major losses and stressful events such as divorce, loss of a job, incarceration, and chronic illness.

Unlike physical illnesses, mental illness has no visible wounds and so is associated with social stigma, isolation, and personal faults. Persons with mental illness contemplating suicide may talk about their distress at the risk of being judged, ignored, and isolated. Warning signs of suicide include withdrawal, talk of death, giving away cherished possessions, and a sudden shift in mood. A severely depressed person may unexpectedly appear better, or a schizophrenic may progressively develop delusions about death prior to a suicide attempt. A suicide attempt or completed suicide is devastating to families, friends, and caregivers who commonly experience remorse and guilt for failing to avert the suicide attempt or death.

## ▶ Diagnostic Tests for Mental Illness

Comprehensive evaluations, including a medical history and physical exam, psychosocial history, mental health exam, and family history, are essential for diagnosis of mental illness. A thorough medical history and physical exam should identify physical illnesses and metabolic and hormonal stresses that masquerade as symptoms of mental illness. The use of multiple informants and obtaining a patient history from family and friends with major timelines of life events can help organize complex and detailed information. Observation of the patient alone or within a family milieu is useful to identify emotional responses, physical appearance and reactions, speech and language abilities, clinical estimate of intelligence, and level of judgment and insight. A number of standardized written questionnaires and rating scales supplement the clinical evaluation by providing a systematic review and standard score of level of behaviors and emotions.

## CHAPTER SUMMARY

Mental illnesses are neurobiological disorders characterized by disturbances in mood, thought, affect, and behavior. Comprehensive physical and psychological evaluations are required to accurately diagnose and treat mental illness. The onset, course, and prognosis of mental illness are determined by biological, psychological, familial, interpersonal, socioeconomic, and cultural variables. Untreated and undertreated mental illness is associated with severe disability, emotional distress, substance abuse, adverse financial consequences, and death by suicide. Medication therapy, psychotherapy, and social counseling methods effectively reduce the symptoms of mental illness. Public health education is helpful to reduce the stigma of mental illness and to promote access to health care.

# DISEASES AT A GLANCE

## Mental Illness

| DISORDER | ETIOLOGY | SIGNS AND SYMPTOMS |
|---|---|---|
| Disruptive behavior disorders | Genetics, biology, environment | Willful disobedience, defiance of authority, aggression |
| Attention deficit hyperactivity disorder | Genetics, biology, environment | Hyperactivity, impulsivity, inattention |
| Mental retardation | Genetics, biology, environment | Social language deficits, below-average intelligence |
| Autistic disorder | Genetics, biology, environment, toxins | Reciprocal language deficits, repetitive stereotypical behaviors |
| Tic disorder | Genetics, biology, environment | Rapid involuntary repetitive movement or vocalization |
| Dementia | Genetics, biology, environment, toxins | Language, memory, and mood deficits |
| Substance use disorders | Genetics, environment | Compulsive use, physical and psychological cravings, tolerance, and withdrawal |
| Schizophrenia | Genetics, biology, environment | Loss of contact with reality, severe disturbance in social functioning, bizarre thoughts, withdrawal from social interactions, hallucinations, delusions |

| DIAGNOSIS | TREATMENT |
|---|---|
| Psychosocial and medical evaluation, psychometric testing; diagnosed in childhood | Cognitive, behavioral psychotherapy<br>Pharmacotherapy: stimulants, atypical antipsychotic medications, mood stabilizers |
| Psychosocial and medical evaluation, psychometric testing; diagnosed prior to the age of 7, with approximately 50% persistence into adulthood | Cognitive, behavioral psychotherapy<br>Pharmacotherapy: stimulants, atypical antipsychotic medications, certain antidepressants |
| Psychosocial and medical evaluation, psychometric testing; diagnosed usually before 3 years of age | Behavioral therapy, occupational therapy, social support services |
| Psychosocial and medical evaluation, psychometric testing; diagnosed usually around 3 years of age | Behavioral therapy, occupational therapy, social support services<br>Pharmacotherapy or other supportive care to manage aggression or self-injurious behavior |
| Psychosocial and medical evaluation, psychometric testing; diagnosed usually before adulthood | Behavioral therapy<br>Pharmacotherapy: certain antidepressants or atypical antipsychotic medications |
| Psychosocial and medical evaluation; diagnosed most commonly after age 60 | Behavioral, cognitive, family psychotherapy; social supportive care services<br>Pharmacotherapy: memory enhancers, atypical antipsychotic medications, antidepressants, and/or mood stabilizers |
| Diagnosis may follow social, medical, or legal consequences imposing psychosocial evaluation | Behavioral therapy, 12-step programs supporting abstinence (such as Alcoholics Anonymous or Narcotics Anonymous)<br>Pharmacotherapy: antidepressants, atypical antipsychotic medications, or mood stabilizers |
| Psychosocial and medical evaluation, psychometric testing, unpredictable behavior | Pharmacotherapy: antipsychotic medications primarily, antidepressants occasionally<br>Behavioral therapy, occupational therapy, social support services |

# DISEASES AT A GLANCE *(continued)*

## Mental Illness

| DISORDER | ETIOLOGY | SIGNS AND SYMPTOMS |
|---|---|---|
| Major depression | Genetics, biology, environment | Prolonged sadness, significant changes in sleep and appetite, irritability, feelings of guilt and anxiety |
| Bipolar disorder | Genetics, biology, environment | Mania (episodic elation, inflated sense of self) alternating with depression |
| Anxiety disorder | Genetics, biology, environment | Inappropriate fear response with avoidance of daily work, family, life, school, and recreational activities |
| Eating disorders | Genetics, social trends, attitudes, and stresses | Anorexia: persistent dieting, starvation, excessive exercise, body weight less than 15% of ideal body weight<br>Bulimia: binge followed by purging behavior, overuse of laxatives, excessive dieting, body weight normal or thin |
| Personality disorders | Environment | Inflexible patterns of behavior with strained relationships; may occur with substance use disorders, reckless sexual behavior, eating disorders and violence |

| DIAGNOSIS | TREATMENT |
| --- | --- |
| Psychosocial and medical evaluation, psychometric testing | Cognitive behavioral therapy, psychotherapy, social supportive care Pharmacotherapy: antidepressants, tranquilizers, sleep aids or sedative medications |
| Psychosocial and medical evaluation, psychometric testing | Cognitive behavioral therapy, psychotherapy, social supportive care<br>Pharmacotherapy: mood stabilizers, atypical antipsychotic medications, sleep aids or sedative medications |
| Psychosocial and medical evaluation, psychometric testing | Cognitive behavioral therapy<br>Pharmacotherapy: antianxiety medications and certain antidepressants |
| Psychosocial and medical evaluation, psychometric testing | Psychosocial therapy, pharmacotherapy |
| Psychosocial and medical evaluation, psychometric testing | Cognitive behavioral therapy, social support, social services<br>Pharmacotherapy for coexisting depression, anxiety, agitation, aggression, delusions, or psychosis |

## RESOURCES

Beers, M. H., & R. Berkow. *The Merck Manual of Diagnosis and Therapy,* 17th ed. John Wiley & Sons, 1999.

Tierney, L. M., M. A. Papadakis, & S. J. McPhee. *Family Medicine: Principals and Practice,* 6th ed. Springer-Verlag, 2003.

First, M. B. *Diagnostic and Statistical Manual Text Revision IV.* American Psychiatric Association, 2000.

Goldman, H. H., et al. *Review of General Psychiatry,* 5th ed. McGraw-Hill, 2000.

World Health Organization: www.who.org

National Institutes of Mental Health: www.nimh.org

National Alliance for the Mentally Ill: www.nami.org

Schreiber, Flora Rheta. *Sybil.* 1973. Provides a full account of the case of Sybil Dorsett and her treatment by Dr. Cornelia Wilbur. After Sybil's death in 1998, her real name was revealed to be Shirley Ardell Mason of Lexington, Kentucky.

# Interactive Activities

## Cases for Critical Thinking

1. J. R. is a 17-year-old male with above average intelligence. As an infant, he was colicky and difficult to put to sleep. He learned to walk around 12 months of age. At home, J. R. seemed to run on a motor: He scurried around the house, frequently bumping into furniture. J. R. had a hearing test at school at 5 years of age because teachers felt that he may have been hard of hearing, but the test was normal. His grades were average during the primary, intermediate, and junior high-school years. By his senior year in high school, J. R.'s grades dropped dramatically. He frequently appeared spacey, irritable, and angry. He preferred to eat lunch alone and spent much time in his room. His parents feared that he was abusing drugs because he had a history of a "poor choice for friends." His high school counselor recommended a psychiatric evaluation for J. R. His parents were offended at this recommendation.

   a. What are the advantages and disadvantages of a full mental health evaluation?
   b. What potential disorders do you suspect J. R. has?
   c. What are the potential causes of his disorders?

2. A. M. is a 10-year-old female with a history of bad school grades and fighting in class. She has a brother with ADHD. Her parents divorced when she was 5 years old, and she has been raised with a nanny because her mother travels frequently with her job. A. M. is very athletic—she is a member of the traveling soccer team and a competitive ballet dancer. She has voiced frustration over her grades, as she feels that although she works hard, she cannot "make the grades." She fears disappointing her mother by quitting dance and soccer, and she feels like a failure. Although A. M. is a very talented dancer, she trembles and feels her heart pound prior to competition. Her appetite has been poor, and she has been observed picking at her food. A. M.'s mother is concerned and has made an appointment with a doctor.

   a. Does A. M. have warning signs of a potential mental illness? What symptoms and behaviors point to a potential problem?
   b. Would you recommend an evaluation for A. M.?
   c. What type of treatments are available for A. M.?

3. D. T. is a 46-year-old male who recently moved his family across the state. His mother recently died of complications from Alzheimer's disease, and he is executor of her estate. D. T. moved his family because of a great job opportunity. Although he loves his job, he regrets moving his family from the town they lived in for 20 years. He has been spending much of his free time alone in his office and has been ignoring his wife and children. D. T.'s father was an alcoholic, and his wife fears that his recent stress may drive him to drink. He has lost interest in sex and recently declined an invitation to a golf outing that he had enjoyed in the past. D. T. has been talking to himself a lot and claims that at times he has seen his mother in his sleep. He awoke abruptly one night from sleep and has been complaining of having nightmares. D. T. sometimes appears frozen, and indifferent to conversations, and behaves as though something is bothering him. His wife feels that D. T. is mourning

the loss of his mother, since his mother was never the person he always longed for. His mother had been abusive to D. T., who was conceived out of wedlock. His mother made sure that he had "proper" upbringing with strict discipline and often punished D. T. rather harshly if he failed to follow directions.

a. What signs of mental illness does D. T. have?
b. What potential diagnosis do you suspect?
c. What recommendations would you give to his wife?

## Multiple Choice

1. Reforms in the treatment of the mentally ill started after the French Revolution with an Austrian physician named _____.
   a. Sigmund Freud          c. Emil Kraepelin
   b. Franz Mesmer           d. Sybil Dorsett

2. Psychiatric diagnoses are categorized in a book named the _____.
   a. PDR                    c. DSM
   b. AMA                    d. Axis

3. Which of the following neurotransmitters is implicated in schizophrenia, depression, and ADHD?
   a. epinephrine
   b. serotonin
   c. gamma aminobutyric acid (GABA)
   d. dopamine

4. Which of the following regarding ADHD is false?
   a. ADHD is limited to children
   b. ADHD is a neurobiological disorder
   c. ADHD is more common in males than in females
   d. there are three subtypes of ADHD

5. Medications that replace _____ are effective in improving memory in persons with Alzheimer's disease.
   a. dopamine               c. acetylcholine
   b. serotonin              d. GABA

6. A false belief that one is being watched or punished is also known as a _____ delusion.
   a. persecutory            c. grandiose
   b. somatic                d. affective

7. Binge eating followed by purging behavior such as self-induced vomiting most commonly occurs in _____.
   a. anorexia nervosa       c. binge eating disorder
   b. bulimia nervosa        d. all of the above

8. Periods of intense mania and depression that last for several weeks is also known as _____.
   a. cyclothymic disorder   c. bipolar II
   b. bipolar I              d. all of the above

9. Adults with bipolar illness may be treated with all of the following types of medications except _____.
   a. sedatives
   b. antidepressant medications
   c. stimulant medications
   d. antipsychotic medications

10. Anxious, irrational thoughts and images are also called _____.
    a. compulsions            c. hallucinations
    b. delusions              d. obsessions

## True or False

_____ 1. Bipolar disorder is a behavioral disorder with extreme highs and lows.

_____ 2. ADHD is an emotional disorder associated with depression, anxiety, and hyperactivity.

_____ 3. Persons of different age groups are at risk for different types of mental illness.

_____ 4. Childhood conduct disorder is also known as childhood antisocial personality.

_____ 5. People with high blood pressure and diabetes have a higher risk for dementia.

_____ 6. Substance abuse is a conscious choice to use drugs or alcohol.

_____ 7. Hallucinations and delusions are symptoms of posttraumatic stress disorder.

_____ 8. Children are at risk for major depression.

_____ 9. Individuals with a schizoid personality disorder are distant, introverted, and tend to hallucinate.

_____ 10. Primary psychiatric diagnoses are indicated in all axes of diagnosis according to the DSM.

## Fill-Ins

1. _____ is the medical specialty that diagnoses and prescribes medical treatment for mental illness.

2. Chemical messengers, or _____, are implicated in mental illness.

3. Mood, thought processes, appetite, movement, heart rate, and blood pressure are regulated by the neurotransmitter _____.

4. Below average intelligence accompanied by deficits in language and adaptive functioning is diagnostic for _____.

5. Rapid stereotyped movements that may be suppressed by conscious effort are known as _____.

6. Alzheimer's disease is mostly due to impaired regulation of _____ neurotransmitters.

7. Core symptoms of drug and alcohol abuse include _____ _____ _____ _____.

8. An individual's emotional state in mental illness is referred to as _____.

9. _____ is due to decreased sunlight exposure during the winter months.

10. Decreased need for sleep, with excessive irritability and grandiosity, is symptomatic for _____.

# MedMedia
# Wrap-Up

**www.prenhall.com/mulvihill**

Remember to visit this website for extra study practice, including exercises, Internet links, news updates, and an audio glossary.

**Activity CD-ROM**

Check out the CD-ROM in the back of this book. You will find games, exercises, puzzles, and videos to help enhance your understanding of this chapter.

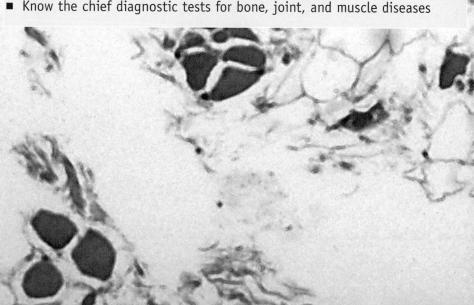

**CHAPTER**

# 16

# Diseases of the Bones, Joints, and Muscles

## Learning Objectives

After studying this chapter, you should be able to

- Understand the normal structure and function of bones, joints, and muscle

- Know the signs, symptoms, and treatment of infectious diseases of bone

- Know how vitamin and mineral deficiencies lead to bone disease

- Know the chief signs and symptoms of neoplasia of bone

- Distinguish rheumatoid arthritis, osteoarthritis, gout, septic arthritis, and bursitis

- Know the causes and treatment of dislocations, sprains, and strains

- Know the causes, treatment, and prevention of carpal tunnel syndrome

- Know the causes and treatment of muscular dystrophy and myasthenia gravis

- Understand age-related changes and disease of bones, joints, and muscles

- Know the chief diagnostic tests for bone, joint, and muscle diseases

## Fact or Fiction?

Rest is best for rheumatoid arthritis.

*Fiction: Unless pain is too severe, daily low-impact exercise maintains mobility and range of motion.*

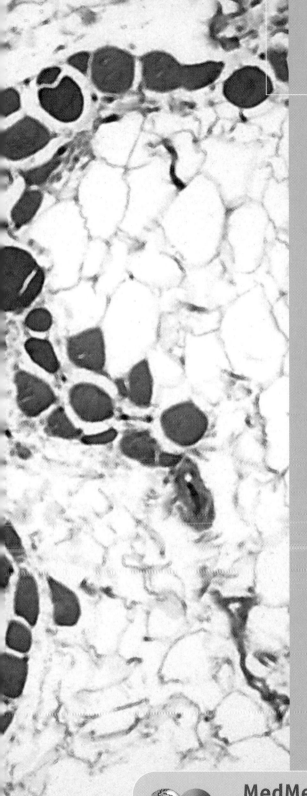

# Disease Chronicle

## Arthritis

**A**rthritis in its various forms has long plagued humans. Lack of understanding of medical science, coupled with a desperate search for relief, produced unusual prescriptions in American traditional and folk medicine. One healer suggested that a person could obtain relief from gout by cutting a hole in a tree, holding the affected body part to it, and sealing the hole with sand, trapping the disease. Another 19th-century prescription required the sufferer to carry a potato in the hip pocket. Treating "like with like" was the basis for treating gout with an earthworm, whose curled shapes resemble gnarled gout-afflicted appendages. How the earthworm was administered is not clear. A home remedy from Texas called for ingestion of wintergreen oil. These ineffective treatments were benign compared to some prescriptions. Citing blood as the culprit, some people were subjected to regular bleedings. Cashing in on the public's misunderstanding of uranium's powers in the 1950s, predatory entrepreneurs recommended baths in uranium pools or ingestion of uranium-laced water. Our understanding and treatment of arthritis has progressed significantly. Still, unscrupulous individuals and companies espouse ineffective and expensive treatments that prey upon vulnerable people.

## MedMedia
**www.prenhall.com/mulvihill**

Use the web address to the left to access the free, interactive Companion Website created for this textbook. It features chapter-specific exercises, Internet links, news links, and an audio glossary. Additionally, explore the CD-ROM that accompanies this book to discover Disease Focus videos and a rich array of activities that accompany this chapter.

## ▶ Interaction of Bones, Muscles, Joints

Because skeletal muscle is attached via tendons to bones, when muscle contracts, or shortens, it moves the skeleton. Muscles that span a joint bring about action at that joint. Groups of muscles may have opposite or antagonistic actions on a joint. For example, one group of muscles extends (straightens) the knee, while another group flexes (bends) the knee. Still other muscles stabilize joints, preventing undesired movements. Bones, joints, and muscles work together. The bones of the skeleton provide the body with a sturdy framework, joints permit movement at portions of the framework, and muscle contraction moves the joints. In this chapter, the principal diseases of bone, joints, and muscles are explained.

## ▶ The Structure and Function of Bone, Joints, and Muscle

Bone may appear inert, but changes constantly occur within it. Bone development, growth, and homeostasis rely on interplay among its constituent minerals, proteins, and living cells. Calcium and phosphate, bone's primary minerals, are embedded in collagen, bone's main protein. The minerals confer hardness and rigidity to bone, while the collagen imparts flexibility. Mature bone cells, osteocytes, along with bone-forming cells, osteoblasts, and bone-resorbing cells, osteoclasts, reside within this bony matrix. The cells receive nutrients by an organized system of blood vessels that course throughout the bone.

Bones are long, flat, or irregularly shaped, but most are covered with a layer of a type of bone tissue called compact bone. The cells, minerals, proteins, and blood vessels of compact bone are arranged in a regular, organized fashion. Another type of bone tissue, spongy bone, contains many bone-marrow-filled spaces. This red-colored marrow is found at the ends of long bones and is the site of blood cell formation.

The long bones found in the arms and legs contain a hollow cavity, the medullary cavity, filled with yellow bone marrow primarily consisting of fat. The growth of long bones occurs at the growth plate, an area of cartilage near each expanded end of the bone (Figure 16–1). At this site, new bone is formed, pushing the ends apart from each other until full growth is achieved, at which time the cartilage turns into bone, a process called ossification. Damage to the growth plate before maturity tends to prevent the bone from reaching its mature length.

The periosteum is a highly vascular layer of fibrous connective tissue that covers the surface of bones. It contains cells that are capable of

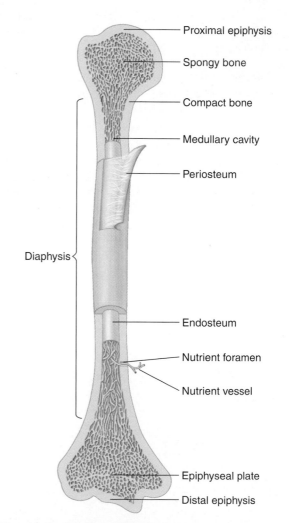

**Figure 16–1** Cut view of long bone.

forming new bone tissue and serves as a site of attachment for tendons or muscles.

Joints are the articulating sites between bones. Various degrees of movement, called *range of motion*, are possible in different kinds of joints. The amount and type of movement at a joint is defined by the shapes of bones and the type of connective tissue holding the bones together at the joint. The shoulder (joint between humerus and scapula) is the most freely movable joint, but it is also the one most easily dislocated.

Articulating bones are held together by ligaments. Dense strands of collagen impart great strength to ligaments. A joint capsule consisting of ligaments and connective tissue surrounds the bone ends. The inner surface of the capsule is lined with a synovial membrane that secretes synovial fluid, which lubricates the joints. Sacs of this fluid, the bursae, are situated near some joints, where they reduce friction during movement. The articulating surfaces of the bone ends are covered with a layer of cartilage, which also reduces friction. A typical joint is illustrated in Figure 16–2.

Skeletal or voluntary muscle tissue is found in muscles that are firmly attached to bones by tendons. Some voluntary muscles, the muscles of facial expression, for example, are attached to soft tissue. Muscles consist of bundles of muscle fibers held together by connective tissue.

When stimulated by nerves at the myoneural junction, muscle fibers contract, and because muscles are attached to bones, the shortening of the muscles moves the bones.

The diseases of muscle described in this chapter are diseases of voluntary muscle. Because muscle action requires nerve stimulation, some nervous system diseases are manifested in muscles. Those diseases are discussed with the nervous system in Chapter 14. This chapter discusses a few muscle diseases that are not directly caused by nervous system disease. Smooth muscle, or involuntary muscle, is a different type of muscle found in the walls of the internal organs and the walls of blood vessels. Cardiac muscle is an involuntary striated muscle and is present only in the heart (Chapter 7). This chapter does not address cardiac or smooth muscle disease.

## ▶ Diseases of Bone

Bone can be affected by disease in various ways. Infectious agents can enter bone through a compound fracture, transmission in the blood, or extension from an adjacent infection. Mineral and vitamin deficiencies prevent proper formation or maintenance of bone structure. Bones atrophy

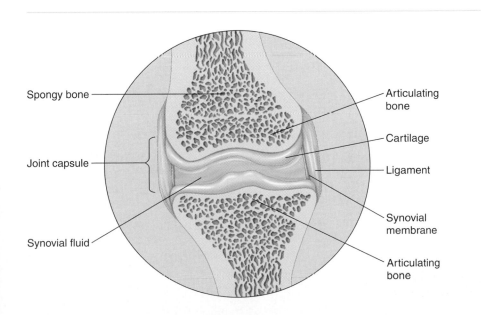

**Figure 16–2**
Typical joint.

Spongy bone

Joint capsule

Synovial fluid

Articulating bone

Cartilage

Ligament

Synovial membrane

Articulating bone

with disuse and fracture, or spontaneously in certain diseases. Tumors can also develop in bone.

## Infectious Diseases of Bone

**Osteomyelitis** is an inflammation of the bone, particularly of the bone marrow in the medullary cavity and the spaces of spongy bone. Osteomyelitis affects principally children and adolescents whose bones are still growing. The long bones—the femur, the tibia, and the humerus—are most frequently affected near their ends at the growth plate.

Osteomyelitis is caused by bacteria, such as staphylococci, that are carried by blood to the bone from some other site in the body, such as infection adjacent to the bone. Bacteria also enter bone through the open wound of a compound fracture. Bone infections may lead to an abscess in the bone, in which case compression of small blood vessels reduces circulation, causing bone necrosis. Infections may spread under the periosteum, lifting sections of it from bone surface, further reducing circulation to bone. In an attempt to heal, bone may be deposited around this area of necrosis.

Local symptoms of bone infection include pain, redness, and heat. Systemic symptoms of chills, fever, and leukocytosis, tachycardia, nausea, and anorexia also occur.

Early antibiotic therapy is an effective treatment and has reduced the incidence of advanced serious cases. Surgery may be required to remove necrotic bone tissue (Figure 16–3).

**Tuberculosis** of bone occurs when bacteria of pulmonary tuberculosis spread to the bones from the lungs. Commonly affected areas are the ends of long bones and knees. Usually seen in children, Pott's disease is tuberculosis of the vertebrae, leading to deformity and paralysis. As in the lungs, tuberculosis of bone leads to cavitation and tissue destruction (Chapter 9). The infection can be treated with antibiotics, although strains of *Mycobacterium tuberculosis* have developed multiple-drug resistance. Surgery may be able to correct bone deformities.

## Bone Disease and Vitamin and Mineral Deficiencies

Vitamins and minerals are key to bone health. Calcium and phosphorus are required in appropriate quantities for proper bone formation and maintenance. However, dietary calcium cannot be absorbed from the digestive tract without vitamin D. Thus, mineral or vitamin D deficiencies may result in soft, malformed, or fragile bones.

**Rickets** is a disease of infancy or early childhood in which the bones do not properly ossify, or harden. The bones of a child with rickets are soft and tend to bend. The weight-bearing bones of the body become deformed: the legs become bent ("bow-legged" or "knock-kneed") and the

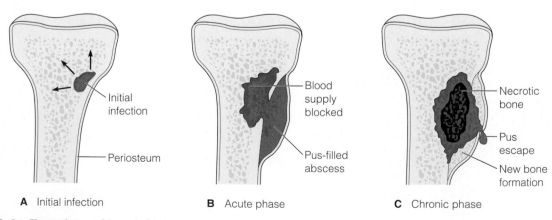

| **A** Initial infection | **B** Acute phase | **C** Chronic phase |

Initial infection
Periosteum

Blood supply blocked
Pus-filled abscess

Necrotic bone
Pus escape
New bone formation

**Figure 16–3** Three phases of bone infection.

vertebral column becomes misaligned. The sternum projects forward, and bony nodules form on the ends of ribs and at wrists, ankles, and knees. The skull is large and square. The pelvic opening in a girl may narrow, leading to problems with childbirth later.

Other symptoms of rickets include flaccid muscles, delayed teething, and a characteristic potbelly. Each of these symptoms can be explained by calcium deficiency. Generally, the disease is caused by a vitamin D deficiency, however, and not by a dietary calcium deficiency. Rickets can be prevented with vitamin D–fortified milk and sunlight. Sunlight converts a substance (dehydrocholesterol) in the skin to vitamin D in the body. This need for sunlight explains the higher incidence of rickets in large, smoky cities where buildings are close together and shut out the sun. Children with rickets respond well to sunlight exposure and treatment with vitamin D concentrate.

Osteomalacia is the softening or decalcification of bones in adults. Symptoms include muscle weakness, weight loss, and bone pain. Bones of the vertebral column, legs, and pelvis become susceptible to bending and fracturing with mild stress.

Osteomalacia is caused by inadequate dietary vitamin D and dietary deficiency of calcium or phosphorus. Osteomalacia is treated with vitamin D supplements and by adding adequate calcium and phosphorous to the diet.

Both rickets and osteomalacia may be secondary to malabsorption syndrome because vitamin D is not absorbed from the intestine.

Osteitis fibrosa cystica is an inflammatory disease in which fibrous nodules and cysts form in bone that becomes porous and decalcified. The bones, particularly the long bones and vertebrae, become deformed and subject to spontaneous fracture.

Hyperparathyroidism (Chapter 13) is usually the cause of osteitis fibrosa cystica. Excessive parathyroid hormone causes bones to lose calcium. The elevated blood calcium deposits in muscles and other soft tissues in the form of insoluble salts. This condition also promotes the formation of kidney stones.

If the high parathyroid hormone levels are caused by a tumor of the parathyroid glands,

## SIDE by SIDE ■ Osteoporosis

▲ X-ray of pelvis in 18-year-old female showing normal bone density. (© B. Bates/Custom Medical Stock Photo.)

▲ X-ray of female pelvis with osteoporosis. Note greatly decreased bone density especially visible in hip bones. (© Custom Medical Stock Photo.)

then removal of these glands may be necessary. Surgery may be required to correct severe bone deformities.

**Osteoporosis** is a disease characterized by porous bone that is abnormally fragile and susceptible to fracture. Weight-bearing bones of the vertebrae and pelvis are especially susceptible, and accumulated compression fractures in these bones cause a decrease in height and bending of the spine (Figure 16–4). Compressed vertebrae press on spinal nerves, causing great pain. Fractures are common in the hip and wrists. No symptoms accompany bone loss until bones weaken and fractures occur. Eighty percent of those affected by osteoporosis are women. Risk factors for osteoporosis include being female, advanced age, and having a small frame (Table 16–1).

Osteoporosis is diagnosed using patient history and bone density tests. No cure exists, so prevention is strongly recommended. A lifelong diet rich in calcium and vitamin D along with weight-bearing exercise stimulates the development of dense and strong bone. Smoking should be avoided, and alcohol and caffeine consumption should be minimized. Bone density screening may identify early osteoporosis. Early diagnosis and appropriate diet and exercise may prevent progression of osteoporosis, but medication may be necessary. The type of medication prescribed depends on the cause of the osteoporosis and other factors. Various medications facilitate calcium uptake in bone and include estrogens, calcitonin, parathyroid hormone, as well as estrogen-receptor modulators and bisphosphonates.

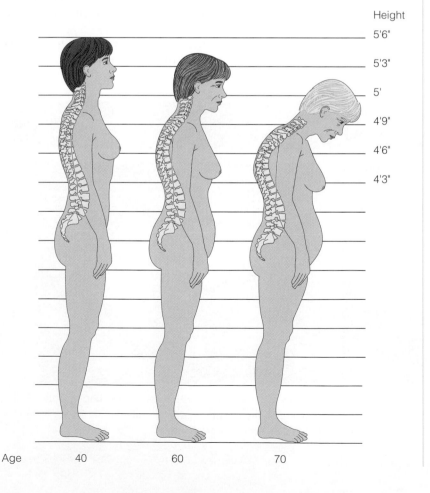

Height

5'6"

5'3"

5'

4'9"

4'6"

4'3"

Age        40              60              70

**Figure 16–4**
Spinal changes caused by osteoporosis.

| Table 16–1 | Risk Factors for Osteoporosis |
|---|---|
| Low bone mass | Low calcium intake |
| Female | Vitamin D deficiency |
| Small frame | Sedentary lifestyle |
| Family history | Cigarette smoking |
| Postmenopausal | Excessive alcohol use |
| Hysterectomy | Caucasian or Asian |
| Amenorrhea | |

## Other Bone Deformities

Paget's disease, or osteitis deformans, results in overproduction of bone, particularly in the skull, vertebrae, and pelvis. The disease begins with bone softening, which is followed by bone overgrowth. The new bone tissue is abnormal and tends to fracture easily. The excessive bony growth causes the skull to enlarge, which often affects cranial nerves; thus vision and hearing are affected. Abnormal bone development causes curvatures in the spinal column and deformities in legs. Another complication of this disease is osteogenic sarcoma. The cause of Paget's disease is unknown, but approximately 20% to 30% of cases are genetically based.

Vertebral column deformities are caused by Paget's disease, tuberculosis, malnourishment, trauma, and various congenital defects. Abnormal lateral curvature is called scoliosis, which occurs to varying degrees of severity and is usually first identified during childhood. It may have a muscular or skeletal origin. Treatment may include bracing or surgery if the defect is severe. Kyphosis, an exaggerated posterior curve of the thoracic spine, occurs more commonly in adults and becomes more noticeable in the elderly (Figure 16–5).

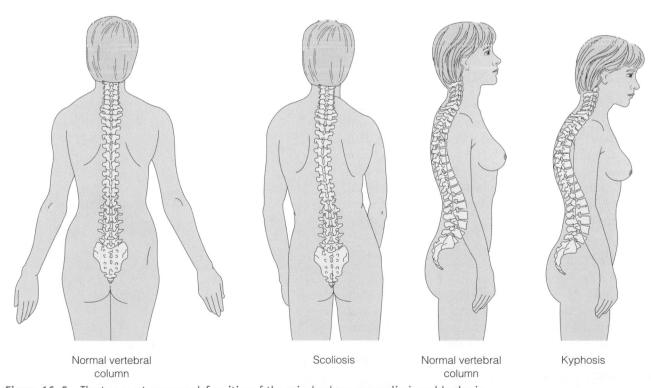

Normal vertebral column     Scoliosis     Normal vertebral column     Kyphosis

**Figure 16–5** The two most common deformities of the spinal column are scoliosis and kyphosis.

## Neoplasia of Bone

Tumors of bone generally cause pain as they progress and make the bone susceptible to fractures. These tumors can be either malignant or benign.

**Benign Bone Tumors**  The most common benign bone tumor is an osteoma. This tumor may give no symptoms, or may appear as a swelling. The tumor will affect joint mobility and cause pain, requiring surgical removal. Giant cell tumors may be benign or malignant. On x-ray, these appear as bubbles. Microscopically, the tumor consists of multinucleated giant cells. These tumors are removed surgically.

**Malignant Bone Tumors**  A primary malignancy of bone is an osteogenic sarcoma. It affects the ends of long bones, frequently at the knee, where enlargement of the bone is observed. It occurs most often in young people. The tumor is first reduced by chemotherapy and then removed surgically. More commonly, malignant bone tumors are secondary tumors that have metastasized from elsewhere. Bone destruction and pain follow. The flat, highly vascular ribs, sternum, and skull are the bones most affected by carcinoma.

## ▶ Diseases of the Joints

Joints are the parts of the skeleton that join bones and thus permit movement. Joints that bear weight—the lower vertebrae, hips and knees—receive a great deal of stress. Diseases of the joints cause pain and limit movement. Muscles, nerves, and bones may all be affected by joint disease.

## Arthritis

Arthritis means inflammation of a joint. Symptoms of arthritis include persistent joint pain and stiffness. Joints may be swollen and may lose mobility and become deformed to the point of losing function. Commonly affected joints include the lower vertebrae, hips, fingers, and knees.

**Rheumatoid Arthritis**  Rheumatoid arthritis is a serious and potentially crippling form of arthritis. It is a systemic disease in which several joints become affected. Symptoms include joint pain and stiffness, particularly on waking. The joints are swollen, red, and warm. The same joints are often affected on both sides of the body. As the disease is systemic, the patient experiences fatigue, weakness, and weight loss. Rheumatoid arthritis begins with an inflammation of the synovial membrane that lines the joints, particularly the small joints of the hands and feet. The membrane thickens and extends into the joint cavity, sometimes filling the space. The inflammation erodes the articular cartilage of the bone ends, causing scar tissue to develop. When this scar tissue turns to bone, the ends of the bones fuse, a condition called ankylosis. The fusion immobilizes and deforms the joint. Figures 16–6 and 16–7 illustrate the crippling swan neck deformity and ulnar deviation characteristic of advanced rheumatoid arthritis in the hands. Rheumatoid nodules may form under the skin, usually near the joints, but they sometimes develop on the white of the eye, too.

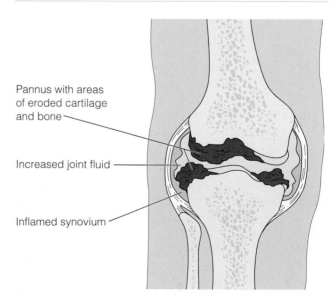

Pannus with areas of eroded cartilage and bone

Increased joint fluid

Inflamed synovium

**Figure 16–6**  Joint inflammation and destruction in rheumatoid arthritis.

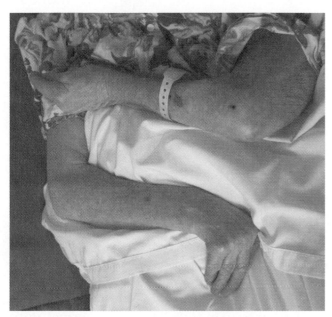

**Figure 16–7** Contractures of rheumatoid arthritis. (Pearson Education/PH College.)

The cause of rheumatoid arthritis is not known, but it appears to be an autoimmune disease. Rheumatoid factors, such as antiglobulin antibodies, combine with immunoglobulin in the synovial fluid to form antibody complexes. Neutrophils are attracted to the joint space and cause destruction. The condition is aggravated by stress, and there is a genetic predisposition toward development of the disease.

Early diagnosis and a good treatment program can reduce pain and the amount of damage done to the joints. A balance between exercise and rest should be achieved. In an acute phase, the joint should be rested to prevent further inflammation. The prescribed exercises help maintain joint function. Exercises for good posture are directed toward removing stress on weight-bearing joints. Anti-inflammatory medications are effective when prescribed by a physician, with aspirin and similar drugs being the most commonly used. Steroids are administered with caution, as they mask the symptoms but do not stop the disease process and have many serious side effects.

**Osteoarthritis** Osteoarthritis is the most common form of arthritis. Unlike rheumatoid arthri-

tis, osteoarthritis may affect only one joint. The individual experiences pain and stiffness in the joint. Muscle tension and fatigue contribute to the aches and pain of osteoarthritis. Arthritis in the lower back may pinch a spinal nerve, such as the sciatic nerve, in which case pain radiates down the back and leg. Affected joints lose their range of motion, and associated muscles become weak.

Degeneration occurs at the articular cartilage of the joint. This cartilage caps the bone surface where bone meets another bone in a joint. This cartilage erodes, exposing the underlying bone, which degenerates and leads to new bone deposits in and around the joint. The bone ends thicken and develop spicules and spurs. Small joints such as the knuckles enlarge and become knobby (Figure 16–8).

Osteoarthritis is probably not associated with routine wear and tear of a joint, as is commonly thought, but rather with joint injury or other

Heberden's node
Bouchard's node

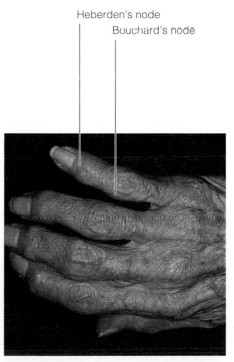

**Figure 16–8** Typical joint changes associated with osteoarthritis. (Courtesy of the American College of Rheumatology.)

chronic irritation. Other than injury, risk factors and causes are not well understood.

Diagnosis of osteoarthritis is made principally by x-rays that show the joint damage and a history of the symptoms. There is no cure for osteoarthritis, but treatment can greatly relieve the pain. A combination of rest and special exercises, medication, and heat applications is generally prescribed. Steroids such as cortisone are not given orally but are sometimes injected into the joint capsule to relieve pain. Surgical replacement of a damaged joint like the hip and knee has become very effective, although factors such as age are important considerations.

**Gout** Gout, often called gouty arthritis, affects the joints of the feet, particularly those of the big toe, and sometimes of the hand, fingers, wrist, or knee. The onset of an acute attack of gout is generally sudden. It sometimes follows a minor injury or excessive eating or drinking, but there may be no accounting for the attack. The affected joints exhibit typical signs of inflammation: pain, heat, swelling, and redness (Figure 16–9). Signs and symptoms may last from days to many weeks. Resolution of an acute attack may be followed by symptom-free periods of 6 months to more than 2 years before recurrence. A chronic form of gout also occurs in which a person experiences persistent arthritis.

Gout can be diagnosed by microscopic examination of aspirated joint fluid, which reveals needle-like urate crystals. High serum level of uric acid is consistent with gout. X-rays of af-

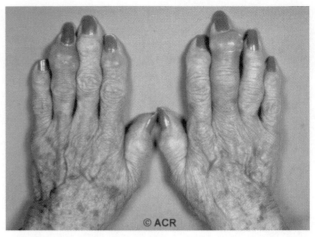

**Figure 16–9** Acute gouty arthritis of the finger joints. (Courtesy of the American College of Rheumatology.)

fected joints may initially appear normal until repeated attacks of chronic gout damages the bone and cartilage at joints.

The cause of gout is unknown, but heredity may be involved. It most frequently affects men over age 40 but also affects postmenopausal women. Excess uric acid in blood results either from a defect in metabolism of purines (a component of nucleic acids), or from abnormal retention of uric acid, or both. The high uric acid level leads to deposits of uric acid crystals in the joints. Uric acid crystals also deposit in the kidneys, stimulating kidney stone formation and irritating the kidney.

Acute gout attacks can be treated with rest, application of hot or cold compresses, anal-

## Prevention ✚ PLUS!

### Bones, Joints, Muscles Benefit from Exercise

In a healthy aging body, muscles lose strength and coordination, bones become thin and brittle, and joints stiffen and lose flexibility. The consequences include greater risk of falls and fractures. These can result in immobility, disability, diminished quality of life, and susceptibility to depression and disease. A vigorous exercise program benefits the bones, joints, and muscles as well as the cardiovascular and respiratory system. However, such a program should not be undertaken without physician guidance. A systematic vigorous program of exercise may not be feasible due to health or may not be appealing. Still, significant physical and psychological benefits can be reaped from daily activities that engage the musculoskeletal system: walking, gardening, doing laundry, and climbing stairs.

gesics, colchicine, and corticosteroids. Chronic gout may be treated with colchicine, which prevents acute attacks, and uricosuric agents such as probenecid that promote excretion of uric acid. If diagnosed early and treated properly, the development of chronic gout can be prevented.

**Septic arthritis** Septic arthritis is considered a medical emergency. It develops as a result of bacterial infection of a joint. Cartilage and bone destruction may lead to ankylosis and life-threatening septicemia (blood-borne bacterial infection). Streptococci and staphylococci cause septic arthritis by invading a joint following trauma or surgery. *Neisseria gonorrhea*, the cause of gonorrhea, may spread to joints via blood from a primary infection site. Antibiotics are required to control the joint infection and to prevent septicemia.

## Bursitis

Bursae are small, fluid-filled sacs located near the joints that cushion and reduce friction on movement. Bursitis is an inflammation of these bursae, and it is a very painful condition. The bursae of the shoulder joint are the most frequently affected, although bursitis can develop at any joint. Repeated irritation or injury of a bursa can cause bursitis. Limitation of movement results from the pain of the inflammation. Treatment includes rest, anti-inflammatories, and moist heat applications. Steroids are sometimes injected into the joint to reduce the inflammatory response.

## Dislocations, Sprains, and Strains

A dislocation is a displacement of bones from their normal position in a joint. Dislocations are most common in the shoulder and finger joints, but they can occur anywhere. The dislocation causes pain and reduced mobility at the involved joint. The bone must be resituated and immobilized to allow healing of torn ligaments and tendons. Congenital dislocations of the hip result from an improperly formed joint, and they are treated in infancy with a cast or surgery.

Sprains result from the wrenching or twisting of a joint such as an ankle that injures the ligaments. Blood vessels and surrounding tissues, muscles, tendons, and nerves may also be damaged. Swelling and discoloration due to hemorrhaging from the ruptured blood vessels occur. A sprain is very painful, and the joint should not be used while it is severely inflamed. Immobilization with a splint or cast might be necessary for more severe sprains. Cold compresses reduce the swelling immediately after the injury, whereas later, heat applications relieve discomfort and speed healing. A "whiplash" is a sprain in which the cervical (neck) ligaments and tissues are injured. Whiplash injuries are often the result of rear-end motor vehicle accidents.

Strains, also called pulled muscles, result from a tearing of a muscle and/or its tendon from excessive use or stretching. Conditioning and warm-up before exercise prevent strains.

## Carpal Tunnel Syndrome

A painful condition of the hand has become quite prevalent in recent years and is known as carpal tunnel syndrome (CTS). It is actually one of a larger class of problems known as repetitive strain injuries (RSI). It usually begins as numbness or tingling in the hand but progresses to pain that can radiate up the arm to the shoulder; the pain is most severe at night. Simple tasks requiring finger movements become difficult. The condition is much more common in women than in men and usually strikes around middle age. Many women report the symptoms during pregnancy, which is attributed to accumulation of fluid within the tissues.

Carpal tunnel syndrome typically develops when the wrists are kept in a bent position for extended periods of time to perform repetitive tasks such as knitting, driving, typing, computing, and piano playing (Figure 16–10). A physician may diagnose carpal tunnel syndrome by requiring certain hand maneuvers. The diagnosis is confirmed by an electromyogram. The test measures the velocity of sensory and motor nerve conduction. If electrical impulses are

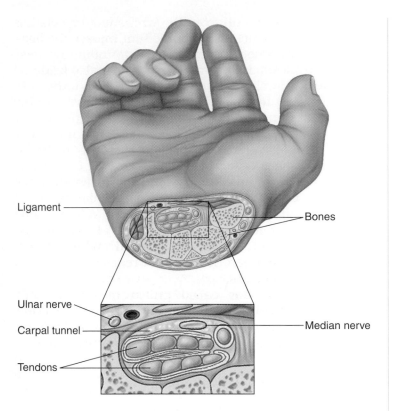

**Figure 16–10**
Cross-section of the wrist showing tendons and nerves involved in carpal tunnel syndrome.

Ligament

Bones

Ulnar nerve

Carpal tunnel

Median nerve

Tendons

slowed as they travel through the carpal tunnel, compression of the nerve is indicated.

Conservative treatments begin with avoiding the repetitive action where possible, at least temporarily. Immobilizing the hand and wrist with a lightweight, molded plastic splint is often adequate for the inflammation to subside. Injection of a steroidal anti-inflammatory drug into the carpal tunnel is sometimes effective. For some individuals, nonsteroidal anti-inflammatory drugs such as aspirin and ibuprofen can reduce symptoms. Surgery may be required to divide the transverse ligament, which is compressing the median nerve. The procedure generally provides permanent relief without affecting hand movement or strength.

## Prevention ✚PLUS!

### Carpal Tunnel Syndrome: An Occupational Hazard

Carpal tunnel syndrome, caused by damage to the median nerve, is a common problem of data processors, computer users, typists, beauticians, and dentists, who often maintain a flexed wrist position. Frequent rest and splinting may help prevent the complications of carpal tunnel syndrome. If surgery is required to relieve pressure on the nerve, a new technique is greatly reducing recovery time and lost work. A tiny video camera enables the surgeon to make two tiny incisions in the wrist and palm, each requiring only one stitch. Recovery is therefore much faster than with the traditional longer incision.

# ▶ Diseases of the Muscles

Skeletal muscle moves the body and provides much of the body's heat. Skeletal muscle function is intimately associated with nervous system function. Muscles cannot function unless they are stimulated by nerves. In Chapter 14, diseases in which the nerves fail to innervate muscles were discussed. Muscles themselves can also be diseased and lose their ability to contract. Another cause of muscle failure is the improper transmission of the impulse for contraction at the myoneural junction, the site at which a nerve ending sends its signal to a muscle cell.

## Muscular Dystrophy (MD)

The term muscular dystrophy includes several forms of the disease, all of which are hereditary. The various forms are transmitted differently and affect different muscles, but all forms result in muscle degeneration, which totally disables the individual.

The most common and serious type is Duchenne, which is caused by a sex-linked gene and affects as many as 33 males per 100,000. Muscular dystrophy can appear at any age, but generally signs appear in the third to fifth year. In Duchenne's muscular dystrophy, a cytoskeletal protein called dystrophin is missing. As a result of this defect, muscle fibers die and are replaced by fat and connective tissue. Because neither of these tissues has the ability to contract, skeletal muscles weaken. A severe form can progress rapidly and affect the muscle of the heart, causing death; other forms progress slowly. In the most severe form of muscular dystrophy, the calf muscles enlarge as a result of fat deposition. The shoulder muscles are weak, which causes the arms to hang limply. A child with this form of muscular dystrophy is very weak and thin, and does not usually live to adulthood.

The diagnosis is based on electromyography, which shows weak muscle contractions. Biopsy of muscle shows abnormal muscle fibers: variation in sizes, fat deposits, and absence of dys-

trophin. Immunologic and molecular biology techniques can diagnose the disease prenatally as well as at birth.

No cure exists. Treatment includes physical and occupational therapy, exercise, and use of orthopedic appliances.

## Myasthenia Gravis (MG)

Myasthenia gravis is a neuromuscular disorder in which neither the nerves nor the muscles are diseased. The failure is in the transmission of the impulse from the nerves to the muscles at the myoneural junction. Lack of stimulation and use leads to muscle atrophy and weakness. Myasthenia gravis affects women more often than men, and the cause is unknown.

The principal symptoms of this disease are fatigue and the inability to use the muscles. The voluntary muscles of the body are affected, including the muscles of facial expression, rendering the person's face expressionless. Eyelid control is lost, and simple actions such as chewing and talking become difficult. The greatest danger in this disease is respiratory failure because the muscles required for respiratory ventilation are unable to contract.

Myasthenia gravis may be classified as an autoimmune disease. Antibodies attach near the myoneural junction and destroy acetylcholine or its receptors. Muscle contraction weakens as a result. Treatment includes drugs that increase acetylcholine levels at the myoneural junction.

The thymus gland, which is involved in the immune response, at least in children, is often enlarged in myasthenia gravis patients. Removal of this gland sometimes brings about a remission but not a cure.

## Tumors of Muscle

Muscle tumors are rare, but when they occur, they are usually highly malignant. A malignant tumor of skeletal muscle is a rhabdomyosarcoma. The tumor requires surgical removal, and the prognosis is poor. The rhabdomyosarcoma metastasizes early and is usually an advanced malignancy when it is diagnosed. Muscle malignancy is rare because muscle cells do not continually divide like blood or skin cells.

# Age-Related Diseases

## Bones

Osteoblast activity declines with age. Because these cells build bone tissue in response to stress, for remodeling or repair, this results in age-related thinning of bones. In addition, aging bone has more minerals and less protein, making the tissue more brittle. Overall, the total amount of bone declines steadily with age. At menopause, bone loss accelerates, making women more susceptible to osteoporosis and its effects. More than 80% of those with osteoporosis are women, and a majority of women over age 60 have osteoporosis.

## Joints

Joint mobility decreases with age because cartilage in movable joints becomes stiffer, ligaments lose flexibility and elasticity, and synovial membranes become fibrous and stiff and produce less synovial fluid. These changes begin at age 20 and become significant by age 30, especially if the joints and muscles are not regularly exercised and stretched. The incidence of arthritis increases with age: While fewer than 20% of young adults have arthritis, 60% of adults over age 60 have some form of arthritis. Most of these cases are osteoarthritis.

## Muscles

Muscles become less sensitive to stimulation with age, meaning that they take longer to contract when stimulated. Recovery following contraction becomes slow, diminishing the ability to sustain repeated contractions and reducing endurance. With age, the number of muscle fibers decreases, and they become shorter and thinner, reducing muscle strength and range of motion. Exercise reduces the rate of these changes and helps maintain muscle mass, strength, and flexibility.

# Diagnostic Tests for Bone, Joint, and Muscle Diseases

X-rays can reveal fractures, joint dislocations, bone deformities, calcification, and other bone damage. MRI (magnetic resonance imaging) uses strong magnetic fields to visualize details of joint anatomy and can show trauma and arthritis damage. CT (computed tomography) scans show details of soft tissues like tendons and ligaments as well as muscle. Arthroscopy is used to visualize the inside of a joint cavity such as the knee. Joint fluid can be aspirated for microscopic and chemical analysis. Electromyography shows muscle function. Biopsy of muscle shows muscle tissue abnormalities.

## CHAPTER SUMMARY

A variety of bacteria cause bone infections like osteomyelitis. Rickets and osteomalacia manifest themselves by soft and deformed bones. Abnormally thin and fragile bone is the principle sign of osteoporosis. Bone is also decalcified in hyperparathyroidism. Bone cancer may be manifested by spontaneous fractures.

The most common joint disease is arthritis, which has several forms. Rheumatoid arthritis is progressive and causes severe joint deformity. Osteoarthritis affects most people to some extent with age. Gouty arthritis is caused by a disorder in purine metabolism. Septic arthritis is potentially serious joint infection that can lead to septicemia. Dislocations, sprains, and strains are painful injuries of joints. A wrist condition that has become very common is carpal tunnel syndrome.

Muscular dystrophy is an inherited sex-linked degenerative disease in which muscles lose the ability to contract. Muscles lose the ability to contract in myasthenia gravis also, but the failure is in the muscle receptors of the neuronal transmitter acetylcholine rather than in the muscles themselves. Tumors are rare in muscles, but when they occur, they are usually highly malignant.

## RESOURCES

Beers, M. H., & R. Berkow. *The Merck Manual of Diagnosis and Therapy,* 17th ed., John Wiley & Sons, 1999.

*Professional Guide to Diseases,* 6th ed. Springhouse, 1998.

Arking, Robert. *Biology of Aging,* 2nd ed. Sinauer Associates, 1998.

# DISEASES AT A GLANCE

## Bones, Joints, and Muscles

| DISEASE | ETIOLOGY | SIGNS AND SYMPTOMS |
| --- | --- | --- |
| Osteomyelitis | Infection by staphylococci | Pain, redness, heat, chills, fever, tachycardia, nausea, weight loss |
| Rickets | Vitamin D deficiency in childhood | Deformation of bones, knock-knee, bow-leg, curved spine, nodular swellings at rib ends and joints, enlarged and square head, flaccid muscles |
| Osteomalacia | Vitamin D deficiency in adults | Muscular weakness, weight loss, pain in bones, deformation of bones, easily fractured bones |
| Osteitis fibrosa cystica | Hyperparathyroidism | Weakened bones, deformation of bones, easily fractured bones, kidney stone formation |
| Osteoporosis | Calcium deficiency, decreased bone density | Decreased height from vertebral compression fractures, curvature of spine, easily fractured bones |
| Paget's disease | Idiopathic, genetic | Enlarged skull, nerve compression curvatures in spine, and deformed legs |
| Bone tumors | Idiopathic; commonly metastatic | Painless lump in bone tissue, fracture without trauma |
| Rheumatoid arthritis | Autoimmunity | Pain and stiffness in joints, swollen, red, warm joints, bilateral involvement, exacerbation and remission, rheumatoid nodules, crippling deformities |
| Osteoarthritis | Idiopathic; may follow joint injury or chronic irritation | Aches, pain, stiffness in joints, limited range of motion, muscle weakness around affected joint, enlarged joints, bone spurs; may involve only one joint |
| Gout | Inherited defect in uric acid metabolism leads to high levels of urate and uric acid deposition in joints | Severe pain, heat, swelling, redness in affected joint; acute onset |
| Septic arthritis | Bacterial infection of joint | Pain, redness, swelling, bone and joint destruction |

| DIAGNOSIS | TREATMENT |
| --- | --- |
| Bone scan, CT scan, MRI, WBC count | Antibiotics, surgery |
| Physical exam, x-ray | Vitamin D–fortified milk, sunlight, cod liver oil |
| Physical exam, x-ray | Vitamin-D-fortified milk, sunshine, cod liver oil, calcium and phosphorous supplements |
| Hypercalcemia, x-ray, bone density scan | Reduce PTH level, orthopedic surgery |
| X-ray and bone scan | Pain relief, fracture treatment, some medical treatment (estrogens, calcitonin, bisphosphonates) |
| Physical exam | Surgical, limited |
| X-ray, biopsy | Surgery |
| Physical exam, presence of rheumatoid factor in blood | Mild exercise, anti-inflammatories, steroid |
| X-ray, history | Pain relief, mild exercise and rest, heat applications, steroids, surgery |
| Uric acid level in blood, x-ray | Analgesics, hot and cold compresses, colchicine, probenecid |
| History, blood and synovial cultures | Antibiotics |

# DISEASES AT A GLANCE (*continued*)

## Bones, Joints, and Muscles

| DISEASE | ETIOLOGY | SIGNS AND SYMPTOMS |
|---|---|---|
| Bursitis | Overuse of joint | Pain at joint especially during use |
| Carpal tunnel syndrome | Repetitive use of wrist | Numbness and tingling of hand, pain radiating to shoulder, limited finger movement, severe at night |
| Muscular dystrophy | Defect in X-linked gene for muscle protein dystrophin | Weakened muscles, muscles may enlarge as fat is deposited; muscles degenerate |
| Myasthenia gravis | Autoimmunity interferes with nerve transmission to muscles | Fatigue, muscle paralysis |

| DIAGNOSIS | TREATMENT |
| --- | --- |
| Physical exam and history | Moist heat, analgesics, steroids, rest |
| Physical exam, electromyography | Splinting hand and wrist, surgery |
| Physical exam, serum enzymes, muscle biopsy | Physical therapy, orthopedic procedures |
| Antibody level, response to anticholinesterase drugs, electromyography | Thymectomy, anticholinesterase drugs, steroids, immune suppression |

# Interactive Activities

## Cases for Critical Thinking

1. A 68-year-old woman visits her physician and reports that her back hurts. Physical exam finds kyphosis and that she has lost height since her last visit a few years ago. What is a likely diagnosis for this case? Name two treatment possibilities that the physician might suggest. Name something that might have helped prevent this condition, especially if it had been initiated and applied at an earlier age.

2. A 55-year-old carpenter reports persistent swelling and pain in the knuckles of his right hand. What information do you need to determine the type of joint disease he has?

3. A 20-year-old woman has worsening pain in her leg below the knee. She says she feels "a little weak and out of sorts" and has stopped her jogging routine. How can you determine whether she has a type of arthritis, or a bone infection, or a fracture, or a joint sprain?

## Multiple Choice

1. Bones are soft in rickets due to a _____ deficiency.
   a. vitamin A          c. vitamin D
   b. vitamin C          d. vitamin K

2. Osteomalacia affects _____.
   a. the joints of young children
   b. the joints of adults
   c. the bones of children
   d. the bones of adults

3. Carpal tunnel syndrome is caused by damage to the _____.
   a. wrist              c. median nerve
   b. fingers            d. forearm muscles

4. Biopsy in addition to electromyography is a diagnostic test for _____.
   a. gout               c. carpal tunnel syndrome
   b. sprain             d. Duchenne's MD

5. _____ is the most common form of arthritis.
   a. Rheumatoid arthritis   c. Septic arthritis
   b. Osteoarthritis         d. Gout

6. Ankylosis and immobility results in severe _____.
   a. rheumatoid arthritis   c. septic arthritis
   b. osteoarthritis         d. gout

7. Colchicine and corticosteroids are used to treat acute cases of _____.
   a. rheumatoid arthritis   c. septic arthritis
   b. osteoarthritis         d. gout

8. Which of these is NOT due to calcium deficiency?
   a. osteoporosis           c. osteogenic sarcoma
   b. osteomalacia           d. rickets

9. Which of these is a type of autoimmune disorder?
   a. rhabdomyosarcoma       c. myasthenia gravis
   b. Duchenne's MD          d. osteitis fibrosa cystica

10. Streptococci and staphylococci are associated with _____.
    a. Pott's disease        c. osteomyelitis
    b. tuberculosis          d. osteoporosis

## True or False

_____ 1. Osteomyelitis affects principally children and adolescents.

_____ 2. Women with large bone mass are most prone to osteoporosis.

_____ 3. An osteoma is a malignant bone tumor.

_____ 4. Rheumatoid arthritis is the most crippling form of arthritis.

_____ 5. Osteomyelitis is a local and systemic infection.

_____ 6. Osteoarthritis is the most common form of arthritis.

_____ 7. Muscular dystrophy is a hereditary disease.

_____ 8. Myasthenia gravis is an infectious disease of the muscles.

_____ 9. Rhabdomyosarcoma is a malignant bone tumor.

_____ 10. There is no cure for osteoarthritis.

## Fill-Ins

1. A special form of tuberculosis that affects the vertebral column of children is called
   _____.

2. A disease of infancy and early childhood in which the bones do not properly ossify, or harden,
   is called _____.

3. The word _____ means increased porosity of the bone, which makes the bone abnormally fragile.

4. A very painful condition caused by deposits of uric acid crystals in the joints is called
   _____.

5. The principle minerals in bone are _____ and _____.

6. Bone is deposited by cells called _____.

7. The _____ membrane becomes inflamed in rheumatoid arthritis.

8. Antibodies against acetylcholine receptors are the cause of _____
   _____.

9. Colchicine is an effective treatment for _____.

10. Vitamin D is required for dietary absorption of _____.

## MedMedia Wrap-Up

**www.prenhall.com/mulvihill**
Remember to visit this website for extra study practice, including exercises, Internet links, news updates, and an audio glossary.

**Activity CD-ROM**
Check out the CD-ROM in the back of this book. You will find games, exercises, puzzles, and videos to help enhance your understanding of this chapter.

# Diseases of the Skin

## Learning Objectives

After studying this chapter, you should be able to

- Describe the normal structure and function of skin
- Describe the key characteristics of major diseases of skin
- Explain the cause of skin diseases
- Name the diagnostic procedures for diseases of skin
- Describe the treatment options for diseases of skin

## Fact or Fiction?

Everyone can get a suntan.

*Fiction: Some people always
burn and never tan, but everyone can develop skin cancer.*

# Disease Chronicle

## Trench Foot

Soldiers in the First World War suffered from trench foot, a fungal infection that thrived in the skin and tissues of feet damaged by chronic exposure to cold, wet, unsanitary conditions. Although healthy skin can resist fungal infections, soldiers stood for hours in waterlogged trenches without removing wet socks or boots, causing their feet to go numb. Reduced circulation caused the skin to turn blue or red, but more importantly, made it difficult to fight infections. Left untreated, gangrene developed and amputation was necessary. British soldiers were ordered to have three pairs of socks with them and to dry their feet and change their socks at least twice per day. Soldiers were also told to cover their dry feet with grease made from whale oil. It is estimated that a battalion at the front used ten gallons of whale oil every day.

## MedMedia
www.prenhall.com/mulvihill

Use the web address to the left to access the free, interactive Companion Website created for this textbook. It features chapter-specific exercises, Internet links, news links, and an audio glossary. Additionally, explore the CD-ROM that accompanies this book to discover Disease Focus videos and a rich array of activities that accompany this chapter.

# ▶ Functions of the Skin

The skin, or the integumentary system, is a vital organ and a protective wrap. As an organ, the skin regulates temperature, senses pain, keeps substances and microorganisms from entering the body, and provides a shield from the harmful effects of the sun.

The skin indicates malfunction within the body through color changes. Cyanosis, a blue coloration of the skin, signals a lack of oxygen and indicates a cardiovascular or pulmonary-problem. Jaundice indicates liver disease, bile obstruction, or hemolysis of red blood cells, in which case an accumulation of the bilirubin in the blood produces the yellowish coloration. An abnormal redness accompanies polycythemia (Chapter 8), carbon monoxide poisoning, and fever. Pallor, or whitening of the skin, may indicate anemia.

Skin color, texture, and folds identify people as individuals. Anything that goes wrong with the skin function or appearance can have important consequences for physical and mental health.

# ▶ Structure of the Skin

Each layer of the skin performs specific tasks. The outermost layer of the skin is the epidermis, consisting of stratified or layered squamous epithelium. The top portion of the epidermis, the stratum corneum, contains keratin. Keratin is a tough, fibrous protein produced by cells called keratinocytes, and it protects the skin from harmful substances. At the bottom of the epidermis are the melanocytes, or the cells that produce melanin. Melanin is the dark pigment of the skin that protects the body from the harmful rays of the sun.

The dermis lies below the epidermis. The dermis is composed of connective tissue that supports blood and lymph vessels, elastic fibers, nerves, hair follicles, sweat glands, and sebaceous or oil glands.

The subcutaneous tissue lies under the dermis and connects the skin to underlying structures. Adipose tissue or fat cells in the subcutaneous tissue help insulate the body from heat and cold. Figure 17–1 shows the structure of the skin.

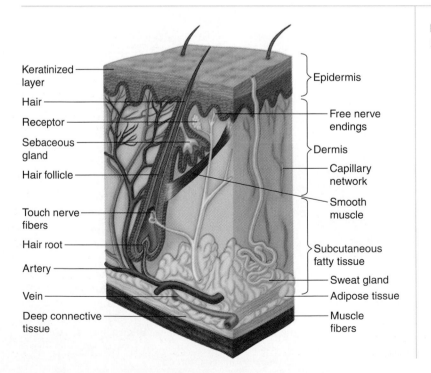

**Figure 17–1**
Structure of the skin.

Keratinized layer
Hair
Receptor
Sebaceous gland
Hair follicle
Touch nerve fibers
Hair root
Artery
Vein
Deep connective tissue

Epidermis
Free nerve endings
Dermis
Capillary network
Smooth muscle
Subcutaneous fatty tissue
Sweat gland
Adipose tissue
Muscle fibers

## ▶ Skin Lesions

Skin diseases are identified and classified according to characteristic lesions. Revealing characteristics of these lesions include the size, shape, color, and location as well as the presence or absence of other signs and symptoms. Pruritus (itching), edema (swelling), erythema (redness), and inflammation usually accompany lesions and are helpful in making a diagnosis.

Lesions may be small, blisterlike eruptions, called vesicles, or larger fluid-containing lesions, called bullae. Lesions containing pus are referred to as pustules, and nodules and tumors are lesions that are hard to the touch. Lesions that are flat are called macular, whereas those that are raised are termed papular. An area of skin reddened by congested blood vessels resulting from injury or inflammation is said to be erythematous. Pruritus, or itching, accompanies many skin diseases, especially those caused by allergies or parasitic infestation. Figure 17–2 shows various skin lesions.

## ▶ Infectious Skin Diseases

Bacteria, viruses, fungi, and parasites may cause infections of the skin. Normal microbes that reside on the skin cause the most common skin infections. Infections from less common microbes may develop in high-risk individuals (immunocompromised or diabetic individuals) and those who reside in nursing homes and hospitals. Most skin infections are not serious unless systemic involvement occurs.

### Bacterial Skin Infections

**Impetigo**   Impetigo is an acute, contagious skin infection common in children. It is caused by streptococci and staphylococci carried in the nose and passed to the skin. The face and hands are most frequently affected. Erythema and oozing vesicles and pustules develop. The vesicles rupture and become covered with a yellow crust. Fever and enlarged lymph nodes may accompany the infection. The lesions should be washed with soap and water, kept dry, and exposed to air. Antibiotic ointment may be used, and oral antibiotics are sometimes prescribed to treat the infection systemically.

**Erysipelas**   Erysipelas is an inflammatory skin infection caused by streptococci. Most commonly, the infections appear on the face, arm, or leg. Sometimes the infection begins where skin is broken. A shiny, swollen, and red rash may develop initially and is often accompanied by small blisters. The erythemastous rash is hot to touch and tender. Fever and chills develop when the infection is severe. Mild erysipelas is self-limiting; however, when the infection is severe, treatment with antibiotics is required.

**Cellulitis**   Cellulitis is a spreading infection of the skin that is most often caused by streptococci. The infection is common on the legs and begins with skin damage. The involved area is generally swollen, red, and tender. Symptoms of the infection may include fever and chills. Prompt treatment with antibiotics prevents the spread of the infection to the blood and vital organs (Figure 17–3).

**Folliculitis, Furuncles, and Carbuncles**   Folliculitis is an inflammation of the hair follicles caused by infection with staphylococci. A small number of pustules develop in the hair follicle. This condition commonly occurs in young men and affects thighs, buttocks, head, and scalp (Figure 17–4). Folliculitis is effectively treated with daily cleansing with an antiseptic soap. Severe cases require treatment with oral antibiotics.

Boils or furuncles are large, tender, swollen, raised lesions caused by staphylococci. The infection appears in hair follicles located on the face, neck, breasts, or buttocks. The core of the furuncle become necrotic and liquefies forming pus (Figure 17–5). Furuncles are effectively treated with application of moist heat, antiseptic skin cleansing, oral antibiotic administration, and incision and drainage.

Carbuncles are clusters of boils. These lesions arise in a cluster of hair follicles. Carbuncles develop and heal more slowly than boils. They

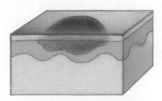

A macule is a discolored spot on the skin; freckle

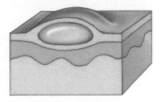

A wheal is a localized, evanescent elevation of the skin that is often accompanied by itching; urticaria

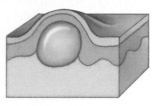

A papule is a solid, circumscribed, elevated area on the skin; pimple

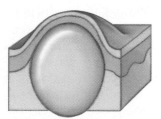

A nodule is a larger papule; acne vulgaris

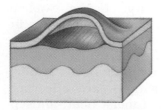

A vesicle is a small fluid filled sac; blister. A bulla is a large vesicle.

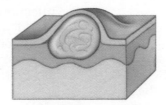

A pustule is a small, elevated, circumscribed lesion of the skin that is filled with pus; varicella (chickenpox)

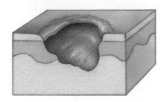

An erosion or ulcer is an eating or gnawing away of tissue; decubitus ulcer

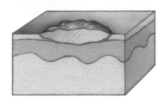

A crust is a dry, serous or seropurulent, brown, yellow, red, or green exudation that is seen in secondary lesions; eczema

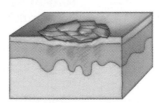

A scale is a thin, dry flake of cornified epithelial cells; psoriasis

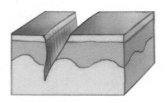

A fissure is a crack-like sore or slit that extends through the epidermis into the dermis; athlete's foot

**Figure 17–2**
Skin signs are objective evidence of an illness or disorder. They can be seen, measured, or felt.

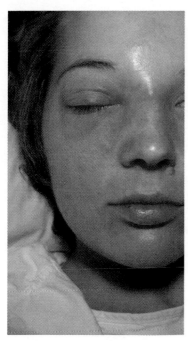

**Figure 17–3** Cellulitis indicated by redness and swelling around the eye. (Courtesy of the CDC/Dr. Thomas F. Sellers/Emory University, 1963.).

appear mostly in men and are commonly located on the back of the neck. Carbuncles are treated with application of moist heat, antiseptic skin cleansing, oral antibiotic administration, and incision and drainage.

## Viral Skin Infections

Many types of viruses invade the skin. The most common viruses cause cold sores or fever blisters and warts.

**Herpes** Herpes is a large family of viruses that cause clusters of fluid-filled vesicles on the skin. The virus remains in the body for life.

Herpes simplex type I causes cold sores or fever blisters. The lesions generally form near the mouth or lips, as in Figure 17–6. The virus may be harbored in the body for a long time with no ill effect, but may suddenly become active. Cold sores frequently form when a person's resistance to infection is low or at a time of emotional stress. They often accompany a respiratory infection such as the common cold, or they develop during menstruation. A bad sunburn sometimes triggers the formation of cold sores. Antiviral drugs are used, and antibiotics are sometimes applied topically to treat secondary bacterial invasion.

Herpes simplex type II causes genital herpes (see Chapter 12 for more information).

Herpes varicella-zoster causes chicken pox, one of the most common childhood infectious diseases. The virus can be transmitted by airborne particles or by direct contact. A rash forms over the face, trunk, and extremities. The rash spots develop into vesicles in a few days,

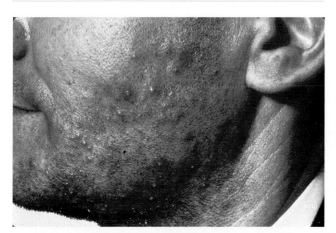

**Figure 17–4** The lesions of folliculitis are pustules surrounded by areas of erythema.

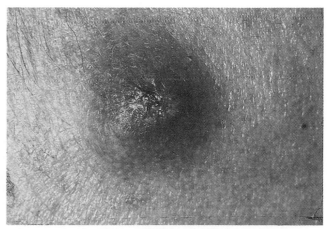

**Figure 17–5** A furuncle (or boil) is a deep, red, painful nodule.

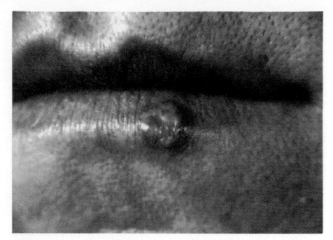

**Figure 17–6** Typical cold sores or fever blisters caused by the virus herpes simplex. (Courtesy of the CDC/Dr. Herrman, 1964.)

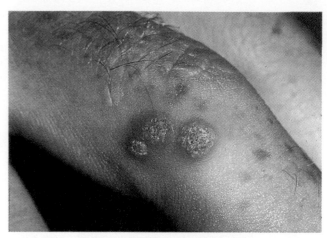

**Figure 17–7** The common wart is a lesion of the skin caused by a virus. It commonly appears as a raised, dome-shaped lesion.

causing intense pruritis. The vesicles break, dry, and become crusty. Treatment is usually symptomatic.

If an adult develops limited immunity to herpes varicella-zoster, the virus may lie dormant for years after recovery from chicken pox. The virus may flare up during periods of stress, diseases, trauma, or immunosuppression, causing painful vesicles called shingles (see Chapter 14).

**Warts** Viruses cause warts, or verucca vulgaris, of the skin. Viral infection of keratinocytes causes them to proliferate, forming a benign neoplasm with a rough, keratinized surface. Warts are most common in children and young adults, developing particularly on the hands. They are often multiple and are contagious, being spread by scratching. Warts sometimes disappear spontaneously, but only a physician can safely remove them via surgery, cryosurgery, or laser. If the virus remains in the body, the warts tend to recur (Figure 17–7).

Warts are not serious or painful except when they form on the soles of the feet. These warts are called plantar warts, and in contrast to warts elsewhere on the body, which appear as an elevation from the skin, plantar warts grow inward. Pressure on the soles of the feet makes them very painful, and they are often difficult to remove permanently.

## Fungal Skin Infections

Fungi, or dermatophytes, that infect the skin tend to live on the dead, top layer of the skin. Fungal infections may or may not cause symptoms. Minor infections cause mild irritation and swelling. Serious infections generally cause itching, swelling, blisters, and severe scales.

Fungi usually reside on moist areas of the body where skin surfaces touch. The skin folds of the breast, groin, and toes are the most common areas affected. Obese people, with excessive skin folds, are more susceptible to fungal infections.

**Tinea** Tinea, or ringworm, is caused by many different fungi and is classified by its location on the body. The fungi particularly reside in warm, moist areas of the body but may also occur with hairy skin on the head, groin, arms, and legs. The fungi can produce symptoms ranging from mild scales cracking skin to painful, raw rashes. Treatment includes keeping the affected area clean and dry, and application of topical antifungal creams, powders, and solutions.

Tinea corporis, or body ringworm, affects smooth areas of skin on the arms, legs, and body. It is characterized by a pink to reddish rash that sometimes forms round patches with clear areas in the center (Figure 17–8).

Scales and fissures on the soles of the feet and between the toes characterize tinea pedis, or athlete's foot (Figure 17–9). A foul odor usually accompanies the lesions. Tinea pedis is highly contagious and is spread by direct contact with contaminated surfaces.

Tinea cruris, or jock itch, generally affects the groin and upper and inner thighs. The fungi cause red, ringlike areas with blisters (Figure 17–10). Tinea cruris develops more frequently during warm weather.

Tinea capitis (Figure 17–11), or scalp ringworm, is highly contagious and most commonly occurs in children. This fungus may produce a mild, scaly rash or a patch of hair loss without a rash.

Tinea unguium, or nail fungus, typically affects toenails, rarely fingernails. This fungus is

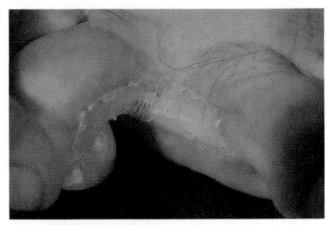

**Figure 17–9** Tinea pedia, or athlete's foot. (Courtesy of the CDC/Dr. Lucille K. Georg, 1964.)

difficult to treat because it resides under the nail. The infection begins at the nail tips, causing white patches and eventually turning the nail brown. The nail thickens and cracks. If left untreated, the fungus may destroy the entire nail and tends to spread to other nails (Figure 17–12).

Tinea barbae causes barber's itch. The fungus affects bearded areas of the face and neck. This fungus may produce deep, inflammatory pustules and crusting around hairs (Figure 17–13).

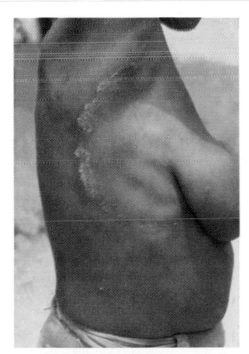

**Figure 17–8** Tinea corporis, or body ringworm. (Courtesy of the CDC/Lucille K. Georg, 1964.)

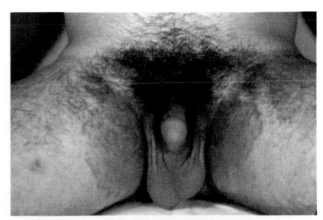

**Figure 17–10** Tinea cruris, or jock itch. (© Custom Medical Stock Photo.)

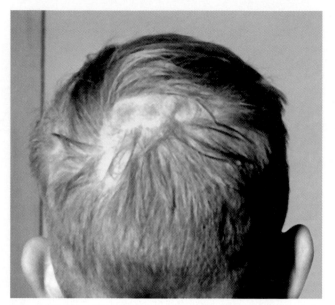

**Figure 17–11** Tinea capitis, or scalp ringworm. (Courtesy of the CDC, 1959.)

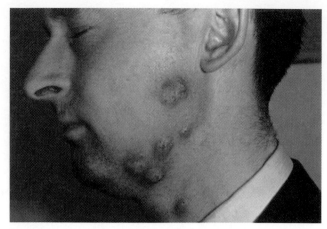

**Figure 17–13** Tinea barbae, or barber's itch. (Courtesy of the CDC, 1975.)

**Candidiasis** Candidiasis is a fungal infection that is caused by the fungus *Candida*. This infection appears on the skin, mucous membranes, or fingernail. Candidiasis on the skin may produce patches of itchy red blisters and pustules. *Candida* growing on the nail bed produces redness and swelling. The nail may turn white or yellow in color and separate from the finger or toe.

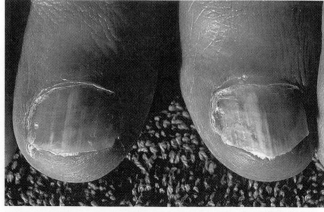

**Figure 17–12** Tinea unguium, or nail fungus. (Courtesy of the CDC/Dr. Edwin P. Ewing, Jr., 1997.)

| Table 17–1 | Ringworm or Tinea Classification and Symptoms |
|---|---|
| **Tinea** | **Symptoms** |
| **Tinea corporis** | Body ringworm; pink to reddish rash sometimes forms round patches with clear areas in the center |
| **Tinea pedia** | Athlete's foot; scales and fissures occur on the soles of the feet and between toes; a foul odor usually accompanies lesions |
| **Tinea cruris** | Jock itch; red, ringlike areas with blisters |
| **Tinea capitis** | Scalp ringworm; mild, scaly rash or patch of hair loss without a rash |
| **Tinea unguium** | Nail fungus; white patches on nails, eventually turn the nail brown; nail thickens and cracks, and may be destroyed |
| **Tinea barbae** | Barber's itch; deep, inflammatory pustules and crusting around hairs |

Vaginal *Candida* infections are common in pregnant women, diabetics, or those who are immunocompromised. Vaginal candidiasis is commonly known as a yeast infection and frequently occurs after antibiotic therapy. Oral antibiotics suppress resident vaginal bacterial flora that normally inhibits overgrowth of *Candida.* Symptoms include a white "cottage cheese"-like discharge from the vagina, accompanied by burning, itching, and redness. Vaginal candidiasis is effectively treated with vaginal antifungal creams or oral antifungal agents (Figure 17–14).

Creamy white patches on the tongue or side of the mouth often characterize a *Candida* infection of the mouth, or thrush. The patches are often painful and can easily be scraped off. Thrush is common in young healthy children, immunosuppressed adults, and diabetics. Long-term treatment of oral thrush with topical liquids or oral antifungals is generally required.

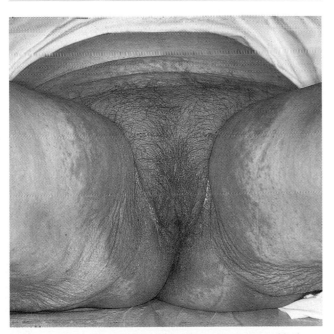

**Figure 17–14** *Candida albicans,* a fungus, causes a skin infection characterized by erythema, pustules, and a typical white substance covering the area.

## Parasitic Infestations

**Pediculosis,** or louse infestations, are classified into three categories: head lice, pubic lice, and body lice.

Head lice are common among schoolchildren, and although annoying, these parasites are not dangerous and do not carry epidemic disease. Lice are spread from head to head directly or indirectly by shared combs, scarves, hats, and bed linen. Itching, the first symptom, results from the saliva of lice as they penetrate the scalp and engorge on human blood. The scratching that follows can open the skin to other invading organisms. Adult head lice are difficult to see, but their white eggs, called nits, can be located on the hair shaft. Treatment includes use of medicated shampoos followed by use of a fine-toothed comb. Over-the-counter medications are also available.

Pubic lice infest pubic hair of both men and women, and are generally spread by sexual contact. The lice do not spread other sexually transmitted diseases. Treatment includes use of a prescription cream (see Chapter 12).

Body lice are most common among underprivileged, transient people. This type of infestation can be prevented with good grooming and hygiene. Body lice can spread serious disease, and they have been responsible for typhus epidemics among soldiers during wartime.

**Scabies,** commonly called "the itch," is a contagious skin disease usually associated with poor living conditions. It is caused by a parasite called a mite. The female mite burrows into skin folds in the groin, under the breasts, and between fingers and toes. As she burrows, she lays eggs in the tunnels, the eggs hatch, and the cycle starts again. The intense itching is caused by hypersensitivity to the mite. Blisters and pustules develop, and the tunnels in the skin appear as grayish lines. Scratching opens the lesions to secondary bacterial infection. Scabies is transmitted by close personal contact and can be linked to a venereal disease. Epidemics of scabies are common in camps and barracks.

To recover from scabies, the mites and eggs must be totally destroyed by hot baths, scrubbing, and medications to eliminate them.

Underwear and bedding that harbor the eggs must be changed frequently and properly laundered, as must be done with lice. The itch may persist while treatment is being administered.

## ▶ Hypersensitivity or Immune Disorders of the Skin

The skin frequently manifests allergic or hypersensitivity reactions. This fact serves as a basis for the patch tests given to determine specific allergies. Some diseases of the skin develop in atopic people, persons with a genetic predisposition to allergies. Others occur in anyone who has been sensitized to an allergen such as poison ivy. Emotional stress frequently triggers or exacerbates an allergy-caused skin disease.

### Insect Bites

Insect bites and stings can produce local inflammatory reactions that may vary in appearance. Acute reactions may appear as hives, whereas more chronic reactions may appear as papules or bullous. See Chapter 2 for more information on allergy to insect bites.

### Urticaria (Hives)

Urticaria, or hives, results from a vascular reaction of the skin to an allergen. The word *urticaria* is derived from a Latin word that means "plants covered with stinging nettles." The lesions are wheals, rounded elevations with red edges and pale centers. Wheals develop most often at pressure points like those under tight clothing, but they may appear anywhere on the skin or mucous membranes.

The allergic response causes damage to mast cells, which then release histamine. Histamine causes blood vessels to dilate and become more permeable. Blood proteins and fluid ooze out of the capillaries into the tissues and result in edema. This irritation to the tissues causes intense itching.

Urticaria is generally treated with steroids, antihistamines, and calamine lotion applied topically to reduce the itching. If the cause of the allergic reaction can be determined, that allergen should be avoided. Foods that are a common cause of hives include certain berries, chocolate, nuts, and seafood. Other allergens, discussed in Chapter 2, frequently cause urticaria in the hypersensitive person. An attack of hives can also be brought on by emotional stress.

### Eczema

Eczema, also called contact dermatitis, is a noncontagious inflammatory skin disorder. Eczema results from sensitization that develops from skin contact with various agents, plants, chemicals, and metals. Poison ivy and poison oak, dyes used for hair or clothing, and metals, particularly nickel, used in costume jewelry are examples of allergens that can cause eczema.

Eczema is a delayed type of allergic response (Chapter 2) in which lymphocytes are sensitized by an antigen, such as poison ivy, and react with it on subsequent exposure. The typical inflammatory reaction occurs: dilated blood vessels, reddened skin, and edema. Vesicles and bullae develop from the excess tissue fluid, and the lesions are very itchy. Scratching causes the vesicles to burst and ooze, and the eczema is thus spread. Scaly crusts form on the ruptured lesions.

Contact dermatitis can affect anyone and is not limited to the genetically allergic person. Skin that has been damaged is more easily sensitized by contact with allergens than is healthy skin. Emotional stress can also be a factor in sensitization. Corticosteroids are sometimes used to reduce the inflammatory reaction. Patients with dermatitis are shown in Figures 17–15 and 17–16.

### Poison Ivy

Contact with poison ivy can cause an extremely itchy rash with blisters and hivelike swelling; the response is a typical example of allergic contact dermatitis. Severity of the condition depends on the amount of plant resin on the skin and the individual's sensitivity to it. Some people are apparently immune to the resin. An ini-

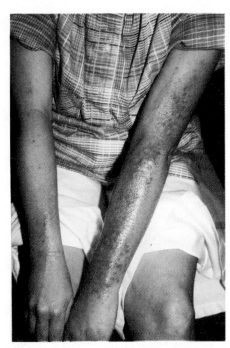

**Figure 17–15** Photodermatitis. (Courtesy of Jason L. Smith, MD.)

tial exposure to the poison ivy plant produces no visible effect but sensitizes the person to subsequent exposure. The rash usually develops a few hours or a few days after contact. Topical cortisone-type cream, gel, or spray are use to reduce inflammation.

## Drug Eruptions

Adverse drug reactions manifest more often on the skin than any other organ system. Topical drug reactions vary in severity from mild pimples over a small area to peeling of the entire skin. Skin reactions may be serious enough to cause anaphylaxis, shock, or death. The most common offending drugs are penicillin, sulfa, anticonvulsants, tetracycline, morphine, codeine, and anti-inflammatory medications. A thorough medical history including current medications can help diagnose the adverse drug reaction and determine the medication that must be changed. Table 17–2 summarizes the most common rashes caused by drugs.

## ▶ Benign Tumors

Benign tumors of the skin are fairly common and usually only a cosmetic problem.

### Nevus (Mole)

A **nevus** is a small, dark skin growth that develops from pigment-producing cells or melanocytes. Moles may be flat or raised and vary in size. Most people have about 10 moles. The moles themselves are usually harmless, but they can become malignant. Sudden changes in moles such as enlargement with an irregular border, darkening, inflammation, and bleeding are warning signs of malignant melanoma. Nevi can be removed by excision or cryosurgery. In cryosurgery, abnormal tissues are destroyed by exposure to extremely cold temperatures. Cold nitrous oxide gas is pumped through a probe. The gas makes the tip of the probe very cold. A physician then touches the tip of the probe to the nevi.

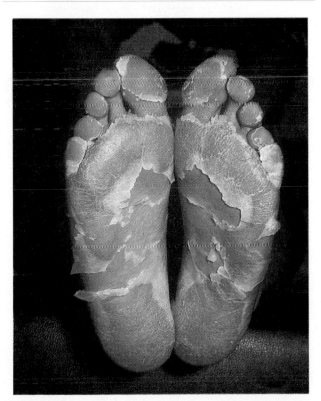

**Figure 17–16** Exfoliative dermatitis is an inflammatory skin disorder causing excessive skin peeling.

## Table 17–2 Common Rashes Caused by Drugs

| Skin Eruption | Description of Lesion | Medication Commonly Associated with Eruption |
|---|---|---|
| Acneiform | • Appear like acne on any part of the body<br>• Unlike common acne, these lesions appear suddenly | Prednisone, oral contraceptives, anticonvulsant medications, lithium |
| Exfoliative dermatitis | • Large areas of skin become erythematous and scaly and slough off (Figure 17-11)<br>• May follow other drug eruptions<br>• Associated with systemic infections and reactions | Sulfa drugs, penicillin, gold compounds, vitamin A |
| Epidermal necrolysis | • Painful red area that may develop blisters (Figure 17-12)<br>• Top layer of skin peels in sheet<br>• Skin appears scalded<br>• Is the most serious skin eruption, 30% of cases result in death from fluid loss or secondary infection | Ibuprofen, penicillin, sulfa drugs |
| Fixed drug eruption | • Caused exclusively by drugs<br>• Red lesions with sharp borders that appear darker in color than the surrounding unaffected skin<br>• Have a propensity to reappear at the same site each time the causative drug is reintroduced | Aspirin, acetaminophen, penicillin, tetracycline, sulfa, codeine, morphine |
| Urticaria | • Hives with intense itching<br>• Sudden onset, resolves within 24 hours after the offending drug has been stopped<br>• Edematous, flat lesions | Aspirin, penicillin, sulfa, codeine, morphine, ibuprofen |
| Maculopapular | • Flat, red lesions involve extensive areas and appear within a week after the causative drug has been started<br>• Pruritus may or may not be present<br>• Resolve 7 to 14 days after the offending drug has been stopped | Ampicilin, amoxicillin, allopurinol, sulfa |
| Photosensitive | • Require the presence of light and the offending drug to occur<br>• Manifest as fluid-filled lesions and sunburn (Figure 17-13) | Sulfa, tetracycline, anticonvulsant medications, antipsychotic medications, ibuprofen, naproxen |
| Purpura | • Characterized by small hemorrhages under the skin<br>• Lesions are purplish in color (Figure 17-14) | Diuretics, penicillin, sulfa, coumadin |
| Stevens-Johnson | • Small hivelike blisters that most commonly occur on mucous membranes<br>• May be accompanied by fever, fatigue<br>• Most common type of severe drug eruption<br>• Mortality is estimated in the range of 5% to 18% | Sulfa, barbiturates, penicillin, lithium |

## SIDE by SIDE ■ Melanoma

▲ Raised nevus, or mole, on forehead. (© Custom Medical Stock Photo.)

▲ Melanoma on calf. (© Custom Medical Stock Photo.)

## Hemangioma

Hemangioma is a benign tumor made of small blood vessels that form a red or purple birthmark. Port-wine stain (Figure 17–17) is a dark red to purple birthmark appearing on the face. Strawberry hemangioma (Figure 17–18) is a strawberry red, rough, protruding lesion on the face, neck, or trunk. Cherry hemangioma (Figure 17–19) is a small, red, dome-shaped lesion. Some hemangioma regress on their own. Treatment options include steroids, interferon, surgery, and laser treatment.

## ▶ Skin Cancer

### Basal Cell Carcinoma

The most common skin cancer is basal cell carcinoma, a slow growing, generally nonmetastasizing tumor. It generally develops on the face of people with light skin who do not tan in the sun but have been exposed to the sun. Figure 17–20 shows a patient with basal cell carcinoma. The lesion begins as a pearly nodule with rolled edges that may bleed and form a crust.

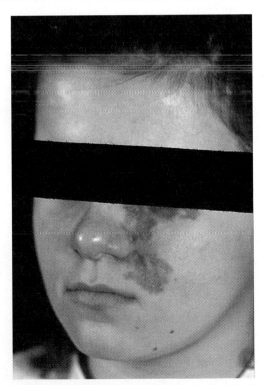

**Figure 17–17** Port-wine hemangioma. (© Custom Medical Stock Photo.)

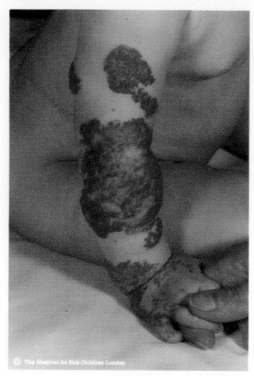

**Figure 17–18**  Strawberry hemangioma. (© NMSB/Custom Medical Stock Photo.)

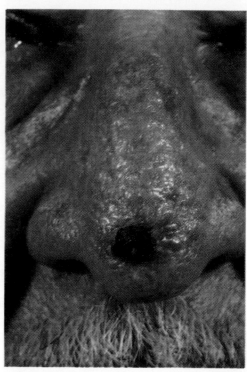

**Figure 17–20**  Basal cell carcinoma. (© Caliendo/Custom Medical Stock Photo.)

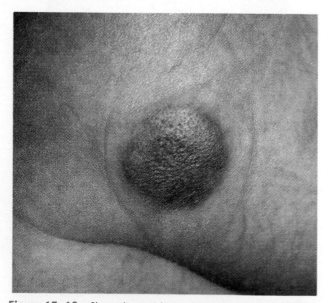

**Figure 17–19**  Cherry hemangioma. (© Logical Images/Custom Medical Stock Photo.)

Ulceration occurs and size increases if it is neglected. This tumor is treated by surgical removal, cauterization, or radiation therapy.

## Squamous Cell Carcinoma

Squamous cell carcinoma is more serious than basal cell carcinoma because it grows more rapidly, infiltrates underlying tissues, and metastasizes through lymph channels. Squamous cell carcinoma is a malignancy of the keratinocytes in the epidermis of people who have been excessively exposed to the sun. The lesion is a crusted nodule that ulcerates and bleeds. This cancer develops in any squamous epithelium of the body, including the skin or mucous membranes lining a natural body opening. It should be completely excised surgically or treated with radiation.

## Kaposi's Sarcoma

Classic Kaposi's sarcoma is a purplish neoplasm of the lower extremities. The lesions are classically described as red-to-purple lesions varying from patches to nodules (Figure 17–21).

The etiological agent of Kaposi's sarcoma is the human herpes virus 8. This cutaneous cancer has been epidemic in persons with AIDS and is one of the indicator diseases for the diagnosis of AIDS (see Chapter 2). Herpes virus has been found within the lesions and may play a part in etiology. Treatment includes surgery, chemotherapy, and radiation.

## Actinic Keratosis

Actinic keratosis is caused by excessive exposure to the sun and is more common in middle-aged, fair-skinned individuals. Multiple wartlike lesions develop on areas of the body exposed to the sun such as the face, arms, and legs. Treatment may include topical medications such as Retin-A and surgical removal of the lesions.

## Malignant Melanoma

The most serious skin cancer is malignant melanoma, which arises from the melanocytes of the epidermis. It is highly malignant and metastasizes early. A malignant melanoma of the skin is seen in Figure 17–22. Melanoma sometimes develops from a mole that changes its size and color and becomes itchy and sore. It is usually excised with the surrounding lymph nodes to

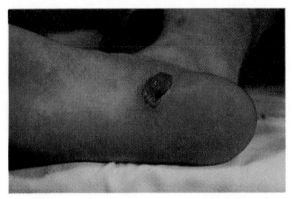

**Figure 17–22** Malignant melanoma is a serious skin cancer that arises from melanocytes.

reduce metastasis. Radiation and chemotherapy follow. Prognosis depends on the depth of infiltration, previous spread, and how completely the tumor is excised. Figure 17–23 shows a malignant melanoma that metastasized to the brain.

Early diagnosis improves prognosis, and one should be vigilant for signs of skin cancer, including the signs and symptoms described above. The general warning signs for cancer are described in detail in Chapter 4.

## ► Sebaceous Gland Disorders

Hyperactivity of the sebaceous glands causes acne and chronic dandruff. Raised, horny, lesions result from an excessive production of keratinocytes.

### Acne (Vulgaris)

Many adolescents suffer at some time or another from acne: blackheads, pimples, and pustules. Acne primarily affects teens; more than 85% experience at least a mild form of acne. Most teens get the mild form, called noninflammatory acne, and just get a few whiteheads and blackheads. Some suffer from inflammatory acne and have a constant breakout of pus-filled pimples and cysts that cause deep pitting and

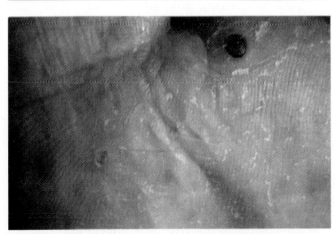

**Figure 17–21** Kaposi's sarcoma on the bottom of the foot. (Courtesy of the CDC/Dr. Steve Kraus, 1981.)

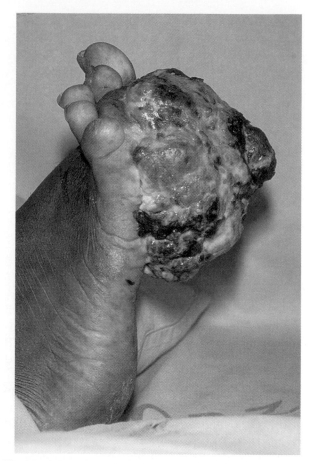

**Figure 17–23** Malignant melanoma on the foot. (© Caliendo/ Custom Medical Stock Photo.)

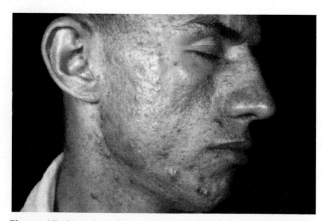

**Figure 17–24** A patient with severe acne. (© Custom Medical Stock Photo.)

scarring. Severe chronic acne, as seen in Figure 17–24, can lead to disfiguring and scarring.

Acne is the result of hormonal changes that occur at puberty. The increased levels of estrogen and testosterone stimulate glandular activity. The sebaceous glands increase their secretions of sebum, the oily fluid that is released through the hair follicles. If the duct becomes clogged by dirt or make-up, the sebaceous secretion accumulates, causing a little bump or whitehead. Sebaceous accumulation at the surface becomes oxidized and turns black, causing the familiar blackhead. Blackheads should not be squeezed or picked because the broken skin offers an entry to bacteria that are always present on the skin surface. Once pyogenic bacteria enter the skin, pus forms and a pimple or pustule results. Squeezing the pimple spreads the infection.

There is no cure for acne, but various treatments can control the lesions. The goal of treatment is to reduce or eliminate outbreaks and to prevent scarring. For mild to moderate acne, a regimen of gentle cleansing with soap, mild exfoliation, and nonprescription benzoyl peroxide lotions often controls mild acne and prevents new outbreaks. If this type of treatment does not work, a physician may prescribe topical lotions containing antibiotics. Low-dose birth control pills are often effective in treating women whose acne worsens around their menstrual period. Light-wave therapy, which uses a narrow-band, high-intensity blue light, may be helpful in treating mild to moderate acne that has not responded to other treatments.

If acne is moderate to severe, oral antibiotics are often prescribed. Topical benzoyl peroxide is often used along with antibiotics because the combination increases their effectiveness and decreases the risk of developing antibiotic resistance. If a patient has acne cysts, treatment may include topical retinoid, a lotion that contains a form of vitamin A; topical antibiotic; oral antibiotic; and benzoyl peroxide. If cystic acne still does not improve, a physician may prescribe an oral retinoid, such as Accutane®. This medication is usually used as a last resort due to some serious but rare side effects and the expense of the medication.

## Prevention ➕ PLUS!

### Warning Signs of Skin Cancer

The earlier skin cancer is diagnosed, the better are the chances for cure. See your physician if you observe any of the following.

### Moles

Dangerous signs are new moles, a change in current moles, lumpy texture, pain, itchiness, scabs, crusts, and bleeding.

### Pigment

Any change in skin pigmentation can be a sign of skin cancer. Look especially for brown or red spots that are rough or scaly in texture.

### Sores

Any sores or scabs that are nonhealing or reoccurring can be skin cancer. These sores are especially common on the face, ears, lips, nose, and hands.

### Scars of Unknown Origin

Some cancers look like scars that are firm to the touch. Beware of scars you know you did not acquire through injury.

### Texture

Any change in skin texture or appearance can be a warning sign. Watch for rough or scaly patches, lumps and bumps, and discolored skin.

## Seborrheic Dermatitis (Chronic Dandruff)

The cause of dandruff is similar to that of acne: the excessive secretion of sebum from the sebaceous glands. The person with seborrheic dermatitis has an oily scalp, and the excessive secretion of sebum forms the familiar scales of dandruff. This condition can spread to the face and ears, and the eyebrows are often affected. Frequent shampooing, particularly with medicated shampoo, is the most effective treatment. Thorough brushing of the hair loosens the dandruff scales so they will wash out easily.

## Sebaceous Cysts

Sebaceous cysts form when a sebaceous gland duct becomes blocked, and the sebum accumulates under the surface of the skin, forming a lump. Sebaceous cysts are not considered serious, but they can rupture, allowing bacteria to enter the body. These cysts can be incised and drained, although they tend to recur, or they can be removed surgically.

## Acne Rosacea

Acne rosacea is a condition that appears during or after middle age in persons with fair skin. Usually the cheeks, chin, and nose develop tiny pimples and broken blood vessels that eventually thicken and give the nose a bulbous appearance. The cause of rosacea is not known, although this condition responds well to topical antibiotic treatment (Figure 17–25).

## ▶ Metabolic Skin Disorder

## Psoriasis

Psoriasis is characterized by red, cracked, and bleeding scales on the scalp, knees, elbows, and trunk, and by an abnormal rate of epidermal cell production and turnover. The root cause of the skin cell pile up is an overzealous immune response, specifically overactive T cells. The scales seen in psoriasis are not the cause, but

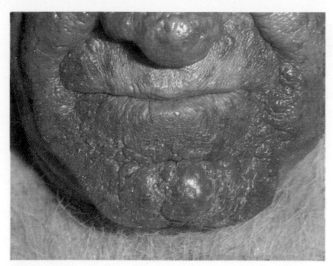

**Figure 17–25** Acne rosacea is more common in the middle-aged to older adult. It causes changes in skin color, enlarged pores, and in some cases, thickening of the soft tissues of the nose.

the effect. Typical lesions in psoriasis are seen in Figure 17–26.

There is no cure for psoriasis, but treatment can improve the condition of the skin and reduce swelling, redness, flaking, and itching. Three basic categories of treatment are used. Topical or external treatments include steroids, coal tar, and anthralin. Phototherapy, which

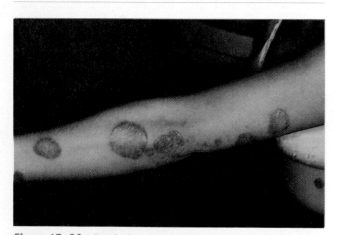

**Figure 17–26** Psoriasis covering the arm of a patient. (Courtesy of the CDC/Dr. N.J. Fiumara, 1976.)

employs lasers and UV light, is generally used for patients with moderate to severe psoriasis who are not responding to topical treatments or who have disease too extensive for topical treatment. Systemic drugs, including the organ-transplant-rejection drug cyclosporine, the cancer drug methotrexate, and oral retinoids, are usually reserved for patients with moderate to severe psoriasis.

## ▶ Pigment Disorders

The main skin pigment, melanin, is interspersed among other cells in the epidermis. Skin color varies from light to dark depending on the number of melanocytes present. Melanin production normally increases with exposure to sunlight, causing tanning.

Hypopigmentation is an abnormally low amount or absence of melanin. The skin may be pale white to various shades of pink caused by blood flowing through it.

### Albinism

Albinism is a rare inherited disorder in which no melanin is formed (Chapter 5). The person has white hair, pale skin, and pink eyes. Because melanin protects the skin from the sun, albinos are prone to sunburn and skin cancer.

### Vitiligo

Vitiligo is a loss of melanin resulting in white patches of skin. The white patches are usually well demarcated and may cover large parts of the body. Hypopigmentation is most striking in dark-skinned persons (Figure 17–27). As in albinism, the unpigmented skin is prone to sunburn. The cause of vitiligo is unknown, and there is no cure for it. Small areas of skin may be covered with tinted make-up, and sunscreen should always be applied to the skin to prevent sunburn. Treatment options include steroids, Psoralen and UV-light therapy, depigmentation therapy, and laser treatments.

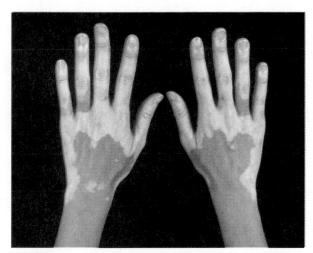

**Figure 17–27** Vitiligo. (© Custom Medical Stock Photo.)

## Ephilis

Ephilis, or freckles, indicate skin damage due to sunburn. The melanocytes in a freckle area are hyper-reactive to sunlight, and the excess melanin they produce causes the freckle. Bleaching creams can be used to lighten freckles.

## Lentigo

Lentigo, or liver spots, are small, brown lesions occurring on the face, neck, and back of the hands (Figure 17–28). Lentigo are not due to aging but are due to excessive sun exposure.

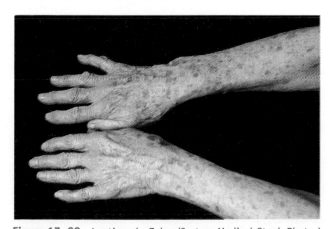

**Figure 17–28** Lentigo. (© Zuber/Custom Medical Stock Photo.)

Bleaching creams can be used to lighten liver spots.

## Melasma

Melasma, also known as chloasma, is triggered by hormonal changes in some women during pregnancy or by oral contraceptives. Patches of darker skin develop on the face, especially over the cheeks. The patches disappear after childbirth or when oral contraceptive use is discontinued.

# ▶ Pressure Injury of Skin

Pressure injuries to the skin occur when pressure decreases bloodflow to an area of the skin.

## Decubitus Ulcer

Decubitus ulcer, or bedsores, usually occur in skin overlying bony projections such as the hips, heels, elbows, and ankles. Shiny, red skin appears over a bony area and eventually develops blisters, erosions, necrosis, and ulceration (Figure 17–29). An infected ulcer becomes foul-smelling and develops a purulent discharge. When individuals are bedridden, they must be turned frequently and repositioned to decrease pressure on tissues and increase bloodflow. Treatments include gelatin sponges, antiseptic irrigation, debriding agents, and antibiotics.

## Corns and Calluses

Corns and calluses are areas of the skin that have grown thick in response to repeated pressure and friction. Corns are small and have a glassy core. They are found on the feet and are usually due to an improperly fitting shoe. Corns can be quite painful, so they may be surgically removed. Calluses are large, are found on the palms of the hands, and are usually due to manual labor. Calluses are not painful; they are protective.

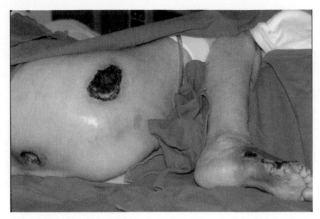

**Figure 17–29** Decubitus ulcer. (© Caliendo/Custom Medical Stock Photo.)

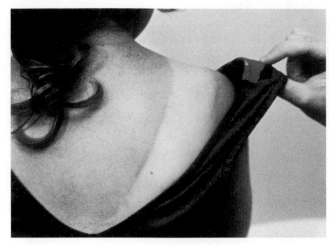

**Figure 17–30** First-degree burn.

## ▶ Thermal Skin Injury

Skin can be injured by excessive heat or cold. The severity of these injuries varies, but they can be life-threatening because of loss of fluids and infection.

### Burns

Fire, steam, hot water, sunlight, chemicals, and electricity can burn skin. Burns are classified on the depth of skin involved. First-degree or superficial burns affect the epidermis and are caused by sunburn or a low intensity flash. The epidermis is red, swollen, and painful. Recovery is complete within a week, and peeling of the dead epidermis occurs (Figure 17–30).

Second-degree or partial thickness burns are caused by scalds or flash flame and affect the dermis or true skin. The epidermis is blistered, red, and broken, and the area is very painful (Figure 17–31). Recovery requires 2 to 3 weeks, and some scarring and depigmentation usually occurs. If infection develops, a major problem with burns, it may convert to a third-degree burn.

Third-degree or full thickness burns result from fire and prolonged exposure to hot liquids. Subcutaneous tissue is affected, and the burn appears pale or charred. Broken skin exposes underlying fat tissue (Figure 17–32). The patient shows symptoms of shock. Healing requires time, and grafting is necessary. Scarring and loss of contour occur.

### Frostbite

Frostbite is the freezing of tissue and is most common on the fingers, toes, and ears. The skin appears white in color and is painless. Treatment for frostbite includes rapid warming in warm water baths. When warmed, the skin turns red and becomes painful. Tissue affected

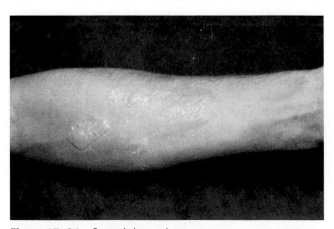

**Figure 17–31** Second-degree burn.

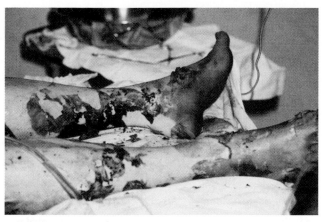

**Figure 17–32** Third-degree burn.

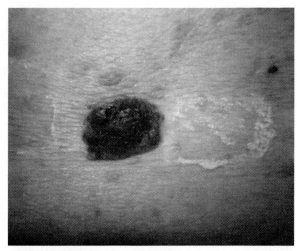

**Figure 17–33** Seborrheic keratosis. (Courtesy of the CDC/Dr. Steve Kraus, 1981.)

by severe frostbite may become necrotic and require surgery or amputation.

## ▶ Age-Related Diseases

The structure and function of skin changes with age. Touch sensation of the skin decreases with age, making burns and frostbite more likely. Xerosis, or dry skin, is a major problem in older adults. The epidermis becomes thinner with age and therefore retains less water. The sweat and sebaceous glands do not function as well, adding to the xerosis. Skin loses some of its elasticity with age due to a decrease in elastic fibers. The skin appears wrinkled and saggy. Nails become thicker and difficult to trim. Hair becomes brittle, thin, gray, and may be lost.

Seborrheic keratosis is a benign overgrowth of epithelial cells that is very common in older adults. The lesions are brown and appear to be pasted on (Figure 17–33). The cause of seborrheic keratosis is unknown, but the lesions do not become malignant. The lesions can be removed by curettage.

Some skin diseases such as psoriasis and seborrheic dermatitis are common in older adults. Older adults with diabetes and bedridden older adults may develop decubitus ulcers.

## ▶ Diagnostic Procedures for Skin Diseases

Skin conditions are usually identified by visual examination. Blood and urine tests may be used to rule out underlying diseases. Scrapings from lesions can be cultured or blood tests for antibodies may be used to identify the causative organism in infectious skin diseases.

In hypersensitivity skin disorders, a complete medical history including prior outbreaks and locations of outbreaks may help identify the allergen. Sensitivity testing or blood tests for antibodies may be used to identify the allergen.

Biopsies are used to diagnose benign tumors and skin caner. Types of biopsies performed include punch, incisional, or total excisional.

## CHAPTER SUMMARY

The skin protects the body from various elements in the environment and is vulnerable to many types of disease. Streptococci and staphylococci cause bacterial infections such as impetigo, erysipelas, cellulitis, and folliculitis. Cold sores and warts result from viral infections. Ringworm and candidiasis are caused by fungus. Parasites such as the louse and mite can infest the skin.

Allergies frequently manifest themselves in the skin. Hives and eczema are examples of skin eruptions caused by hypersensitivity to various antigens, insect bites, or drugs.

Neoplasia of the skin cells ranges from the common mole to malignant melanoma. Hyperactivity of the seba-ceous glands results in acne, sebaceous cysts, and seborrheic dermatitis. Change in melanin is evidence of pigment disorders. Hyperactivity in epidermal cell production results in characteristic silvery lesions of psoriasis. Pressure and thermal changes can cause injury to skin.

## RESOURCES

The American Academy of Dermatology: www.aad.org

The National Institute of Arthritis and Musculoskeletal and Skin Disorders: www.niams.nih.gov

Mayo Clinic: www.mayo.edu

American Cancer Society: www.cancer.org

# Interactive Activities

## Cases for Critical Thinking

1. A 4-year-old girl has red lesions with crust under her nose and on her cheek. According to her mother, the lesions appeared shortly after she developed a cold. On examination, the doctor notes the girl's glands are still swollen. What is your diagnosis?

2. A 25-year-old man complains of intense jock itch. On examination, the doctor observes raised lesions on his penis and red circular patches on his groin. He lives in a transient hotel, and his hygiene is poor. What are the possible causes for this rash? What diagnostic tests should the doctor order?

3. A 39-year-old woman notices a mole on the tip of her ear that has recently started to bleed. She has a fair complexion and suntan lines on her shoulder. What are possible diagnoses? What diagnostic tests should be ordered?

## Multiple Choice

1. Bacterial infections on the skin are caused by _____.
   a. tinea          c. staphylococci
   b. herpes simplex  d. candida

2. Round elevations of the skin with red borders and pale centers are lesions called _____.
   a. acne    c. wheals
   b. macules  d. fissures

3. Sulfa, tetracycline, and antipsychotic medications can cause a _____ reaction on the skin upon exposure to sunlight.
   a. photosensitive  c. urticarial
   b. exfoliative     d. purpura

4. A _____ carcinoma grows rapidly and metastasizes through lymph channels.
   a. basal cell     c. melanocyte
   b. squamous cell  d. malignant

5. In pallor, the skin appears _____.
   a. blue  c. white
   b. red   d. brown

6. The outer layer of the skin is the _____.
   a. epidermis  c. subcutaneous tissue
   b. dermis     d. adipose tissue

7. Small, blisterlike eruptions are called _____.
   a. pustules  c. vesicles
   b. pruritis  d. popular

8. Folliculitis is an inflammation of _____.
   a. sebaceous glands  c. hair follicles
   b. sweat glands      d. furuncles

9. Pediculosis is a _____ infection.
   a. parasitic  c. viral
   b. bacterial  d. fungal

10. _____ is the oily fluid that is released through the hair follicles.
    a. Macular  c. Sebum
    b. Keratin  d. Wheals

# DISEASES AT A GLANCE

## Skin

| DISEASE | ETIOLOGY | SIGNS AND SYMPTOMS |
| --- | --- | --- |
| Impetigo | Streptococci, staphylococci | Erythema, oozing, vesicles, pustules that crust, fever, swollen lymph nodes |
| Erysiples | Streptococci | Shiny, swollen red rash that is tender and hot to touch; fever; chills |
| Cellulitus | Streptococci | Red, swollen, tender lesions follow skin damage; fever; and chills |
| Folliculitis | Staphylococci | Inflammation of hair follicle, pustules appear |
| Furuncles | Staphylococci | Boil or large, tender, swollen pus-filled lesion |
| Carbuncles | Staphylococci | A cluster of furuncles (boils) |
| Herpes | Herpes virus family | Small, painful vesicles |
| Warts | Viruses | Benign neoplasms with rough, keratinized surface |
| Tinea | Fungi | Mild scales, cracking skin, painful raw rash |
| Candidiasis | *Candida* fungus | Body: itchy, red blister, pustules<br>Nail: redness, swelling, nail may turn white or yellow and separate from the finger or toe<br>Vaginal: white cottage-cheese discharge with burning, itching, and redness<br>Mouth: Creamy white, painful patches |
| Pediculosis | Lice | Itching |

| DIAGNOSIS | TREATMENT |
| --- | --- |
| Visual examination, culture | Antibiotics |
| Visual examination, culture | Antibiotics |
| Visual examination, culture | Antibiotics |
| Visual examination, culture | Daily cleansing with antiseptic soap, antibiotics |
| Visual examination, culture | Moist heat, antiseptic, skin cleansing, antibiotics, incision and drainage |
| Visual examination, culture | Moist heat, antiseptic, skin cleansing, antibiotics, incision and draining |
| Visual examination, culture | Self-limiting, antiviral drugs |
| Visual examination, culture | Removal by cryosurgery, laser, surgery |
| Visual examination, culture | Antifungals |
| Visual examination, culture | Antifungals |
| Visual examination | Medicated shampoo |

# DISEASES AT A GLANCE *(continued)*

## Skin

| DISEASE | ETIOLOGY | SIGNS AND SYMPTOMS |
|---|---|---|
| Scabies | Mite | Itching, blisters, pustules |
| Urticaria (hives) | Hypersensitivity | Wheal lesions with rounded elevations and red, pale centers |
| Eczema | Inflammation | Red, itchy lesions, edema |
| Poison ivy | Poison ivy plant | Itchy rash with blisters and hivelike swelling |
| Drug eruptions | Adverse drug reactions | Varies (see Table 17–1) |
| Nevus (mole) | Benign tumor | Small, dark skin growth |
| Hemangioma | Benign tumor | Red or purple birthmarks |
| Basal cell carcinoma | Sun exposure | Slow-growing, pearly nodule, rolled edges; lesion bleeds, forms crust |
| Squamous cell carcinoma | Sun exposure | Crusted nodule, ulcerates and bleeds, infiltrates underlying tissue |
| Kaposi's sarcoma | Human herpes virus 8 | Red to purple lesions varying from macules to nodules |
| Actinic keratosis | Sun exposure | Multiple wartlike lesions |
| Malignant melanoma | Sun exposure | Mole changes in size and color; irregular border; bleeds, itches |
| Acne (vulgaris) | Hormonal changes, increased sebum production | Whiteheads, blackheads, cysts |
| Seborrheic dermatitis | Excessive sebum production | Oily scalp, dandruff scales |
| Sebaceous cysts | Blocked sebaceous gland duct | Lump under skin surface |

| DIAGNOSIS | TREATMENT |
|---|---|
| Visual examination | Hot baths, scrubbing, medication |
| Visual examination | Steroids, antihistamines, calamine lotion |
| Visual examination | Steroids |
| Visual examination | Cortisone |
| Visual examination, medical history | Change medication |
| Visual examination, biopsy | Cryosurgery, excision |
| Visual examination | Steroids, interferon, surgery, laser treatments |
| Visual examination | Surgical removal, cauterization, radiation therap |
| Visual examination, biopsy | Surgical removal, radiation therapy |
| Visual examination, biopsy | Surgery, chemotherapy, radiation |
| Visual examination, biopsy | Retin-A, surgical removal |
| Visual examination, biopsy | Surgical removal, radiation, chemotherapy |
| Visual examination | Antibiotics, comedolutic agents, accutane |
| Visual examination | Medicated shampoo |
| Visual examination | Incision and drainage, removal |

# DISEASES AT A GLANCE (*continued*)

## Skin

| DISEASE | ETIOLOGY | SIGNS AND SYMPTOMS |
|---|---|---|
| Acne rosacea | Unknown | Reddened skin, broken blood vessels; nose, cheek, and chin develop bulbous appearance |
| Psoriasis | Unknown | Round, red lesions with silvery scales |
| Albinism | Hereditary | White hair, pale skin, pink eyes |
| Vitiligo | Unknown | White, well-demarcated areas of skin without melanin |
| Ephilis (freckles) | Sun damage | Excess melanin production |
| Lentigo (liver spots) | Sun exposure | Small, brown lesions on the face, neck, back of hands |
| Melasma | Hormonal changes | Patches of darker skin over the cheeks |
| Decubitus ulcer | Pressure decreases blood flow to an area of the skin | Shiny red skin over bony area, blisters, erosions, necrosis, ulceration, purulent discharge if infected |
| Corns and calluses | Pressure, improperly fitting shoes, manual labor | Areas of skin that grow thick |
| Burns | Fire, steam, hot water, sunlight, chemicals, electricity | First-degree: red, swollen, painful epidermis<br>Second-degree: blistered, painful epidermis<br>Third-degree: pale or charred skin with exposed underlying fat tissue |
| Frostbite | Cold | White, painless skin; when warmed, skin becomes red and painful |
| Seborrheic keratosis | Benign tumor | Brown lesions that appear to be pasted on |

| DIAGNOSIS | TREATMENT |
|---|---|
| Visual examination | Antibiotics |
| Visual examination, biopsy | Creams, steroids, UV-light treatment, anticancer medication |
| Visual examination | Sunscreen |
| Visual examination | Steroids, psoralen and UV-light treatment, depigmentation therapy, laser treatments |
| Visual examination | Bleaching cream |
| Visual examination | Bleaching cream |
| Visual examination | Self-limiting, after childbirth or when oral contraceptive use is discontinued |
| Visual examination | Gelatin sponges, antiseptic irrigation, debriding agents, antibiotics |
| Visual examination | None: surgical removal of corns may be necessary |
| Visual examination | First-degree: none<br>Second-degree: none<br>Third-degree: grafting |
| Visual examination | Rapid warming, warm water baths, surgery, amputation |
| Visual examination | Curettage |

## True or False

_____ 1. Impetigo is caused by a virus.

_____ 2. Basal cell carcinoma metastasizes rapidly.

_____ 3. Fever blisters are examples of a bacterial infection.

_____ 4. Seborrheic dermatitis is a malignant skin tumor.

_____ 5. Warts are benign neoplasms.

_____ 6. A mole is a nevus.

_____ 7. Ringworms are viral infections.

_____ 8. Erythema is whitening of the skin.

_____ 9. The cause of seborrheic dermatitis is excessive secretion of sebum.

_____ 10. The cause of acne rosacea is fungus.

## Fill-Ins

1. _____ is the dark pigment of the skin that protects the body from the harmful rays of the sun.

2. _____ is a tough, fibrous protein that protects the skin from harmful substances.

3. The _____ is composed of connective tissue that supports blood and lymph vessels and elastic fibers.

4. _____ _____ are large, tender, swollen, raised lesions caused by staphylococci.

5. _____ is a contagious skin disease usually associated with poor living conditions.

6. _____ is a superficial recurring idiopathic skin disorder characterized by an abnormal rate of epidermal cell production and turnover.

7. Urticaria, also known as _____, results from a vascular reaction of the skin to an allergen.

8. A person with seborrheic dermatitis has an oily scalp, and the excessive secretion of sebum forms scales of _____.

9. _____ is loss of melanin resulting in white patches of skin.

10. Lesions containing pus are referred to as _____.

 **MedMedia Wrap-Up**

 **www.prenhall.com/mulvihill**
Remember to visit this website for extra study practice, including exercises, Internet links, news updates, and an audio glossary.

 **Activity CD-ROM**
Check out the CD-ROM in the back of this book. You will find games, exercises, puzzles, and videos to help enhance your understanding of this chapter.

# Glossary

**Abruptio placentae.** Premature separation of the placenta from the uterus prior to or during birth.

**Acetylcholine.** Neurotransmitter of the parasympathetic nervous system.

**Achlorhydria.** A condition in which hydrochloric acid is absent in the stomach.

**Achondroplasia.** An autosomal dominant disorder of defective cartilage formation in the fetus.

**Achondroplastic dwarfism.** A condition caused by defective cartilage formation that results in improper bone development.

**Acidosis.** The condition in which the production of acids lowers the body's pH.

**Acne.** Blackheads, pimples, and pustules that result from hormonal changes that occur most often during puberty.

**Acne rosacea.** Tiny pimples and broken blood vessels on the cheeks, chin, and nose of some fair-skinned people.

**Acquired immunodeficiency syndrome (AIDS).** The deadly disease caused by HIV that destroys an individual's immune system, making the victim remarkably susceptible to infection.

**Acrodermatitis enteropathica.** A rare autosomal recessive disorder that results in defective malabsorption of zinc.

**Acromegaly.** The condition that results if an excessive production of growth hormone occurs after puberty.

**Actinic keratosis.** Wartlike lesions found on areas of the body that receive excessive sun exposure.

**Activated lymphocytes.** White blood cells that have been stimulated by antigens that include B and T cells.

**Active immunity.** A type of artificial immunity; the person is given a vaccine or toxoid as the antigen, and he or she forms antibodies to counteract it.

**Acute.** A disease is that has a sudden onset and a short duration.

**Adenocarcinomas.** Cancerous glandular tumors.

**Adenohypophysis.** The anterior and larger portion of the hypophysis; it is glandular and in direct communication with the hypothalamus of the brain.

**Adenoma.** A benign tumor of glandular tissue that often develops in the breast, thyroid gland, or mucous glands of the intestinal tract.

**Adhesions.** Connective tissue fibers that anchor adjacent structures together; a kinking of the intestines.

**Adipose.** Fat tissue.

**Adrenalin.** A hormone of the sympathetic nervous system; the most vital therapy in treatment of allergy and can be self-injected in an emergency.

**Adrenal virilism.** Expression of secondary male sexual characteristics in females caused by a testosterone-secreting adrenal gland neoplasm.

**Adrenocorticotropic hormone (ACTH).** The tropic that affects the adrenal cortex.

**Affect.** Emotional state or feeling tone used to describe ones emotional expression.

**Agglutinate.** Clumping or aggregation, as occurs in some antibody-antigen reactions.

**Albinism.** An autosomal recessive disorder in which no melanin is formed, causing a person to have white hair, pale skin, and pink eyes.

**Albuminuria.** The presence of the plasma protein albumin in urine.

**Aldosterone.** The principle hormone from the adrenal cortex that causes sodium retention and potassium secretion by the kidneys.

**Alleles.** Alternative forms of a gene.

**Allergens.** Agents that initiate an allergic response.

**Allergy.** Abnormal immunologic response to allergens such as pollens, dust, dog hair, and certain foods.

**Alpha cells.** Glucagon-secreting cells of the endocrine pancreas.

**Alpha-feto-protein.** Fetal protein found in maternal blood, and sometimes detected in adults with various cancers.

**Alveoli.** Small air sacs in the lungs where gas exchange occurs.

**Alzheimer's disease.** A common form of dementia unique to humans usually over age 65.

**Amenorrhea.** The absence of menstruation.

**Amniocentesis.** A diagnostic test for hereditary diseases performed on fetal cells withdrawn from amniotic fluid.

**Amoeboids.** A type of protozoa that moves with pseudopodia.

**Amygdala.** Almond-shaped structure located deep within the brain.

**Amylase.** A digestive enzyme, which breaks down carbohydrates.

**Amyotrophic (ALS).** Also known as Lou Gehrig's disease, a chronic, terminal, degenerative disease of the motor nervous system.

**Analgesics.** Medications that reduce pain.

**Anaphylactic shock.** A severe inflammation brought on by a severe antigen-antibody reaction such as occurs in an incompatible blood transfusion.

**Anaphylaxis.** The condition of anaphylactic shock, which is a life-threatening state in which blood pressure drops and airways become constricted.

**Anatomy.** Study of the normal structure of the body.

**Androgenital syndrome.** A form of hyperadrenalism caused when the male hormone is secreted in excess.

**Androgens.** The sex hormone in males.

**Anemia.** A condition caused by a reduction of oxygen-carrying hemoglobin.

**Aneurysm.** A localized dilation caused by a weakening in the wall of a blood vessel.

**Angina pectoris.** The temporary chest pain or sensation of chest pressure caused by transient oxygen insufficiency.

**Angiocardiography.** An x-ray of the heart and great vessels in which a contrast indicator (dye) is injected into the cardiovascular system.

**Angioma.** A type of benign tumor composed of blood vessels, such as red birthmark or "port-wine" stain.

**Angioplasty.** A procedure by which a balloon-tip catheter is inserted into the coronary arteries and expanded to break and crush the plaques.

**Ankylosis.** Scar tissue formation at bone ends that can turn to bone, causing the ends to fuse.

**Anorexia nervosa.** A disease of psychoneurotic origin in which the aversion to food leads to emaciation and malnutrition found to be most common in teenage girls.

**Anorexia.** A loss of appetite.

**Antibiotic resistance.** Resistance arising when bacteria adapt to antibiotics and the adaptation becomes common in the bacterial population, rendering the antibiotics ineffective.

**Antibiotics.** Drugs used to treat bacterial infections.

**Antibodies.** Proteins secreted by plasma cells that aid in defense against infectious agents.

**Anticoagulant.** Medication used to prevent intravascular clotting.

**Antidiuretic hormone.** One of two hormones secreted by the posterior pituitary.

**Antigen.** A substance, usually foreign to the body, which triggers the immune response.

**Antihistamine.** A drug to counteract the unpleasant effects caused by the release of histamines in the body due to allergies. It has a drying effect on the mucous membranes of the mouth and throat.

**Anuria.** The total stoppage of urine production.

**Anxiety disorder.** Includes a number of disorders in which the primary feature is abnormal or inappropriate anxiety that interferes with daily work, school, recreational, and family activities. Includes several subtypes: panic disorder, generalized anxiety disorder, phobic disorders, social phobia, obsessive-compulsive disorder, and posttraumatic stress disorder.

**Aorta.** The largest artery that carries blood away from the heart to the arteries.

**Aortic stenosis.** The narrowing of the valve leading into the aorta.

**Aphasia.** Loss of speech.

**Aphonia.** Inability to produce sounds from the larynx.

**Aplasia.** Developmental failure leading to the absence of a structure or tissue.

**Apnea.** Temporary cessation of breathing.

**Apoptosis.** Cell death or cell deletion by fragmentation into membrane particles, which are phagocytosed by other cells.

**Arrhythmia.** A deviation from the normal rhythm of the heartbeat.

**Arteriosclerosis.** Progressive hardening of blood vessels, especially arteries.

**Arthritis.** The inflammation of a joint.

**Ascites.** Fluid that develops as a result of liver failure and accumulates in the peritoneal cavity.

**Aspermia.** Caused when there is no formation or emission of sperm due to the absence of the gonadotropic hormones in a male before puberty.

**Asthma.** A disease caused by increased responsiveness of the tracheobronchal tree to various stimuli, which tends to cause dyspnea and wheezing.

**Astrocytoma.** Basically benign, slow-growing tumors of the brain.

**Atherosclerosis.** The accumulation of fatty material under the inner lining of the arterial wall.

**Atresia.** The absence or closure of a normal body opening or tubular structure.

**Atrophic.** A degenerating, wasting condition.

**Atrophy.** The decrease in size or function of an organ.

**Attention deficit hyperactivity disorder (ADHD).** Neurobiological disorder characterized by prominent symptoms of innattention, hyperactivity, and impulsivity.

**Aura.** A warning signal such as the symptoms that precede an epileptic seizure.

**Auscultation.** Listening with a stethoscope for sounds within the body, such as heart valve sounds or the lungs, during an exam.

**Autistic disorder.** Developmental disorder of reciprocal language and social interactions, with stereotypical behavior.

**Autoantibodies.** Antibodies produced against self-antigens.

**Autoimmune diseases.** Failure of immune tolerance; activated T cells and antibodies attack the body's own tissue.

**Autosomes.** Name for 44 of the 46 chromosomes.

**B lymphocytes.** Lymphocytes that produce antibodies in cell-mediated immunity.

**Bacilli.** Rod-shaped bacterial cells.

**Bacteria.** A single-celled organism with simple structure and lacking a nucleus.

**Bartholin's glands.** Mucus-secreting glands situated at the vaginal entrance.

**Basal cell carcinoma.** Most common form of skin cancer.

**Basal ganglia (basal nuclei).** Nerve cell bodies deep within the white matter of the brain, which help control position and unconscious movements.

**Basophils.** A type of white blood cell that promotes inflammation and participates in allergic responses.

**Benign.** The term used to describe a noncancerous neoplasm or tumor.

**Benign prostatic hyperplasia.** Enlargement of the prostate gland in older men.

**Beriberi.** Thiamine deficiency includes dry or wet syndromes, cerebral beriberi, and Wernicke-Korsakoff syndrome.

**Beta cells.** Insulin-secreting cells of the endocrine pancreas.

**Beta human chorionic gonadotropin.** Hormone secreted during pregnancy.

**Bile.** Substance secreted by the liver and necessary for fat digestion; consists of water, bile salts, cholesterol, and bilirubin.

**Biliary calculi.** Gallstones; consist mainly of cholesterol, bilirubin, and calcium.

**Biliary cirrhosis.** A form of cirrhosis resulting from cholecystitis.

**Bilirubin.** A colored pigment produced when hemoglobin breaks down.

**Binary fission.** Process in which bacteria reproduce by splitting in half.

**Binge.** Eating excessive amounts of food within a restricted period of time.

**Biopsy.** Procedure in which a small sample of a tissue is surgically removed and examined microscopically for abnormalities.

**Bipolar disorder.** Mood disorder associated with shifts from depression to mania. Includes three subcategories: bipolar I, bipolar II, and cyclothymic disorder.

**Blunted conduct.** Dull behavior bearing no relationship to social signals; may occur in persons with schizophrenia.

**Bowman's capsule.** A sac containing the glomerular capillaries; also called glomerular capsule.

**Bradycardia.** Heart rate of 60 beats per minute or less.

**Bradykinesia.** Slowness of movement.

**Bradykinin.** Substance released by damaged tissue that promotes inflammation.

**Bronchi.** Passageway that leads from the trachea to the lung.

**Bronchioles.** Small soft tissue tubules with smooth muscle wrappings that connect small bronchi to alveolar structures.

**Bronchitis.** Inflammation of the bronchi; may be acute or chronic.

**Bronchogenic carcinoma.** Most common type of lung cancer that arises from the bronchial tree.

**Bronchopneumonia.** Type of pneumonia that may develop as a result of small bronchi becoming obstructed because of infection or aspirated gastric contents.

**Bulbourethral glands.** A pair of glands that secrete into the urethra as it enters the penis.

**Bulimia nervosa.** A gorge-purge syndrome, the opposite of, yet similar to, anorexia nervosa.

**Bundle of His.** The specialized tissue in heart muscle capable of sending the impulse for contraction to the ventricles.

**Bursae.** Sacs of fluid situated near the joint to reduce friction on movement.

**Bursitis.** Inflammation of the bursae.

**Cachexia.** Condition caused when a patient becomes weak and emaciated in appearance due to the rapid growth of a malignant tumor; also accompanies many chronic diseases like cancer, HIV/AIDS, and tuberculosis.

**Calcium.** Mineral essential for bone and tooth structure and for cell physiology.

**Capsid.** Protein coat of viruses.

**Carbuncles.** Clusters of boils.

**Carcinogens.** Various chemicals that promote cancer development.

**Carcinoma in situ.** Premalignant lesion, the earliest stage of cancer in which the underlying tissue has not yet been invaded.

**Carcinoma.** Type of cancer affecting epithelial tissues, skin, and mucous membranes lining body cavities. Also, the malignancy of glandular tissue such as the breast, liver, and pancreas.

**Cardiac catheterization.** Procedure in which a catheter is passed into the heart through appropriate blood vessels to sample the blood in each chamber for oxygen content and pressure.

**Cardiac cycle.** The alternate contraction and relaxation of atria and ventricles.

**Cardiac sphincter.** Muscular gateway between the esophagus and stomach.

**Cardiogenic shock.** The result of extensive myocardial infarction, it is often fatal, but drugs to combat it are sometimes effective.

**Cardiopulmonary resuscitation (CPR).** Pertains to both heart and lung assistance by emergency or trained personnel to rhythmically compress chest and breathe into victim's airway until medical services can be provided.

**Carotene.** A plant pigment from which vitamin A is derived.

**Caseous.** The term used to describe soft and cheese-like lung tissue in tuberculosis.

**Casts.** Molds of kidney tubules consisting of coagulated protein and blood.

**Cataracts.** Clouding of the eye lens to the point of opacity.

**Catatonic.** Motor disturbance that may occur in persons with schizophrenia.

**Cell walls.** A rigid layer of organic material surrounding delicate cell membranes of bacteria.

**Cell-mediated immunity.** Protection from infection provided by T cells.

**Cellulitis.** Spreading skin infection caused by streptococci.

**Cerebrospinal.** A term pertaining to the brain and spinal cord; cerebrospinal fluid bathes these organs.

**Cerebrovascular accident (CVA).** A stroke.

**Chancre.** An ulceration on the genitals in the primary stage of syphilis.

**Chemotaxis.** The attraction of white blood cells to the site of inflammation.

**Chemotherapy.** Systemic administration of medications to kill malignant cells.

**Chlamydial infection.** STD caused by *Chlamydia trachomatis.*

**Cholecystectomy.** The surgical removal of the gallbladder.

**Cholelithiasis.** The formation or presence of gallstones.

**Cholesterol.** A fatty substance found in animal cell membranes.

**Choriocarcinoma.** Malignant tumor of the placenta.

**Chorionic gonadotropin hormone.** The hormone that indicates a positive pregnancy test.

**Chorionic villus sampling.** Genetic test involving the removal of cells from the villi through the cervix.

**Chromosome.** A molecule of DNA found in the human cell. Each human cell contains 46 chromosomes divided into 23 pairs.

**Chronic.** A disease that may begin insidiously and be long-lived.

**Chronic fatigue syndrome.** A disease that produces flulike symptoms, including severe and persistent fatigue, muscle and joint pain, and fever.

**Chronic obstructive pulmonary disease (COPD).** The term used to describe a number of conditions, including chronic bronchitis and emphysema, in which the exchange of respiratory gases in ineffective.

**Chronic ulcerative colitis.** A serious inflammation of the colon, the origin of which is unknown.

**Chymotrypsin.** A digestive enzyme that digests protein.

**Cilia.** The hairlike projections found in the mucous membrane that lines the respiratory tract.

**Ciliates.** A type of protozoa that moves using hairlike cilia.

**Cirrhosis.** A chronic destruction of liver cells and tissues with a nodular, bumpy regeneration.

**Coarctation.** A narrowing, or stricture, of the aorta that provides blood to the entire body.

**Cocci.** Spherical, round bacterial cells.

**Collagen.** A fibrous protein found in connective tissues, causing wounds to heal poorly.

**Colostomy.** An artificial opening in the abdominal wall with a segment of the large intestine attached.

**Communicable.** An infectious disease transmitted from human to human.

**Co-morbid.** The occurance of two or more concurrent mental illnesses or conditions.

**Compact bone.** Dense bone issue surrounding most bones.

**Complications.** Diseases that develop in a patient already suffering from a disease.

**Compression sclerotherapy.** A treatment for varicose veins in which a strong saline solution is injected into specific sites within the vessel tract.

**Computerized tomography (CT scan).** A diagnostic imaging technique used to make diagnosis and determine the location of lesions or growths inside the body.

**Concussion.** A transient disorder of the nervous system resulting from a violent blow on the head or from a fall.

**Conduct disorder.** Disruptive behavior disorder diagnosed in children.

**Congenital diseases.** Diseases that appear at birth or shortly after but are not caused by genetic or chromosomal abnormalities.

**Conjunctiva.** The membrane that lines the eyelids and covers the eyeball.

**Conn's syndrome.** A form of hyperadrenalism in which aldosterone is excreted in excess.

**Contagious.** An infectious disease transmitted from human to human.

**Contusion.** An injury, or bruise, to brain tissue without a breaking of the skin at the site of the trauma.

**Cor pulmonale.** A serious heart condition in which the right side of the heart fails as a result of long-standing chronic lung disease.

**Coronary arteriography.** The selective injection of contrast material into coronary arteries for a film recording of blood vessel action.

**Corpus luteum.** The structure that develops from the ovarian follicle after ovulation.

**Cortisol.** The principle hormone in the group of steroid hormones, also known as hydrocortisone; stress increases production of cortisol.

**Cortisone.** A hormone of the adrenal gland that has anti-inflammatory properties.

**Creatinine.** Nitrogen-containing waste products of protein metabolism.

**Cri du chat syndrome.** A hereditary disease resulting from the deletion of part of the short arm of chromosome 5.

**Cretinism.** A congenital thyroid deficiency in which thyroxine is not synthesized.

**Crohn's disease.** An inflammatory disease of the intestine in which the intestinal walls become thick and rigid.

**Cryptorchidism.** The failure of the testes to descend from the abdominal cavity, where they develop during fetal life, to the scrotum.

**CT scan.** Computed tomography scan; 3-D computer aided x-ray.

**Cushing's syndrome.** A condition resulting from excessive levels of glucocorticoid hormones.

**Cyanosis.** Blue color in the body tissues.

**Cyclins.** Cell cycle proteins.

**Cyst.** A sac or capsule containing fluid; usually harmless.

**Cystic fibrosis.** A disease that affects all the exocrine glands of the body, the glands of external secretion usually affecting children.

**Cystitis.** An inflammation of the urinary bladder, commonly called a bladder infection.

**Cystocele.** Urinary bladder is displaced into the vagina.

**Cystoscope.** An endoscope (lighted scope) through which the interior of the urinary bladder is made visible for observation.

**Cytotoxic T cells.** T cells, often called *killer cells* because of their capability to kill invading organisms.

**Decubitus ulcers.** Bedsores that typically occur on the bony areas of the body.

**Defibrillator.** A machine that delivers electrical shocks used to re-establish normal heart rhythm.

**Delirium tremens.** A medical emergency caused by heavy drinking over a long period of time; may occur after withdrawal from heavy alcohol intake.

**Delusion.** False beliefs associated with various mental illnesses.

**Dementia.** Organic loss of intellectual functions.

**Deoxyribonucleic acid (DNA).** The blueprint for protein synthesis within the cell.

**Dermatitis.** A noncontagious skin disorder.

**Dermatophytes.** Fungi that infect the skin and tend to live on the dead, top layer.

**Desensitize.** A procedure for causing tolerance to allergens so that they do not trigger allergic reactions.

**Diabetes insipidus.** A disease that results from a deficiency of ADH.

**Diabetes mellitus.** An endocrine disease in which the beta cells fail to secrete insulin or target cells fail to respond to insulin.

**Diabetic nephropathy.** A kidney disease resulting from diabetes mellitus.

**Diagnosis.** The determination of the nature of a disease based on many factors, including signs, symptoms, and, often, laboratory results.

**Diaphragm.** Primary muscle for inspiration that divides the thorax and abdominopelvic cavities.

**Diastole.** The period of the heartbeat when the heart relaxes and fills with blood.

**Diethylstilbestrol (DES).** A synthetic hormone used in the 1950s and early 1960s to prevent spontaneous abortion.

**Discoid.** The mild form of lupus erythematosus in which red, raised, itchy lesions develop.

**Disease.** A state of functional disequilibrium that may be resolved by recovery or death.

**Disinfection.** Reducing the risk of infection or contamination.

**Diuretic.** A substance that causes the kidneys to excrete water. Diuretics can lower blood pressure.

**Diverticula.** Little pouches or sacs formed when the mucosal lining pushes through the underlying muscle layer.

**Diverticulitis.** Inflammation of the diverticula, usually occurring in the colon or small intestines.

**Dominant.** A gene that is expressed when inherited.

**Dopamine.** A neuronal transmitter substance.

**Doppler echocardiography.** Instrument that uses echoes of moving blood columns to produce images of the vessel wall outline; the velocity of the blood is measured and the degree of carotid stenosis is determined.

**Down syndrome.** Trisomy 21.

**Duodenal ulcers.** Ulcers of the small intestine caused by an excessive secretion of hydrochloric acid and *Helicobacter pylori* infection.

**Duodenum.** First section of the small intestine; receives digested material from stomach.

**Dysentery.** An acute inflammation of the colon, a colitis.

**Dysmenorrhea.** Painful or difficult menses.

**Dyspareunia.** Painful sexual intercourse.

**Dysphagia.** Difficult or painful swallowing.

**Dyspnea.** Air hunger resulting in labored or difficult breathing.

**Dysthymia.** Chronic, persistent depression for a period of at least 2 years.

**Dystrophin.** A skeletal protein that is missing in Duchenne's muscular dystrophy.

**Dystrophy.** Muscle degeneration that disables an individual.

**Dysuria.** Painful urination.

**Ecchymoses.** Hemorrhagic spots that develop on the skin and in mucous membranes, causing discoloration.

**Echocardiography.** A noninvasive procedure (ultrasound cardiography) that utilizes high-frequency sound waves to examine the size, shape, and motion of heart structures.

**Eclampsia.** Convulsions and coma that follow untreated pregnancy-induced hypertension.

**Ectopic pregnancy.** A pregnancy in which the fertilized ovum implants in a tissue other than the uterus, most commonly in the fallopian tubes.

**Eczema.** A noncontagious inflammatory skin disorder.

**Edema.** Swelling caused by leakage of plasma into tissues.

**Electrocardiogram (ECG).** An electrical recording of the heart action that aids in the diagnosis of coronary artery disease, myocardial infarction, valvular heart disease, and some congenital heart diseases.

**Electroencephalogram (EEG).** A recording of brain waves.

**Electrolyte balance.** The proper balance of salts, like potassium, and calcium.

**Electromyogram (EMG).** A testing procedure used to diagnose muscle and nerve disorders.

**Embolism.** A circulating blood clot.

**Emphysema.** A crippling, noncontagious disease of chronic lung obstruction and destruction.

**Encephalitis.** The inflammation of the brain and meninges, caused by a viral infection.

**Encephalomyelitis.** Acute inflammation of the brain and spinal cord.

**Endarterectomy.** A common surgical procedure used to treat a blockage in an artery by removing the thickened area of the inner vascular lining.

**Endemic.** Describes a disease which always occurs at low levels in a population.

**Endocarditis.** Inflammation within the heart.

**Endocardium.** A smooth delicate membrane that lines chambers of the heart.

**Endometriosis.** A disease in which endometrial tissue from the uterus becomes embedded elsewhere.

**Endoscope.** An instrument consisting of a hollow tube with a lens and light system used to view the inner surface of the digestive tract.

**Endoscopic sclerotherapy.** A procedure used to guide a retractable needle device through an area such as the esophagus to seal off vessels such as esophageal varices with a hardening agent.

**Endoscopy.** Imaging technique using flexible tubing mounted with camera and surgical tools.

**Endospores.** Structures produced by bacteria and formed to cope with harsh environmental conditions.

**Endotoxin.** A potent toxin from certain bacteria that causes life-threatening shock.

**Eosinophila-myalgia syndrome.** Multisystem disease with pain, fatigue, and elevations of circulating blood eosinophils.

**Eosinophils.** White blood cells that kill parasites and are involved in allergic responses.

**Ephylis.** Freckles.

**Epidemic.** The occurrence of a disease in unusually large numbers over a specific area.

**Epididymis.** A coiled tube that lies along the outer wall of the testis and leads into the vas deferens.

**Epididymitis.** Inflammation of the epididymis.

**Epidural.** A hemorrhage between the dura mater and the skull.

**Epilepsy.** A group of uncontrolled cerebral discharges that recur at random intervals.

**Epinephrine.** The hormone secreted by the adrenal medulla in emergency situations or during periods of high stress; also used as a drug to dilate bronchioles in some asthma attacks.

**Erysipelas.** An inflammatory skin infection caused by streptococcus bacteria. Most commonly, the infections appear on the face, arm, or leg.

**Erythema.** A reddened area of skin.

**Erythematous.** An area of skin reddened by congested blood vessels resulting from injury or inflammation.

**Erythrocytes.** Red blood cells.

**Erythropoiesis.** The process of red cell formation that takes place in the red marrow of flat bones such as the sternum, hip bones, ribs, and skull bones.

**Erythropoietin.** A hormone synthesized principally by the kidney that stimulates red blood cell development.

**Esophageal varices.** Varicose veins of the esophagus.

**Esophagitis.** Inflammation of the esophagus caused by acid reflux.

**Essential trace minerals.** Minerals required in the diet in very low amounts.

**Estrogen.** The sex hormone in females.

**Etiology.** The cause of a disease.

**Exacerbation.** The period of a chronic disease when signs and symptoms recur in all their severity.

**Exocrine glands.** The glands of external secretion. They secrete mucus, perspiration, and digestive enzymes.

**Exophthalmos.** The condition in which the eyeballs protrude outward, characteristic of a person with Graves' disease.

**Extradural.** A hemorrhage between the dura mater and the skull.

**Familial hypercholesterolemia.** An autosomal dominant disorder caused by a mutation in the gene encoding the receptor for low-density lipoproteins.

**Familial polyposis.** A hereditary disease in which numerous polyps develop in the intestinal tract.

**Female arousal-orgasmic dysfunction.** Lack of sexual desire or response in a female.

**Fibrillation.** Quivering or spontaneously uncoordinated contraction of muscle fibers, such as heart ventricles.

**Fibrin.** A plasma protein essential for blood-clotting.

**Fibroblasts.** Connective tissue cells that produce fibers to aid in healing damaged tissue.

**Fibrocystic disease.** The formation of numerous fluid-filled lumps in the breast.

**Fimbriae.** Fingerlike projections at the outer ends of the fallopian tubes, they propel ova into the tube.

**Flagella.** Whip-like cell appendages used for locomotion.

**Flagellates.** A type of protozoa that moves using whiplike appendages called flagella.

**Flatus.** Intestinal gas.

**Flatworm.** A wormlike animal that has a flattened body.

**Fluoroscopy.** A diagnostic procedure that permits visualization of the lungs and diaphragm during respiration.

**Folliculitis.** Inflammation of hair follciles caused by staphylococci.

**Foramen ovale.** A small opening that allows blood from the right side of the heart to enter the left directly, bypassing the nonfunctional fetal lungs.

**Fragile X syndrome.** A sex-linked disorder associated with mental retardation. It is identified by a break, or weakness, on the long arm of the X chromosome.

**Free radicals.** The molecules that may cause disease by injuring cells.

**Friable.** Easily broken nodules or vegetations.

**Fulminating.** Having a rapid or severe onset.

**Functional.** Condition is one in which there is no organic change.

**Furuncles.** Large, tender, swollen raised lesions, boils, caused by staphylococci.

**Gaba aminobutyric acid (GABA).** Inhibitory neurotransmitter associated with various mental illnesses, sleep, mood, and behavior.

**Galactosemia.** An autosomal recessive disorder in which the enzyme necessary to convert galactose, a sugar derived from lactose in milk, to glucose is lacking.

**Gangrene.** Condition in which bacteria infects and destroys dead tissue.

**Gastric ulcers.** Ulcers of the stomach.

**Gastritis.** Inflammation of the stomach caused by irritants such as aspirin, excessive coffee, tobacco, alcohol, or an infection.

**Gastroesophageal reflux disease.** Regurgitation of acidic stomach contents onto the esophagus.

**Gastroscopy.** A procedure in which a camera is attached to a gastroscope, and the entire inner stomach is photographed.

**Genes.** Found in chromosomes, each is responsible for the synthesis of one protein.

**Genital herpes.** STD caused by herpes simplex virus type II.

**Genital warts.** STD causes by the human papilloma virus.

**Gigantism.** Usually the result of a tumor of the anterior pituitary.

**Glioblastomas.** Highly malignant, rapid-growing tumors of the brain.

**Glioma.** A sarcoma of neuroglial tissue or glial cells.

**Glomerular capsule.** Structure surrounding the glomerular capillaries of the nephron.

**Glomerulonephritis.** A degenerative inflammation of the glomerulus of a nephron, which usually follows a prior streptococcal infection.

**Glomerulus.** A tuft of capillaries situated inside the glomerular capsule of a nephron.

**Glucagon.** A hormone that works antagonistically to insulin and is released when the blood sugar level falls below normal.

**Glucagon.** Hormone secreted by endocrine pancreas that raises blood glucose.

**Glucocorticoids.** The group of steroid hormones that helps regulate carbohydrate, lipid, and protein metabolism.

**Glycogen.** A form of glucose that is stored in the liver and muscle.

**Glycosuria.** The condition in which excess glucose is excreted in the urine, a major sign of diabetes mellitus.

**Gonadotropins.** Hormones of the anterior pituitary that regulate sexual development and function.

**Gonorrhea.** STD caused by *Neiserria gonorrhea*.

**Gout.** Often called "gouty arthritis," it affects the joints of the feet, particularly those of the big toe, and is very painful.

**Graafian follicles.** Ovarian follicles stimulated at the beginning of each monthly cycle so that they begin to grow and develop by a pituitary gonadotropic hormone.

**Gram stain.** The staining technique that permits the identification of bacteria.

**Grandiose delusion.** A false belief of having special power, influence, or wealth.

**Gynecomastia.** A condition in which the breasts become enlarged.

**Hallucination.** Disturbance in sensory perception in sight, sound, touch, or smell.

**Health.** A state of relative equilibrium in which the body's many organ systems function adequately and are free from disease.

**Heart block.** Impulses are prevented from flowing from the atria to the ventricles because of a damaged route (e.g., MI), and thus the heart rate and EKG are altered.

**Heart murmurs.** Characteristic sounds of the heart that indicate the presence of valve defects.

**Helicobacter pylori.** A bacterium associated with ulcers.

**Helper T cells.** T cells that help the immune system by increasing the activity of killer cells and stimulating the suppressor T cells.

**Hemangioma.** Benign tumor made of small blood vessels that forms a red or purple birthmark.

**Hematemesis.** Vomiting of blood.

**Hematocrit.** The ratio of red-blood-cell-volume to whole blood.

**Hematoma.** A bruise caused by an injection.

**Hematuria.** Blood in the urine.

**Hemiplegia.** Paralysis on one side of the body.

**Hemodialysis.** Treatment for kidney failure; blood removed from the body is cleansed of metabolic waste, restored to physiological balance, and returned to the body.

**Hemoglobin.** A protein containing iron; serves as the oxygen-carrier protein that enables red blood cells to carry oxygen from the lungs to all body tissues.

**Hemolysis.** The rupture of red blood cells.

**Hemolytic streptococci.** A type of bacteria that cause a variety of infectious diseases, including infections of throat, skin, ear, and heart valves.

**Hemolyze.** Lysis of erythrocytes.

**Hemophilia.** Sex-linked inherited coagulation disorder cause by a deficiency of clotting factors.

**Hemoptysis.** Coughing blood.

**Hemorrhage.** A large loss of blood in a short period of time, either internally or externally

**Hemorrhoids.** Varicose veins of the rectum or anus.

**Hemostasis.** Reduced bloodflow.

**Heparin.** An anticoagulant.

**Hepatic coma.** Develops in the final stages of advanced liver disease; it is caused by an accumulation of ammonia in the blood, which has a toxic effect on the brain and may cause death.

**Hepatocarcinoma.** Cancer of the liver.

**Hereditary hemorrhagic telangiectasia.** Abnormal dilation of small vessels causing the appearance of red-violet lesions on the face, lips, oral, and nasal mucosa.

**Hermaphrodites.** Individuals who have both testes and ovaries.

**Heterozygous.** A person having two different alleles of a certain gene.

**Hiatal hernia.** The protrusion of part of the stomach through the diaphragm at the point where the esophagus joins the stomach.

**High-density lipoproteins (HDL).** The smallest lipoprotein particles containing the smallest amount of triglycerides. This HDL component is called good cholesterol.

**Hippocampus.** Structure of the brain that processes and stores information to memory.

**Hirsutism.** Term to describe the condition in which hair develops on the face of a woman.

**Histamine.** A substance that causes the capillary walls to become more permeable.

**Hodgkin's disease.** A type of lymphoma, distinguished by the presence of characteristic *Reed-Sternberg* cells in affected lymph nodes.

**Homeostasis.** The maintenance of a steady state within the body.

**Homozygous.** A person having the same two alleles of a particular gene.

**Horizontal transmission.** The route by which an infectious disease is transmitted directly from an infected human to a susceptible human.

**Hormones.** Chemical messengers secreted by endocrine glands.

**Human chorionic gonadotropin (HCG).** Hormone secreted by the chorionic villi after implantation of the fertilized ovum in the uterus.

**Human immunodeficiency virus (HIV).** The causative agent of AIDS; a retrovirus—that is, it carries its genetic information as RNA rather than DNA.

**Human papilloma virus (HPV).** The type of virus responsible for genital warts that seems to be the causative agent in uterine cervical carcinoma.

**Humoral immunity.** Protection from infection provided by antibodies.

**Huntington's chorea.** A progressive degenerative disease of the brain that results in the loss of muscle control.

**Hydatidiform mole.** A benign tumor of the placenta, consisting of multiple cysts and resembling a bunch of grapes.

**Hydrocephalus.** The accumulation of cerebrospinal fluid in the brain.

**Hydrocortisone.** Anti-inflammatory agent.

**Hydrolithotripsy.** A procedure using sonic vibrations to crush kidney stones while the patient is immersed in a tank of water.

**Hydronephrosis.** A condition when the kidney is extremely dilated with urine.

**Hydroureters.** The condition caused when the ureters above a kidney obstruction dilate.

**Hymen.** A membranous fold that partly or completely closes the vaginal opening.

**Hyperactive.** The term used to describe when a gland produces an excessive amount of its secretion.

**Hypercalcemia.** A condition in which too much calcium occurs in the blood.

**Hyperemesis gravidarum.** Excessive vomiting during pregnancy.

**Hyperemia.** Increased bloodflow to an injured area, causing heat and redness associated with inflammation.

**Hyperglycemia.** A condition resulting from deposits of calcium in organs such as kidneys, heart, lungs, and the walls of the stomach.

**Hyperkalemia.** An excess of potassium, which causes muscle weakness and can slow the heart to the point of cardiac arrest.

**Hypernephroma.** Carcinoma of the kidney; causes enlargement of kidney and destroys the organ.

**Hyperpituitarism.** Conditions associated with hypersecretion of the pituitary, usually manifested as the effects of excessive growth hormone, which retards the normal closure of bones at puberty.

**Hypersensitivity.** An abnormal immune response and sensitivity to allergens such as pollens, dust, dog hair, and certain foods.

**Hypertension.** High blood pressure.

**Hypertrophy.** Abnormal enlargement of an organ.

**Hypoactive.** The term used to describe when a gland fails to secrete its hormone or secretes an inadequate amount.

**Hypoalbuminemia.** An albumin deficiency.

**Hypochromic.** Red blood cells appear lighter than normal, caused by an iron deficiency.

**Hypophysis.** Another name for the pituitary gland. It has two parts, each of which acts as a separate gland.

**Hypothalamus.** The homeostatic center for the body, located just superior to the pituitary; controls thirst, temperature, and other functions, as well release of pituitary hormones.

**Hypovolemic shock.** Results from fluid volume loss after severe hemorrhage or loss of plasma in burn patients.

**Hypoxia.** Decreased concentration of oxygen in the blood due to low oxygen availability or blockages that prevent oxygen diffusing into the bloodstream.

**Icterus.** Jaundiced, yellow coloration.

**Idiopathic.** Term used to describe a disease for which the cause is not known.

**Idiopathic hypereosinophilic syndrome.** Mulitsystem disease associated with persistent increases in blood eosinophils.

**Immunity.** The ability of the body to defend inself against infectious agents, foreign cells, and abnormal body cells.

**Immunoglobulin.** Antibodies.

**Impetigo.** An acute, contagious skin infection common in children, most frequently affecting face and hands.

**Impotence.** Inability to achieve and maintain an erection sufficient for sexual intercourse.

**In situ.** In position; not disturbing surrounding tissues.

**Incidence.** The number of new cases of a disease in a population.

**Incontinence.** Inability to retain urine or feces due to loss of sphincter control or because of cerebral or spinal lesions.

**Infarct.** Dead tissue that occurs due to lack of blood flow in any organ or area, such as a coronary blockage in a heart vessel.

**Infectious diseases.** Diseases caused by pathogenic microorganisms.

**Infestations.** Infections involving wormlike animals called helminths.

**Inflammatory exudate.** Fluid composed of plasma and white cells that escape from capillaries.

**Influenza.** A viral infection of the upper respiratory system.

**Initiation.** The first stage of cancer in which there is a genetic change in a cell, an altering of the DNA by some agent, chemical, radiation, or an oncogenic virus.

**Insulin.** A hormone that is secreted when the blood sugar level rises.

**Insulin shock.** Hypoglycemic shock that results from too much insulin, not enough food, or excessive exercise.

**Interferon.** A group of substances that stimulates the immune system.

**Intravenous pyelogram.** Allows the visualization of the urinary system by means of contrast dyes injected into the veins, followed by an x-ray examination.

**Intrinsic factor.** Produced in the stomach, it carries vitamin $B_{12}$ to the small intestine, where it is absorbed into the bloodstream.

**Intussusception.** A type of organic obstruction in which a segment of intestine telescopes into the part forward of it.

**Irritable bowel.** A functional condition of the colon with diarrhea, constipation, abdominal pain, and gas.

**Irritable colon.** A functional disorder of the colon that results in diarrhea and cramping.

**Ischemia.** A deficiency of blood supply to any organ.

**Isolation.** Keeping an infected person in the hospital or staying at home in bed when suffering from a disease as a way of controlling the transmission of infectious diseases.

**Jaundice.** A yellow-orange discoloration of the skin, tissues, and the whites of the eyes caused when bilirubin (an orange pigment) accumulates in the plasma.

**Kaposi's sarcoma.** Purple neoplasm of the lower extremities.

**Karyotype.** The normal chromosomal composition of the nucleus of the cell that is characteristic of each species.

**Keloid.** The healing that occurs after surgery or a severe burn, consisting of a hard, raised scar.

**Keratin.** Protein in the epidermis produced by cells called keratinocytes; protects the skin from harmful substances.

**Ketone bodies.** Substances produced in diabetics' blood when insulin levels are low.

**Kidney dialysis.** Treatment for kidney failure; removes metabolic waste from blood and restores it to physiological balance.

**Klinefelter's syndrome.** A condition in which there is an extra sex chromosome resulting in a karyotype of 47,XXY.

**Kupffer cells.** Specialized cells that line the blood spaces within the liver. They engulf and digest bacteria and other foreign substances, thus cleansing the blood.

**Kwashiorkor.** Protein-calorie malnutrition that results from early weaning from breast milk.

**Laparoscopy.** A procedure in which an illuminated tube is inserted through a small incision or opening, used to diagnose endometriosis.

**Larynx.** The voice box located at the entrance of the trachea.

**Latent infection.** A condition caused when viruses insert themselves in cells and do not reproduce.

**Legionnaire's disease.** A lung infection caused by the bacterium *Legionella pneumophila;* characterized by flulike symptoms.

**Leiomyomas.** Benign tumors of the smooth muscle of the uterus, known as fibroid tumors.

**Lesion.** An abnormal tissue structure or function. May be the result of a wound, injury, or pathologic condition.

**Lethargy.** A condition of drowsiness.

**Leukemia.** A cancer of white blood cells in which the bone marrow produces a large number of abnormal white blood cells.

**Leukocytes.** White blood cells.

**Leukocytosis.** The excessive production of white cells.

**Leukorrhea.** White, foul-smelling vaginal discharge.

**Ligaments.** The substance that holds bones together.

**Lipase.** A digestive enzyme that breaks down lipid or fat.

**Lipoma.** Tumor that develops in adipose or fat tissue.

**Lipoproteins.** A water-soluble lipid fat. It is packaged into particles that contain blood proteins, which do mix with water.

**Lithotripsy.** A procedure using sonic vibrations to crush kidney stones; the patient is not immersed in water for the procedure.

**Low-density lipoproteins (LDL).** The larger lipoprotein particles containing triglycerides.

**Lumbar puncture.** A procedure (spinal tap) used to diagnosis meningitis in which a hollow needle is inserted into the spinal canal between vertebrae near the L-4, or lumbar region, to obtain and analyze cerebrospinal fluid.

**Lumen.** The inner space of a hollow organ such as a blood vessel or intestine.

**Lumpectomy.** Surgery to remove only the tumor from the breast.

**Lymphadenopathy.** Enlarged lymph nodes.

**Lymphatic system.** An important part of the body's immunity, it consists of modes, organs, and a complex network of thin-walled capillaries carrying lymph fluid to help to maintain the internal fluid environment of the body.

**Lymphocytes.** A type of white blood cell consisting of T lymphocytes and B lymphocytes.

**Lymphocytic.** The type of leukemia that results from cancer of the lymphocytic stem cells, which are found both in the bone marrow and in the lymph nodes.

**Lymphomas.** Several types of malignancies of the lymphatic system.

**Lyse.** The infecting of cells by viruses.

**Macular.** Flat lesions on the skin.

**Magnetic resonance imaging (MRI).** A diagnostic-imaging technique that uses the behavior of protons when placed in powerful magnetic fields to make images of organs and tissues.

**Major depression.** Mood disorder associated with sadness, hopelessness, and despair.

**Malabsorption.** The inability of a person to absorb substances from the small intestines.

**Malignant melanoma.** The most serious skin cancer; arises from the melanocytes.

**Malignant.** Term used to describe a neoplasm or tumor that spreads and possibly causes death.

**Malnutrition.** Suboptimal supply of nutrients that results in decreased tissue mass and energy stores needed for proper growth and development.

**Mammography.** Diagnostic x-ray for breast tissue that can detect small, early cancers.

**Mania.** An overly energetic elevated or irritable mood.

**Marfan syndrome.** An autosomal dominant disorder that results from the dysfunction of the gene that codes for the connective tissue protein fibrillin.

**Marasmus.** Protein-calorie malnutrition caused by near starvation.

**Mast cells.** Cells found in connective tissue; they contain heparin, serotonin, bradykinin, and histamine.

**Mastectomy.** Surgery to remove the breast due to cancer.

**Mastoiditis.** Inflammation of the air cells in the mastoid process of the temporal bone.

**Medullary cavity.** A hollow cavity found in the long bones of the arms and legs that is filled with yellow bone marrow primarily consisting of fat.

**Melanin.** The dark pigment of the skin that protects the body from the harmful rays of the sun.

**Melanocytes.** Cells at the bottom of the epidermis that produce melanin.

**Melanoma.** Skin cancer.

**Melasma.** Patches of dark skin on the cheeks that develop due to hormonal changes.

**Melena.** Stool with a dark, tarry appearance caused by blood from the upper part of the digestive tract.

**Memory cells.** B lymphocytes that do not become plasma cells but remain dormant until reactivated by the same antigen.

**Menarche.** The onset of menstruation, the beginning of a woman's reproductive life, occurring generally between ages 10 and 15.

**Meninges.** Three coverings that protect the delicate nerve tissue of the spinal cord and brain.

**Meningioma.** A benign brain tumor that occurs in the membranes that surround the brain.

**Meningitis.** An acute inflammation of the first two meninges that cover the brain and spinal cord.

**Meningocele.** A form of spina bifida noticeable at birth; the spinal cord is not involved in this defect.

**Meningomyelocele.** A form of spina bifida in which the nerve elements protrude into the sac and are trapped, thus preventing proper placement and development.

**Menopause.** The cessation of menstrual periods, the ending of a woman's reproductive life, which usually begins in the late 40s or early 50s.

**Menorrhagia.** Excessive or prolonged bleeding during menstruation.

**Metastasis.** The spread of cancer to distant sites within the body.

**Metastasize.** To invade by metastasis.

**Metrorrhagia.** Bleeding between menstrual periods or extreme irregularity of the cycle.

**Mineralocorticoids.** A group of steroid hormones that regulate salt balance in the body.

**Mitral stenosis.** Occurs when the mitral valve opening is too small and the cusps that form the valve become rigid and fuse together.

**Mitral valve.** The valve between the left atrium and left ventricle; it has two flaps, or cusps, that meet when the valve is closed.

**Mixed cancers.** Cancer consisting of cells of different origins or tissue types.

**Monocyte.** A type of white blood cell that aids in clearing pus.

**Morbidity.** The number who become sick or disabled from a disease per 100,000.

**Mortality.** The number who die from a disease per 100,000 who have the disease.

**Mucosa.** Secretes excessive mucus, causing a runny nose and congestion.

**Mucus.** A thick, watery secretion.

**Mutagens.** Chemicals introduced to the lungs by cigarette smoking.

**Mutations.** Changes in DNA structure that may be inherited and cause disease.

**Myasthenia gravis.** An autoimmune neuromuscular disorder characterized by muscular fatigue that develops with repetitive muscle use and improves with rest.

**Mycelia.** Filaments in fungi specialized for absorption of nutrients.

**Mycoses.** Infectious diseases caused by fungi.

**Myelin.** A lipid covering that insulates the fibers of sensory and motor neurons.

**Myelocele.** The most severe form of spina bifida.

**Myelogenous.** The type of leukemia in which the cancer originates in the bone marrow.

**Myelomonocytic leukemia.** A type of myelogenous leukemia of malignant monocytes.

**Myocardial infarction.** A true heart attack.

**Myocardium.** The cardiac muscle found in the chamber walls of the heart.

**Myoma.** A tumor of the muscle that develops in smooth or involuntary muscle.

**Myxedema.** The condition of severe hypothyroidism, an inadequate level of thyroxine.

**Natural killer cells.** A type of leukocyte that destroys cells with abnormal membranes.

**Necrotic.** Dead tissue due to lack of blood.

**Negative feedback.** Homeostatic control mechanism.

**Neoplasm.** A mass of new cells that grows in a haphazard fashion with no useful function; a tumor.

**Nephron.** The functional unit of the kidney.

**Neurofibrillatory tangle.** Abnormal collection of protein in the brain associated with Alzheimer's disease.

**Neurogenic shock.** Condition due to generalized vasodilation resulting from decreased vasomotor tone.

**Neuron.** Nerve cell.

**Neurotransmitter.** Chemical messengers that communicate in the synapse between nerve cells, or neurons.

**Neutropenia.** A reduction of circulating neutrophils, or white blood cells.

**Neutrophils.** White blood cells that fight against invading agents or injury.

**Nevus.** A small, dark skin growth that develops from pigment-producing cells, or melanocytes; a benign tumor.

**Nitroglycerin.** Medication used to dilate coronary arteries, permitting adequate bloodflow.

**Noncommunicable.** Infectious diseases that are not transmitted directly by humans.

**Nondisjunction.** The failure of two chromosomes to separate as the gametes, either the egg or the sperm, are being formed.

**Nonspecific defenses.** Defenses that are effective against any foreign agent that enters the body.

**Norepinephrine.** Neurotransmitter of the sympathetic nervous system.

**Notifiable diseases.** Diseases under surveillance that must be reported by physicians to the Centers for Disease Control and Prevention.

**Nucleic acid analogues.** Anti-viral medications.

**Nutrient.** Chemical compound consumed in food that are required for vital cellular processes.

**Nystagmus.** Involuntary, rapid movement of the eyeball, characteristic of multiple sclerosis.

**Obesity-hypoventilation syndrome.** Also called pickwickian syndrome, a condition of recurrent episodes of apnea during sleep caused by airway occlusion due to excess weight or obesity.

**Obesity.** A nutritional disorder in which an abnormal amount of fat accumulates in adipose tissue.

**Obstructive sleep apnea syndrome.** Respiratory complication often associated with obesity.

**Occult blood.** Blood detected in stool by means of a chemical test but not apparent to the naked eye.

**Oliguria.** A reduced production of urine.

**Oncogene.** Any gene having the potential to induce a cancerous transformation.

**Oppositional defiant disorder.** Disruptive behavior disorder diagnosed in childhood.

**Orchitis.** Inflammation of the testes; can follow an injury or viral infection such as mumps.

**Organic obstructions.** A material blockage that prevents the contents of the intestinal tract from moving forward.

**Ossification.** Process by which bone tissue is formed.

**Osteitis fibrosa cystica.** In this disease, fibrous nodules and cysts form in the bones, which become very porous and decalcified.

**Osteoarthritis.** The most common form of arthritis, a chronic disease that accompanies aging and may affect only one joint.

**Osteoblasts.** A cell that works within the bone to form bone tissue.

**Osteoclasts.** A cell that works within the bone and resorbs bone.

**Osteocytes.** Mature cells in bone tissue.

**Osteogenic sarcoma.** A primary malignancy of the bone.

**Osteoma.** The most common benign tumor of the bone.

**Osteomalacia.** A bone disease in adults caused by the lack of vitamin D, which results in a softening of the bones.

**Osteomyelitis.** An inflammation of the bone, particularly of the bone marrow in the medullary cavity and in the spaces of spongy bone.

**Osteoporosis.** The increased porosity of the bone.

**Outbreak.** The sudden occurrence of a disease, in unexpected numbers in a limited area, which then subsides.

**Oxytocin.** One of two hormones secreted by the posterior pituitary; it causes smooth muscle, particularly that of the uterus, to contract and initiates milk secretions.

**Paget's disease.** A rare cancer involving inflammatory changes that affect the nipple and the areola.

**Pallor.** Whitening of the skin.

**Pancreatic islets.** Endocrine cells of the pancreas.

**Pancreatitis.** A potentially life-threatening inflammation of the pancreas.

**Pandemic.** Describes an epidemic that has spread to include several large areas worldwide.

**Papanicolaou test.** Screening test for cervical cancer based on observations of cells in obtained in biopsies of cervix.

**Papilloma.** Also known as a polyp, an epithelial tumor that grows as a projecting mass on the skin or from an inner mucous membrane; the common wart is an example.

**Pap smear.** A diagnostic technique for identifying cancer in the cervix by scraping cells from the cervix and examining them microscopically.

**Papular.** Lesions on the skin that are raised.

**Paralytic obstructions.** Caused when the contents of the intestinal tract are unable to move forward due to a decrease in peristalsis, preventing propulsion of intestinal contents.

**Parathormone.** The hormone secreted by the parathyroids.

**Paresis.** A general paralysis associated with organic loss of brain function; results in death if untreated.

**Paresthesia.** Numbness, burning, or tingling sensation resulting from nerve injury.

**Passive immunity.** Doses of preformed antibodies from immune serum of an animal, usually a horse. This type of immunity is short-lived but acts immediately.

**Patent ductus arteriosus (PDA).** A common congenital disease in which the ductus arteriosus remains open and blood intended for the body flows from the aorta to the lungs, overloading the pulmonary artery.

**Pathogenesis.** The source or cause of an illness or abnormal condition and its development.

**Pathogens.** Microorganisms that cause disease.

**Pathology.** The branch of medicine that studies the characteristics, causes, and effects of disease.

**Pathology.** Study of disease.

**Pediculosis.** Louse infestations that are classified into three categories: head lice, pubic lice, and body lice.

**Pellagra.** Niacin deficiency.

**Pelvic inflammatory disease (PID).** Inflammation of the female reproductive organs due to bacterial, viral, fungal, or parasitic invasion.

**Peptic ulcers.** Ulcers of the stomach and small intestine due, in part, to the action of pepsin, a proteolytic enzyme secreted by the stomach.

**Perforation.** An ulcer breaks through the intestinal or gastric wall, causing sudden and intense abdominal pain.

**Pericardium.** The double membranous sac that encloses the heart.

**Periosteum.** A highly vascular layer of fibrous connective tissue that covers the surface of bones.

**Peristalisis.** Muscle contractions that propel food during the digestive process.

**Peritoneal dialysis.** Treatment for kidney failure; fluid added to peritoneal cavity draws metabolic waste from the blood and restores it to physiological balance.

**Peritonitis.** Inflammation of the lining of the abdominal cavity, usually results when the digestive contents enter the cavity, because this material contains numerous bacteria.

**Pernicious anemia.** A vitamin $B_{12}$ deficiency.

**Persecutory delusion.** False belief that one is being followed, watched, or plotted against.

**Personality disorder.** Mental disturbance characterized by inflexible patterns of behavior that affect interpersonal relationships. Includes three major categories or clusters based on symptoms: paranoid, schizoid (cluster A), antisocial, borderline, histrionic, narcissistic (cluster B), and avoidant, dependent, obsessive-compulsive (cluster C).

**Petechiae.** Tiny red or purple spots caused by minute blood vessels that rupture in the skin.

**Phagocyte.** Leukocytes that take in and destroy foreign material.

**Phagocytosis.** White blood cells take in and destroy foreign material.

**Pharyngeoplasty.** Surgical removal of the uvula to alleviate obstructive sleep apnea.

**Pharynx.** The throat.

**Phenylketonuria.** Also called PKU, caused by an autosomal recessive allele that lacks a specific enzyme that converts one amino acid, phenylalanine, to another, tyrosine.

**Pheochromocytoma.** A neuroendocrine tumor of the adrenal gland.

**Phlebitis.** An inflammation of a vein, usually in the leg.

**Phosphate.** Compound containing phosphorous essential for bone and tooth structure as well as cell physiology.

**Physiology.** Study of the normal function of the body.

**Pipestem colon.** Term used to describe the colon in patients suffering from chronic ulcerative colitis; colon appears straight and rigid.

**Placenta.** The interdigitation of embryonic and maternal tissue.

**Placenta previa.** Abnormal positioning of the placenta in the lower uterus, often near the cervical opening.

**Plantar warts.** Serious, painful warts that form on the soles of the feet.

**Plaque.** Fatty deposits in the walls of arteries.

**Plasma cells.** Cells that develop from B cells and produce antibodies.

**Platelets.** Clotting elements of blood.

**Pleura.** A double membrane consisting of two layers that encases the lungs.

**Pleural cavity.** The space between the two layers of the pleura containing a small amount of fluid that lubricates the surfaces, preventing friction as the lungs expand and contract.

**Pleurisy.** The inflammation of the pleural membranes occurring as a complication of various lung diseases like pneumonia or tuberculosis.

**Pneumonia.** An acute inflammation of the lung in which air spaces in the lungs become filled with an inflammatory exudate.

**Poliomyelitis.** An infectious disease of the brain and spinal cord caused by a virus.

**Polydactyly.** An autosomal dominant disorder that causes extra fingers or toes.

**Polydipsia.** Extreme thirst.

**Polymorphs.** White blood cells specialized to fight against invading agents or injury.

**Polyp.** Benign epithelial tumor.

**Polyuria.** The excessive production of dilute urine.

**Postpartum depression.** Subcategory of depression that occurs 2 weeks to 6 months following the birth of a child.

**Premature ejaculation.** Ejaculation during foreplay or immediately after beginning intercourse.

**Premenstrual dysphoric disorder.** Subcategory of depression with cyclical symptoms prior to menstruation.

**Premenstrual syndrome (PMS).** A group of severe symptoms—emotional, physical, and behavioral—that are associated with the menstrual cycle.

**Prevalence.** The number of existing cases of a disease.

**Primary atypical pneumonia.** Also known as "walking pneumonia," it is caused by a variety of microorganisms, including viruses and unusual bacterium called *Mycoplasma pneumoniae.*

**Primary follicle.** A single layer of cells that surround each ovum.

**Proctoscope.** An instrument consisting of a hollow tube with a lighted end used by physicians to observe the lining of the colon.

**Prognosis.** The predicted course and outcome of a disease.

**Progression.** The third stage of cancer development.

**Prolapse.** A falling or dropping down of an organ or internal structure, such as the uterus or rectum.

**Promotion.** The second stage of cancer development in which altered cells proliferate and resemble benign neoplasms, which can either regress to normal-appearing tissue or evolve into cancer.

**Prostate.** Produces alkaline fluid to help neutralize vaginal pH.

**Prostatitis.** Inflammation of the prostate.

**Prothrombin.** An enzyme synthesized by the liver with the aid of vitamin K that initiates the chain reaction in the blood-coagulation process.

**Pruritis.** Itching that accompanies many skin diseases.

**Pseudopodia.** Cell membrane extensions used for locomotion of phagocytosis.

**Psoriasis.** A superficial, recurring idiopathic skin disorder characterized by an abnormal rate of epidermal cell production and turnover.

**Psychiatric.** Pertaining to mental health.

**Psychiatry.** Medical field that studies and treats mental illness.

**Psychology.** Study of human behavior.

**Puerperal mastitis.** Bacterial infection of the breast.

**Puerperal sepsis.** An infection of the endometrium after childbirth or an abortion.

**Puerperium.** The time period after childbirth when the endometrium is open and particularly susceptible to infection.

**Pulmonary edema.** A buildup of fluid in the lungs, causing shortness of breath.

**Pulmonary stenosis.** The first cause of cyanosis in which the valve opening that leads into the pulmonary artery is too small and an inadequate amount of blood reaches the lungs to be oxygenated.

**Purging.** Self-induced, willful elimination of consumed food by vomiting or misuse of laxatives or diuretics.

**Purkinje fibers.** The specialized heart tissue that conducts the impulse for contraction to the myocardium of the ventricles.

**Purpura simplex.** A condition of easy bruising.

**Purpura.** Small hemorrhages into the tissue beneath the skin or mucous membranes.

**Pustules.** Lesions containing pus.

**Pyelitis.** An inflammation of the renal pelvis, the juncture between the ureter and the kidney, caused by *E. coli* or other pus-forming bacteria.

**Pyelonephritis.** A suppurative inflammation of the kidney and renal pelvis.

**Pyloric sphincter.** The sphincter muscle through which food passes from the stomach into the small intestine.

**Pyloric stenosis.** A congenital obstruction of the intestinal tract.

**Pyogenic.** Bacteria that cause pus.

**Pyuria.** This condition is caused when abscesses in the kidney rupture and pus enters the renal pelvis and then appears in urine.

**Quarantine.** The separation of persons who may or may not be infected from healthy people until the period of infectious risk is passed.

**Rabies.** An infectious disease of the brain and spinal cord caused by a virus that is transmitted by the saliva, urine, or feces of an infected animal.

**Rales.** Abnormal respiratory sounds detected with a stethoscope.

**Raynaud's disease.** The condition in which small arteries or arterioles in the fingers and toes constrict.

**Recessive.** Term used to describe an allele that manifests itself when the person is homozygous for the trait.

**Rectocele.** Protrusion of the rectum into the vagina.

**Reflux.** The back-flow of the acid contents of the stomach causing inflammation of the esophagus.

**Regional enteritis.** An inflammatory disease of the intestine that most frequently affects young adults, particularly females.

**Regurgitated.** Passage of stomach contents into the esophagus.

**Relapse.** Occurs when a disease returns weeks or months after its apparent cessation.

**Remission.** The period of a chronic disease when signs and symptoms subside.

**Renal pelvis.** The juncture between the kidneys and the ureters; final urine from all collecting ducts empties here.

**Renin.** Secreted by cells that convert angiotensinogen to angiotensin, an active enzyme to help elevate blood pressure.

**Reservoirs.** The sources of a pathogen and a potential source of disease.

**Respiratory epithelium.** A mucous membrane that lines the entire respiratory tract.

**Resuscitation.** Assisting or reviving respiration to a person with a myocardial infarction.

**Reticulocyte.** The late stage of erythrocyte development.

**Reye's syndrome.** A potentially devastating neurologic illness that sometimes develops in young children after a viral infection.

**Rh factor.** Antigen on erythrocyte, used for blood typing.

**Rhabdomyosarcoma.** A malignant tumor of the skeletal muscle.

**Rheumatoid factor.** Antibodies in blood that are associated with rheumatoid arthritis.

**Rhodopsin.** The pigment that absorbs light in the rods of the retina.

**Rickets.** A disease of infancy and early childhood in which the bones do not properly ossify, or harden, generally caused by a vitamin D deficiency.

**Roundworm.** A wormlike animal that is relatively round in cross-section.

**Salpingitis.** An inflammation of the fallopian tubes.

**Sarcoma.** A less common type of cancer that spreads rapidly and is highly malignant.

**Scabies.** A contagious skin disease associated with poor living conditions.

**Schizophrenia.** Mental illness characterized by social withdrawal, delusions, hallucinations, and unpredictable behavior.

**Scleroderma.** A chronic, progressive autoimmune disorder of the skin.

**Sclerosis.** An abnormal hardening of a tissue.

**Sclerotherapy.** Use of sclerosing or hardening agents to treat diseases like hemorrhoids or esophageal varices.

**Scurvy.** Disease due to vitamin C deficiency.

**Seasonal affective disorder.** Subcategory of major depression associated with decreased sunlight exposure during the winter months.

**Sebaceous glands.** Oil glands located within the dermis.

**Seborrheic dermatitis.** The excessive secretion of sebum from the sebaceous glands; chronic dandruff.

**Seborrheic keratosis.** Benign overgrowth of epithelial cells common in older adults.

**Sebum.** Oily fluid released through the hair follicles.

**Secondary pneumonia.** A pneumonia that develops as a secondary disorder from other diseases that weaken the lungs or the body's immune system.

**Seizures.** An uncontrolled nervous-system activity manifested by uncoordinated motor action.

**Seminal vesicle.** Produce fructose to nourish sperm.

**Seminiferous tubules.** Highly coiled tubules contained within the testes in which sperm develop.

**Septic embolism.** An embolism that contains infected material from pyogenic bacteria.

**Sequela.** The aftermath of a particular disease, such as permanent damage to the heart after rheumatic fever.

**Serotonin.** One of many neurotransmitters involved in regulating mood, emotions, and behavior.

**Sex-linked inheritance.** Diseases transmitted on the sex chromosomes.

**Serum.** Liquid portion of the blood.

**Shingles.** An acute inflammation of nerve cells caused by the chicken pox virus, herpes zoster.

**Sickle cell anemia.** An autosomal recessive disorder, in which the hemoglobin is abnormal, resulting in deformed, sickle-shaped red blood cells.

**Signs.** The objective evidence of disease observed on physical examination, such as abnormal pulse or fever.

**Sinoatrial node.** The pacemaker of the heart, it is a small patch of tissue that initiates the heartbeat.

**Skeletal muscle.** Striated muscle attached to bone and that is under conscious control.

**Somatic.** False belief that something physical is occuring in one's body.

**Spastic colon (irritable colon).** A functional condition of the colon with diarrhea and cramping.

**Specific defenses.** Defenses that are effective against particular identified foreign agents.

**Spider veins.** Small, dense, red networks of veins.

**Spina bifida.** A condition in which one or more vertebrae fail to fuse, leaving an opening in the vertebral canal. The word *bifid* means a cleft, or split into two parts, which is the condition of the vertebra in spina bifida.

**Spirilla.** Spiral-shaped bacterial cells.

**Spirochetes.** Corkscrew-shaped bacterial cells.

**Spirometer.** A simple instrument used to measure the movement of air in and out of the lungs.

**Spirometry.** A diagnostic procedure that measures and records changes in gas volume in the lungs, determining ventilation capacity and flow rate.

**Splenomegaly.** An enlarged spleen.

**Spongy bone.** Bone tissue with blood-filled spaces; found at ends of bones or in flat bones like those of the skull.

**Spores.** Microscopic fungal reproductive structures that can induce allergies.

**Sporozoans.** A form of protozoa; a single-celled, not mobile, eukaryotic microorganism.

**Sprains.** The result of the wrenching or twisting of a joint such as an ankle that injures the ligaments.

**Spurs.** Spicules of abnormal new bone development.

**Squamous cell carcinoma.** A malignancy of the keratinocytes in the epidermis.

**Staghorn calculus.** A kidney stone that becomes so large it fills the renal pelvis completely, blocking the flow of urine.

**Standard precautions.** Precautions such as gloves required of medical personnel when handling patients or bodily fluids.

**Stasis.** Slow bloodflow that may lead to thrombosis or cause infection; slow urine flow that may promote kidney stones.

**Status asthmaticus.** Life-threatening form of an asthma attack.

**Stenosis.** Constriction or narrowing of a passage or orifice.

**Stent.** Rigid structure surgically inserted into arteries in order to hold them open.

**Stomatitis.** Inflammation of the lining of the mouth often caused by bacteria or fungi.

**Strabismus.** The condition of crossed eyes.

**Strains.** Pulled muscles that result from a tearing of a muscle and/or its tendon from excessive use or stretching.

**Streptococci.** A type of bacterium associated with infections of the ear, throat, skin, and heart valves.

**Stroke.** The term used broadly to include cerebral hemorrhages and blood-clot formation within cerebral blood vessels.

**Subarachnoid.** A tear in the surface membrane of the brain by a skull fracture.

**Subdural.** A hemorrhage under the dura mater; from large venous sinuses of the brain rather than an artery.

**Substance use disorders.** Includes alcohol and drug abuse and addiction.

**Suppressor T cells.** The type of T cell that controls the immune response.

**Suppurative.** A type of inflammation associated with pus formation.

**Symptoms.** An indication of disease perceived by the patient, such as pain, dizziness, and itching.

**Syncope.** Fainting caused by insufficient blood supply to the brain.

**Syndrome.** Combination of symptoms.

**Synovial fluid.** Lubricating and shock-absorbing fluid found within joints.

**Synovial membrane.** The membrane that lines the joints.

**Syphilis.** STD caused by *Treponema pallidum.*

**Systemic lupus erythematosus (SLE).** An autoimmune disease that not only affects the skin but also causes the deterioration of collagenous connective tissue.

**Systole.** The period of the heartbeat when the heart contracts and pumps the blood.

**T lymphocytes.** Provide cell-mediated immunity and are processed by the thymus gland.

**Tachycardia.** Heart rate of 100 beats per minute or more.

**Tay-Sachs.** An autosomal recessive disorder caused by the absence of the A enzyme.

**Tachypnea.** Rapid respiration rate.

**Tendons.** Connective tissue that attaches skeletal or voluntary muscles firmly to bones.

**Terminal.** A disease ending in death.

**Tetanus toxoid.** A type of immunization that protects from the disease tetanus.

**Tetany.** A sustained muscular contraction.

**Tetralogy of Fallot.** One of the most serious congenital defects consisting of four (*tetra*) abnormalities.

**Thalassemia.** Group of inherited blood disorders in which there is deficient synthesis of one or more alpha or beta chains required for proper formation and optimal performance of the hemoglobin molecule.

**Thrombi.** Blood clots.

**Thrombocytopenia.** A disease of platelets resulting in gastrointestinal and urogenital hemorrhages as well as severe nosebleeds.

**Thrombolytic.** Agents that dissolve blood clots.

**Thrombophlebitis.** Thrombus formation in deep veins.

**Thrombosis.** The forming of blood clots on blood vessel walls.

**Thrombus.** A blood clot that forms in a blood vessel.

**Thyroxine.** One of the thyroid hormones.

**Tic.** Sudden, rapid, involuntary stereotyped movement or vocalization.

**Tinea.** Fungal skin infection.

**Toxic shock syndrome (TSS).** Caused by infection with *Staphylococcus aureus.*

**Toxoid.** A chemically altered toxin that stimulates an immune response.

**Trachea.** The "windpipe," which connects the larynx to the primary bronchi of the lungs.

**Tracheotomy.** Emergency procedure to maintain airway by cutting a hole in the trachea.

**Trachoma.** A chronic contagious form of conjunctivitis causing hypertrophy of the conjunctiva.

**Transformation.** A change from one tissue to another.

**Tremors.** A shakiness, particularly of the hands.

**Trichomonas vaginalis.** A parasite that can be transmitted by sexual intercourse; one causative agent of vaginitis.

**Trichomoniasis.** STD caused by the protozoan *Trichomonas vaginalis.*

**Tricuspid valve.** The valve between the right atrium and right ventricle. It has three cusps.

**Triglycerides.** A lipid fat that is not water-soluble and therefore cannot mix with blood plasma.

**Triiodothyronine.** A thyroid hormone.

**Trisomy 21.** The condition of having chromosome 21 in triplicate, causing Down syndrome.

**Tubercles.** Lesions that are formed when tissue infected with tuberculosis heals with fibrosis and calcification, walling off the bacteria for months or many years.

**Tuberculosis.** A chronic infectious disease characterized by necrosis of vital lung tissue, which can affect other body systems as well.

**Tumor marker.** Abnormal levels or substances found in the blood of cancer patients; used to monitor the presence of cancer and the extent of disease.

**Tumor.** A mass of new cells that grows in a haphazard fashion with no control or useful function.

**Turner's syndrome.** The condition caused when one of the sex chromosomes is missing, resulting in a karyotype of 45,XO.

**Ultrasound cardiography.** Shows the anatomy of arteries, particularly the carotid bifurcation and the internal carotid artery.

**Ultrasound.** Imaging technique utilizing low-frequency sound waves.

**Upper respiratory infections.** Disorders of the nose and throat, including common infections and allergies.

**Urea.** Nitrogen-containing waste products formed in the liver.

**Uremia.** A toxic condition of blood; the end result is kidney failure.

**Ureterocele.** Cyst-like dilation of the ureter near its opening to the urinary bladder.

**Ureters.** Muscular tubes that pass urine from the kidney to the urinary bladder.

**Urethra.** The single tube through which urine empties to the outside from the urinary bladder.

**Urethritis.** Inflammation of the urethra.

**Urinalysis.** A simple diagnostic procedure that examines a urine specimen physically, chemically, and microscopically.

**Urinary calculi.** Stones formed primarily in the kidney when certain salts in the urine form a precipitate and grow in size.

**Urticaria.** Known as hives, results from a vascular reaction of the skin to an allergen.

**Uterine prolapse.** Uterus dropping downward into the vagina.

**Uvula.** Soft structure hanging from free edge of the soft palate in midline above the root of the tongue.

**Vaccine.** A low dose of dead or deactivated bacteria or virus that stimulates an immune response.

**Valvular insufficiency.** Occurs when a valve opening is too large and does not prevent backflow.

**Vas deferens.** A duct that passes through the inguinal canal into the abdominal cavity of males.

**Vascular dementia.** Degenerative memory disorder most often caused by physical insults to the brain.

**Vasopressin.** One of two hormones secreted by the posterior pituitary, also called antidiuretic hormone.

**Vectors.** Animals that transmit pathogenic microorganisms to humans.

**Vegetations.** Small nodular structures composed of bacteria and clots that form along the edge of cusps in a valve opening.

**Venae cavae.** The two largest veins of the body.

**Ventricular fibrillation.** Occurs when a series of uncoordinated impulses spread over the ventricles, causing them to twitch or quiver rather than contract.

**Verruca vulgaris.** Warts caused by viruses affecting the keratinocytes of the skin, causing them to proliferate.

**Vertical transmission.** The route by which an infectious disease is transmitted from one generation to the next.

**Vesicles.** Small, blisterlike eruptions on the skin.

**Vibrios.** Comma-shaped bacterial cells.

**Vitiligo.** A loss of melanin resulting in white patches of skin, which are usually well demarcated and may cover large parts of the body.

**Voluntary muscle.** Striated muscle attached to bone and that is under conscious control.

**Volvulus.** A condition in which the intestine is twisted on itself.

**Wernicke's encephalopathy.** A brain disease, often associated with chronic alcoholism, in which the patient becomes mentally confused and disoriented and may suffer delirium tremens.

**Wheals.** Rounded elevations on the skin known as lesions, with red edges and pale centers, extremely pruritic, or itchy.

**Wheezing.** The sound of labored breathing as a result of narrowed tubes in the lungs.

**Wilms' tumor.** A malignant tumor of the kidney that develops in very young children.

# Answers to Interactive Activities

## CHAPTER 1

### Multiple Choice

1. a. sign
2. a. acute
3. d. etiology
4. a. homeostasis
5. b. exacerbation

### True or False

1. False
2. True
3. False
4. True
5. True

### Fill-Ins

1. prognosis
2. lesions
3. idiopathic
4. relapse
5. remission

## CHAPTER 2

### Multiple Choice

1. e. all of the above
2. b. allergy
3. b. Plasma cells
4. a. innate immunity
5. a. long lived
6. e. casual contact
7. b. nonspecific defense
8. c. cytotoxic T cells
9. d. cortisol
10. d. chemotaxis

### True or False

1. False
2. True
3. False
4. False
5. False
6. True
7. True
8. True
9. True
10. True

### Fill-Ins

1. helper $T_4$
2. antigen
3. memory cells
4. Cytotoxic
5. vaccine
6. Immunity
7. Nonspecific
8. histamine
9. lymphatic system
10. phagocytosis

## CHAPTER 3

### Multiple Choice

1. b. pandemic
2. a. cannot grow on their own
3. b. *Plasmodium*
4. c. cell walls
5. d. malaria
6. a. bacteria
7. d. flagella
8. b. capsid
9. c. fungal
10. d. ringworm

## True or False

1. False
2. True
3. True
4. True
5. False
6. True
7. True
8. True
9. False
10. True

## Fill-Ins

1. pathogenic microorganisms
2. Vaccination
3. arthropods
4. Epidemiology
5. Standard Precautions
6. vectors
7. reservoir
8. tick
9. incidence
10. Schistosoma

# CHAPTER 4

## Multiple Choice

1. b. adenoma
2. d. melanoma
3. c. metastasis
4. a. DNA
5. b. Cachexia
6. c. once a month
7. a. cyclins
8. c. chemotherapy

## True or False

1. True
2. False
3. True
4. True
5. False
6. True
7. True
8. True

## Fill-Ins

1. 15
2. beta human chorionic gonadotropin, alpha feto protein
3. angiomas

4. TNM
5. endoscopy
6. biopsy
7. cyclins
8. Initiation

# CHAPTER 5

## Multiple Choice

1. b. XY
2. b. 46
3. a. Recessive
4. c. men have one X chromosome
5. c. red and green
6. b. autosomal recessive
7. b. 50
8. c. 50
9. c. heterozygous
10. c. autosomes

## True or False

1. True
2. True
3. False
4. False
5. False
6. False
7. False
8. True
9. True
10. True

## Fill-Ins

1. Congential
2. Hermaphrodites
3. Recessive
4. Genes
5. Alleles
6. Polydactyly
7. Nondisjunction
8. 23
9. karyotype
10. meiosis

# CHAPTER 6

## Multiple Choice

1. b. folic acid
2. c. beriberi
3. c. coronary artery disease
4. a. Cushing's syndrome
5. d. body mass index

6. c. carotene
7. a. the skin
8. c. vitamin K
9. b. potassium
10. a. chloride

## True or False

1. True
2. False
3. True
4. True
5. True
6. False
7. True
8. False
9. True
10. True

## Fill-Ins

1. A, D, E, and K.
2. RDA
3. cultural, social, and religious
4. fluoride
5. Vitamin E and vitamin C
6. niacin
7. calcium, phosphorus, and magnesium
8. Inflammatory bowel disease and Crohn's disease
9. Bile
10. Insulin, glucose

## CHAPTER 7

### Multiple Choice

1. a. right ventricle
2. d. (2), (4), (6), (7)
3. c. Pulmonary stenosis
4. b. Ventricular fibrillation
5. b. coarctation of the aorta
6. b. atherosclerosis
7. a. veins
8. c. aneurysm
9. b. pulmonary artery
10. a. constriction

### True or False

1. True
2. False
3. False
4. True
5. True
6. True

7. False
8. False
9. False
10. False

## Fill-Ins

1. Cardiac ultasonography
2. hypertrophy
3. pulmonary lungs
4. aorta
5. constriction
6. systole
7. embolism
8. unknown
9. aspirin
10. defibrillator

## CHAPTER 8

### Multiple Choice

1. a. hematocrit
2. d. all the above
3. c. clotting factors
4. d. all of the above
5. b. is shorter in duration
6. a. iron deficiency
7. a. leukemia
8. b. bilirubin
9. d. all of the above
10. c. pain and inflammation

### True or False

1. True
2. True
3. False
4. False
5. True
6. True
7. True
8. True
9. False
10. False

### Fill-Ins

1. leukocytes
2. erythrocytes
3. oxyhemoglobin
4. hemoglobin S
5. iron, protein chains
6. myelogenous leukemia
7. bacterial, fungal
8. platelets

9. eosinophilia myalgia syndrome
10. quantitative, qualitative

## CHAPTER 9

### Multiple Choice

1. d. emphysema
2. c. asthma
3. c. emphysema
4. c. tuberculosis
5. c. asthma
6. a. pneumonia
7. b. emphysema
8. d. bacteria
9. a. cilia
10. d. laryngitis

### True or False

1. True
2. False
3. False
4. True
5. False
6. False
7. False
8. True
9. False
10. True

### Fill-Ins

1. Mantoux skin test
2. sinusitis
3. cigarette smoking
4. spirometry
5. viruses
6. pleurisy
7. lobar
8. emphysema
9. cilia
10. cystic fibrosis

## CHAPTER 10

### Multiple Choice

1. b. inflammation of stomach mucosa
2. b. ulcerative colitis
3. b. celiac disease/malabsorption syndrome
4. d. diverticulitis
5. d. prognosis is good with an 85% cure rate
6. c. most often caused by diabetes
7. b. chronic alcoholism

8. a. cirrhosis
9. a. *Candida albicans*
10. c. cholecystitis

### True or False

1. False
2. True
3. False
4. True
5. True
6. False
7. False
8. False
9. False
10. True

### Fill-Ins

1. amoebic dysentery
2. Crohn's disease
3. hernia
4. endoscope
5. C
6. cholelithiasis
7. bile duct
8. ascites
9. mouth
10. large intestine

## CHAPTER 11

### Multiple Choice

1. d. diabetes mellitus
2. a. pyelonephritis
3. c. pyelitis
4. d. uremia
5. b. usually exhibit dysuria, urgency, and frequency
6. a. peritoneal dialysis
7. b. incontinence
8. a. protein
9. c. decreased plasma protein
10. b. aging

### True or False

1. False
2. True
3. True
4. True
5. True
6. True
7. True

8. False
9. False
10. True

## Fill-Ins

1. Pyuria
2. Diabetic nephropathy
3. kidney stones
4. Lithotripsy
5. Polycystic kidney
6. oliguria
7. nocturia
8. bacteria
9. obstruction
10. IVP

## CHAPTER 12

### Multiple Choice

1. c. uterine leiomyomas
2. d. caused by *Treponema pallidum:* genital warts
3. d. secondary syphilis is characterized by lesions that form in several organs
4. a. gonorrhea
5. b. salpingitis
6. b. cystocele
7. b. dysmenorrhea
8. c. cryptorchidism
9. d. hydatidiform mole
10. b. abruptio placentae

### True or False

1. True
2. False
3. False
4. False
5. True
6. False
7. False
8. True
9. False
10. False

### Fill-Ins

1. fibrocystic
2. orchitis
3. chlamydia
4. cervical cancer.
5. Premature ejaculation
6. Trichomoniasis
7. I, II

8. Leukorrhea
9. Menopause
10. Puerperal mastitis

## CHAPTER 13

### Multiple Choice

1. c. anterior pituitary
2. b. parathormone
3. b. Addison's disease
4. b. Cushing's disease
5. c. diabetes insipidus
6. a. Graves' disease
7. d. adrenal
8. a. Addison's disease
9. d. glucose
10. c. thryoxine

### True or False

1. True
2. False
3. False
4. False
5. False
6. True
7. False
8. True
9. True
10. True

### Fill-Ins

1. gigantism
2. acromegaly
3. oxytocin, vasopressin
4. Addison's disease
5. pheochromocytoma
6. islet cells
7. acidosis
8. anterior pituitary
9. growth hormone
10. eunuchism

## CHAPTER 14

### Multiple Choice

1. b. virus
2. d. all of these
3. d. heart rate and breathing
4. b. meningitis
5. a. is caused by a virus
6. c. damaged myelin sheath

7. b. TPA
8. c. epilepsy
9. a. no dopamine
10. c. conjunctivitis

## True or False

1. True
2. True
3. False
4. True
5. False
6. True
7. False
8. True
9. False
10. False

## Fill-Ins

1. Tetanus
2. electromyography
3. Multiple sclerosis
4. Essential tremor
5. L-dopa
6. Cluster
7. trigeminal neuralgia
8. Bell's palsy
9. ALS
10. Myelocele

# CHAPTER 15

## Multiple Choice

1. b. Franz Mesmer
2. c. DSM
3. d. dopamine
4. a. ADHD is limited to children
5. c. acetylcholine
6. a. persecutory
7. b. bulimia nervosa
8. b. bipolar I
9. c. stimulant medications
10. d. obsessions

## True or False

1. False
2. False
3. True
4. True
5. True
6. True
7. False

8. True
9. False
10. False

## Fill-Ins

1. Psychiatry
2. neurotransmitters
3. dopamine
4. mental retardation
5. tic disorders
6. acetylcholine
7. compulsive use, cravings, tolerance and withdrawal
8. affect
9. Seasonal affective disorder
10. mania

# CHAPTER 16

## Multiple Choice

1. c. vitamin D
2. d. the bones of adults
3. c. median nerve
4. d. Duchenne's MD
5. b. Osteoarthritis
6. a. rheumatoid arthritis
7. d. gout
8. c. osteogenic sarcoma
9. c. myasthenia gravis
10. c. osteomyelitis

## True or False

1. False
2. False
3. False
4. True
5. True
6. True
7. True
8. False
9. True
10. True

## Fill-Ins

1. Pott's disease
2. rickets
3. osteoporosis
4. gout
5. calcium, phosphate
6. osteoblasts
7. synovial

8. mysasthenia gravis
9. gout
10. calcium

## CHAPTER 17

### Multiple Choice

1. c. staphylococci
2. c. wheals
3. a. photosensitive
4. b. squamous cell
5. c. white
6. a. epidermis
7. c. vesicles
8. c. hair follicles
9. a. parasitic
10. c. Sebum

### True or False

1. False
2. False
3. False
4. False
5. True
6. True
7. False
8. False
9. True
10. False

### Fill-Ins

1. Melanin
2. Keratin
3. dermis
4. Boils or furuncles
5. Scabies
6. Psoriasis
7. wheals
8. dandruff
9. Vitiligo
10. pustules

# SINGLE PC LICENSE AGREEMENT AND LIMITED WARRANTY

**READ THIS LICENSE CAREFULLY BEFORE OPENING THIS PACKAGE.** BY OPENING THIS PACKAGE, YOU ARE AGREEING TO THE TERMS AND CONDITIONS OF THIS LICENSE. IF YOU DO NOT AGREE, DO NOT OPEN THE PACKAGE. PROMPTLY RETURN THE UNOPENED PACKAGE AND ALL ACCOMPANYING ITEMS TO THE PLACE YOU OBTAINED THEM. *THESE TERMS APPLY TO ALL LICENSED SOFTWARE ON THE DISK EXCEPT THAT THE TERMS FOR USE OF ANY SHAREWARE OR FREEWARE ON THE DISKETTES ARE AS SET FORTH IN THE ELECTRONIC LICENSE LOCATED ON THE DISK:*

**1. GRANT OF LICENSE and OWNERSHIP:** The enclosed computer programs and data ("Software") are licensed, not sold, to you by Pearson Education, Inc. ("We" or the "Company") and in consideration of your purchase or adoption of the accompanying Company textbooks and/or other materials, and your agreement to these terms. We reserve any rights not granted to you. You own only the disk(s) but we and/or our licensors own the Software itself. This license allows you to use and display your copy of the Software on a single computer (i.e., with a single CPU) at a single location for academic use only, so long as you comply with the terms of this Agreement. You may make one copy for back up, or transfer your copy to another CPU, provided that the Software is usable on only one computer

**2. RESTRICTIONS:** You may not transfer or distribute the Software or documentation to anyone else. Except for backup, you may not copy the documentation or the Software. You may not network the Software or otherwise use it on more than one computer or computer terminal at the same time. You may not reverse engineer, disassemble, decompile, modify, adapt, translate, or create derivative works based on the Software or the Documentation. You may be held legally responsible for any copying or copyright infringement which is caused by your failure to abide by the terms of these restrictions.

**3. TERMINATION:** This license is effective until terminated. This license will terminate automatically without notice from the Company if you fail to comply with any provisions or limitations of this license. Upon termination, you shall destroy the Documentation and all copies of the Software. All provisions of this Agreement as to limitation and disclaimer of warranties, limitation of liability, remedies or damages, and our ownership rights shall survive termination.

**4. LIMITED WARRANTY AND DISCLAIMER OF WARRANTY:** Company warrants that for a period of 60 days from the date you purchase this SOFTWARE (or purchase or adopt the accompanying textbook), the Software, when properly installed and used in accordance with the Documentation, will operate in substantial conformity with the description of the Software set forth in the Documentation, and that for a period of 30 days the disk(s) on which the Software is delivered shall be free from defects in materials and workmanship under normal use. The Company does not warrant that the Software will meet your requirements or that the operation of the Software will be uninterrupted or error-free. Your only remedy and the Company's only obligation under these limited warranties is, at the Company's option, return of the disk for a refund of any amounts paid for by you or replacement of the disk. THIS LIMITED WARRANTY IS THE ONLY WARRANTY PROVIDED BY THE COMPANY AND ITS LICENSORS, AND THE COMPANY AND ITS LICENSORS DISCLAIM ALL OTHER WARRANTIES EXPRESS OR IMPLIED, INCLUDING WITHOUT LIMITATION, THE IMPLIED WARRANTIES OF MERCHANTABILITY AND FITNESS FOR A PARTICULAR PURPOSE. THE COMPANY DOES NOT WARRANT, GUARANTEE OR MAKE ANY REPRESENTATION REGARDING THE ACCURACY, RELIABILITY, CURRENTNESS, USE, OR RESULTS OF USE, OF THE SOFTWARE.

**5. LIMITATION OF REMEDIES AND DAMAGES:** IN NO EVENT, SHALL THE COMPANY OR ITS EMPLOYEES AGENTS, LICENSORS, OR CONTRACTORS BE LIABLE FOR ANY INCIDENTAL, INDIRECT, SPECIAL, OR CONSEQUENTIAL DAMAGES ARISING OUT OF OR IN CONNECTION WITH THIS LICENSE OR THE SOFTWARE INCLUDING FOR LOSS OF USE, LOSS OF DATA, LOSS OF INCOME OR PROFIT, OR OTHER LOSSES, SUSTAINED AS A RESULT OF INJURY TO ANY PERSON, OR LOSS OF OR DAMAGE TO PROPERTY, OR CLAIMS OF THIRD PARTIES, EVEN IF THE COMPANY OR AN AUTHORIZED REPRESENTATIVE OF THE COMPANY HAS BEEN ADVISED OF THE POSSIBILITY OF SUCH DAMAGES. IN NO EVENT SHALL THE LIABILITY OF THE COMPANY FOR DAMAGES WITH RESPECT TO THE SOFTWARE EXCEED THE AMOUNTS ACTUALLY PAID BY YOU, IF ANY, FOR THE SOFTWARE OR THE ACCOMPANYING TEXTBOOK BECAUSE SOME JURISDICTIONS DO NOT ALLOW THE LIMITATION OF LIABILITY IN CERTAIN CIRCUMSTANCES, THE ABOVE LIMITATIONS MAY NOT ALWAYS APPLY TO YOU.

**6. GENERAL:** THIS AGREEMENT SHALL BE CONSTRUED IN ACCORDANCE WITH THE LAWS OF THE UNITED STATES OF AMERICA AND THE STATE OF NEW YORK, APPLICABLE TO CONTRACTS MADE IN NEW YORK, AND SHALL BENEFIT THE COMPANY, ITS AFFILIATES AND ASSIGNEES. HIS AGREEMENT IS THE COMPLETE AND EXCLUSIVE STATEMENT OF THE AGREEMENT BETWEEN YOU AND THE COMPANY AND SUPERSEDES ALL PROPOSALS OR PRIOR AGREEMENTS, ORAL, OR WRITTEN, AND ANY OTHER COMMUNICATIONS BETWEEN YOU AND THE COMPANY OR ANY REPRESENTATIVE OF THE COMPANY RELATING TO THE SUBJECT MATTER OF THIS AGREEMENT. you are a U.S. Government user, this Software is licensed with "restricted rights" as set forth in subparagraphs (a)-(d) of the Commercial Computer-Restricted Rights clause at FAR 52.227-19 or in subparagraphs (c)(1)(ii) of the Rights in Technical Data and Computer Software clause at DFARS 252.227-7013, and similar clauses, as applicable.

Should you have any questions concerning this agreement or you wish to contact the Company for any reason, please contact in writing: Prentice-Hall, New Media Department, One Lake Street, Upper Saddle River, NJ 07458.